Clinical Trials in Optic Nerve Disease Treatment

Jeffrey N. Weiss

Clinical Trials in Optic Nerve Disease Treatment

Springer

Jeffrey N. Weiss
Parkland, FL, USA

ISBN 978-3-031-58814-3 ISBN 978-3-031-58815-0 (eBook)
https://doi.org/10.1007/978-3-031-58815-0

This Springer imprint is published by the registered company Springer Nature Switzerland AG
The registered company address is: Gewerbestrasse 11, 6330 Cham, Switzerland

For the patients that have allowed us the privilege to serve.

Preface

This book is a compendium of the worldwide ocular stem cell, gene therapy, and other studies treating Optic Nerve Disease that are registered with Clinicaltrials.gov. Clinicaltrials.gov is the largest website listing of clinical research studies in the world. The information presented is accurate as of September 2023. I have divided the studies into multiple categories: Recruiting, Completed, Active/Not-Recruiting, Not Yet Recruiting, Withdrawn, Terminated, and Unknown. Regarding study location, United States locations are listed first, followed by other countries in alphabetical order.

I have rectified the mischaracterization of studies, to only include those that truly belong within each category, and to correct spelling and grammar, so as to produce a consistent and easy-to-read format. The Study and the Clinical Trial number are provided in order to make it easier for the reader to obtain further information.

I hope that by providing this reference, the field of optic nerve disease treatment will be advanced.

Parkland, FL, USA Jeffrey N. Weiss

Contents

Chapter 1
Introduction to Optic Nerve Disease

Optic Nerve

The optic nerve (OND) is considered the second cranial nerve of the peripheral nervous system but technically it is part of the central nervous system and not the peripheral nervous system. The myelin covering the nerves is produced by oligodendrocytes, not the Schwann cells of the peripheral nervous system. It is formed during the seventh week of embryonic development by the diencephalon. Peripheral nerves are insheathed by epineurium, perineurium, and endoneurium, the optic nerve is covered by meningeal layers, dura, arachnoid, and pia mater. Unlike the peripheral nervous system, the optic nerve has only limited regenerative capability.

The optic nerve begins in the retina, at the ganglion cells, and contains between 770,000 and 1.7 million nerve fibers. Axons from the temporal retina form a papillomacular bundle around the fovea and enter the temporal optic nerve head. Nasal axons directly enter the nasal optic nerve. Retinal and optic nerve fibers are unmyelinated, gaining the myelin sheath when entering the intraorbital area, through the lamina cribrosa.

Axons leave the orbit in the optic canal, posterior-medially to the optic chiasm, where fibers from the temporal visual field cross, or decussate. The temporal hemiretinal fibers represent the nasal visual field. Most axons terminate in the lateral geniculate nucleus, continuing as the optic radiations to the visual cortex in the occipital lobe of the brain. Axons also terminate in the pretectal area, and are concerned with reflexive eye movements.

There is a normal variation in the size of the optic disc opening. The optic nerve diameter increases in the orbit, and further increases in the cranial space.

Optic Neuropathy

The type and amount of visual loss is dependent on the location of the damage to the optic nerve. Damage anterior to the chiasm causes visual loss in the eye on the same side as the damage. Damage at the optic chiasm affects the bitemporal visual fields.

J. N. Weiss, *Clinical Trials in Optic Nerve Disease Treatment*,
https://doi.org/10.1007/978-3-031-58815-0_1

Damage posterior to the optic chiasm within the optic tract produces the loss of the visual field on the side opposite the area of damage.

There are multiple causes of optic nerve damage, including:

Glaucoma

A simple definition of glaucoma is that the intraocular pressure damages the optic nerve. There are many causes. Retinal ganglion damage initially produces the loss of peripheral vision, accounting for the insidious nature of the condition. Central vision loss is a late finding.

Optic Neuritis

Inflammation of the optic nerve leads to the destruction of the surrounding myelin sheath. Symptoms include pain on eye movement, an afferent pupillary defect, the loss of color vision, and visual loss. Most commonly diagnosed in young adults, especially females, generally resulting from multiple sclerosis.

Compressive Optic Neuropathy

Common causes include tumors, inflammatory processes, and infections. Optic disc swelling and the loss of vision may result.

Traumatic Optic Neuropathy

The intracanalicular portion of the optic nerve is the most common site of injury. Damage may be caused by both direct and indirect injury.

Infiltrative Optic Neuropathy

Sarcoidosis is the most common cause of optic nerve infiltration. Other primary causes include: cavernous hemangiomas, capillary hemangiomas, and gliomas. Secondary causes include: leukemia, lymphoma, metastatic carcinoma, and nasopharyngeal carcinoma. Fungi, viruses, and bacteria may also be sources of infiltration.

Nutritional Optic Neuropathy

Most patients will exhibit obvious signs of malnutrition, however vitamin B12 deficiency and pernicious anemia may be observed in well-nourished individuals as well as in those patients who have undergone gastric bypass surgery.

Toxic Optic Neuropathy

The most common worldwide cause of this condition is a result of methanol toxicity, a life-threatening condition. Causes include: ethylene glycol (antifreeze), ethambutol, and tobacco use, in the presence of malnutrition.

Hereditary Optic Neuropathy

Leber Hereditary Optic Neuropathy (LHON) most commonly affects young males. It is the most common inherited mitochondrial disease. One eye is initially affected, followed by visual loss in the other eye generally months later. There are many genes associated with this condition. There are other rare syndromes which include optic neuropathy as a feature.

Dominant Optic Atrophy (DOA)
A slowly progressive, bilaterally symmetrical optic neuropathy inherited in an autosomal dominant manner. It generally presents in the first decade of life.

Optic Nerve Hypoplasia (ONH)
The optic disc appears small as a result from the underdevelopment of the optic nerve. This is a congenital optic nerve abnormality often associated with developmental delay, brain malformations, and endocrinopathies.

Further Reading

Anderson DR, Quigley HA. The optic nerve. In: Adler's physiology of the eye. 9th ed. Mosby-Year Book; 1992. p. 616–40.

Atkins EJ, Newman NJ, Biousse V. Lesions of the optic nerve. Handb Clin Neurol. 2011;102:159–84. https://doi.org/10.1016/B978-0-444-52903-9.00012-1.

Becker M, Masterson K, Delavelle J, Viallon M, Vargas MI, Becker CD. Imaging of the optic nerve. Eur J Radiol. 2010;74(2):299–313. https://doi.org/10.1016/j.ejrad.2009.09.029. Epub 2010 Apr 21

Biousse V, Newman NJ. Ischemic optic neuropathies. N Engl J Med. 2015;372(25):2428–36. https://doi.org/10.1056/NEJMra1413352. Erratum in: N Engl J Med. 2015 Dec 10;373(24):2390

Drakon AK, Kosova JV, Sheludchenko VM, Korchazhkina NB. Sovremennye sposoby terapii razlichnykh form atrofii zritel'nogo nerva [Modern treatment of different forms of optic nerve atrophy]. Vestn oftalmol. 2021;137(5. Vyp. 2):340–5. Russian. https://doi.org/10.17116/oftalma2021137052340.

Golnik KC. Congenital optic nerve anomalies. Curr Opin Ophthalmol. 1998;9(6):18–26. https://doi.org/10.1097/00055735-199812000-00004.

Jonas JB, et al. Human optic nerve fiber count and optic disc size. Invest Ophthalmol Vis Sci. 1992;33(6):2012–8. PMID 1582806

Miller NR. The optic nerve. Curr Opin Neurol. 1996;9(1):5–15. https://doi.org/10.1097/00019052-199602000-00003.

Selhorst JB, Chen Y. The optic nerve. Semin Neurol. 2009;29(1):29–35. https://doi.org/10.1055/s-0028-1124020. Epub 2009 Feb 12

Sofferman RA, Harris P. Mosher award thesis. The recovery potential of the optic nerve. Laryngoscope. 1995;105(7 Pt 3 Suppl 72):1–38.

Chapter 2
Stem Cell Studies in Optic Nerve Disease Treatment

Recruiting

United States

Stem Cell Ophthalmology Treatment Study II (SCOTS2)

ClinicalTrials.gov ID NCT03011541

Sponsor MD Stem Cells
Information provided by MD Stem Cells (Responsible Party)
Last Update Posted 2023-06-06

Brief Summary
This study will evaluate the use of autologous bone marrow-derived stem cells (BMSC) for the treatment of retinal and optic nerve damage or disease.

Detailed Description
Eyes with loss of vision from retinal or optic nerve conditions generally considered irreversible will be treated with a combination of injections of autologous bone marrow-derived stem cells isolated from the bone marrow using standard medical and surgical practices. Retinal conditions may include degenerative, ischemic or physical damage (examples may include macular degeneration, hereditary retinal dystrophies such as retinitis pigmentosa, Stargardt, nonperfusion retinopathies, postretinal detachment). Optic nerve conditions may include degenerative, ischemic or physical damage (examples may include optic nerve damage from glaucoma, compression, ischemic optic neuropathy, optic atrophy). Injections may include retrobulbar, subtenon, intravitreal, intraocular, subretinal, and intravenous. Patients will be followed for 12 months with serial comprehensive eye examinations including relevant imaging and diagnostic ophthalmic testing.

J. N. Weiss, *Clinical Trials in Optic Nerve Disease Treatment*,
https://doi.org/10.1007/978-3-031-58815-0_2

Official Title
Bone Marrow-Derived Stem Cell Ophthalmology Treatment Study II

Conditions
Retinal Disease
Age-Related Macular Degeneration
Retinitis Pigmentosa
Stargardt Disease

Intervention/Treatment
Procedure: Arm 1

Study Start (Actual)
2016-01

Primary Completion (Estimated)
2024-07

Study Completion (Estimated)
2025-07

Enrollment (Estimated)
500

Study Type
Interventional

Phase
Not Applicable

Other Study ID Numbers
SCOTS2

Eligibility Criteria
Inclusion Criteria

- Have objective, documented damage to the retina or optic nerve unlikely to improve OR.
- Have objective, documented damage to the retina or optic nerve that is progressive AND have less than or equal to 20/30 best-corrected central visual acuity in one or both eyes AND/OR an abnormal visual field in one or both eyes.
- Be at least 3 months postsurgical treatment intended to treat any ophthalmologic disease and stable.
- If under current medical therapy (pharmacologic treatment) for a retinal or optic nerve disease be considered stable on that treatment and unlikely to have visual function improvement (for example, glaucoma with intraocular pressure stable on topical medications but visual field damage).
- Have the potential for improvement with BMSC treatment and be at minimal risk of any potential harm from the procedure.
- Be over the age of 18.

- Be medically stable and able to be medically cleared by their primary care physician or a licensed primary care practitioner for the procedure.
- Medical clearance means that in the estimation of the primary care practitioner, the patient can reasonably be expected to undergo the procedure without significant medical risk to health.

Exclusion Criteria

- Patients who are not capable of an adequate ophthalmologic examination or evaluation to document the pathology.
- Patients who are not capable or not willing to undergo follow-up eye exams with the Principal Investigator or their ophthalmologist or optometrist as outlined in the protocol.
- Patients who are not capable of providing informed consent.
- Patients who may be at significant risk to general health or to the eyes and visual function should they undergo the procedure.

Ages Eligible for Study

18 Years and older (Adult, Older Adult)

Sexes Eligible for Study

All

Accepts Healthy Volunteers

No

General Publications

- Weiss JN, Levy S, Benes SC. Stem Cell Ophthalmology Treatment Study: bone marrow-derived stem cells in the treatment of non-arteritic ischemic optic neuropathy (NAION). Stem Cell Investig 2017; 4:94. http://sci.amegroups.com/article/view/17421/17703

Abstract Background: Ten patients with bilateral visual loss due to sequential nonarteritic ischemic optic neuropathy (NAION) underwent autologous Bone Marrow-Derived Stem Cell (BMSC) therapy within the Stem Cell Ophthalmology Treatment Study (SCOTS). SCOTS is an Institutional Review Board approved clinical study utilizing autologous BMSC in the treatment of optic nerve and retinal diseases that meet inclusion criteria.

Methods: The average age of the patients treated was 69.8 years. The average duration of visual loss in eyes treated was 9.8 years and ranged from 1 to 35 years. Affected eyes were treated with either retrobulbar, subtenons, and intravenous BMSC or, following vitrectomy, intraoptic nerve. The primary outcome was visual acuity as measured by Snellen or converted to LogMAR.

Results: Following a therapy in SCOTS, 80% of patients experienced an improvement in Snellen binocular vision ($P = 0.029$) with 20% remaining stable; 73.6% of eyes treated gained vision ($P = 0.019$) and 15.9% remained stable in the postoperative period. There was an average of 3.53 Snellen lines of vision improvement per eye with an average 22.74% and maximum 83.3% improvement in LogMAR acuity per eye. The average LogMAR change in treated eyes was a gain of 0.364 ($P = 0.0089$). Improvements typically manifested no later than 6 months postprocedure.

Conclusions: The use of BMSC in the Stem Cell Ophthalmology Treatment Study achieved meaningful visual improvements in a significant percentage of the NAION patients reported. Improvements typically manifested no later than 6 months postprocedure. Duration of visual loss did not appear to affect the ability of the eyes to respond to treatment. Possible mechanisms by which visual improvement occurred may include BMSC paracrine secretion of proteins and hormones, transfer of mitochondria, release of messenger RNA or other compounds via exosomes or - stem cells.

Keywords Nonarteritic ischemic optic neuropathy (NAION); Optic neuropathy; Stem cells; Bone marrow-derived stem cells (BMSC); Blindness; Visual loss

- Weiss JN, Levy S, Malkin A. Stem Cell Ophthalmology Treatment Study (SCOTS) for retinal and optic nerve diseases: a preliminary report. Neural Regen Res. 2015 Jun;10(6):982–988. https://www.ncbi.nlm.nih.gov/pmc/articles/PMC4498363/

Abstract In this report, we present the results of a single patient with optic neuropathy treated within the Stem Cell Ophthalmology Treatment Study (SCOTS). SCOTS is an Institutional Review Board approved clinical trial and is the largest ophthalmology stem cell study registered at the National Institutes of Health to date—www.clinicaltrials.gov Identifier NCT 01920867. SCOTS utilizes autologous bone marrow-derived stem cells in the treatment of optic nerve and retinal diseases. Pre- and posttreatment comprehensive eye exams were independently performed at the Wilmer Eye Institute at the Johns Hopkins Hospital, USA. A 27-year-old female patient had lost vision approximately 5 years prior to enrollment in SCOTS. Pretreatment best-corrected visual acuity at the Wilmer Eye Institute was 20/800 Right Eye (OD) and 20/4000 Left Eye (OS). Four months following treatment in SCOTS, the central visual acuity had improved to 20/100 OD and 20/40 OS.

- Weiss JN, Levy S, Malkin A. Stem Cell Ophthalmology Treatment Study (SCOTS) for retinal and optic nerve diseases: a preliminary report. Neural Regen Res. 2015 Jun;10(6):982–988. https://www.ncbi.nlm.nih.gov/pmc/articles/PMC4498363/

Abstract We present the results from a patient with relapsing optic neuropathy treated within the Stem Cell Ophthalmology Treatment Study (SCOTS). SCOTS is an Institutional Review Board approved clinical trial and has become the largest ophthalmology stem cell study registered at the National Institutes of Health to date (www.clinicaltrials.gov Identifier NCT 01920867). SCOTS utilizes autologous bone marrow-derived stem cells (BMSCs) for treatment of retinal and optic nerve diseases. Pretreatment and posttreatment comprehensive eye exams of a 54-year-old female patient were performed both at the Florida Study Center, USA and at

The Eye Center of Columbus, USA. As a consequence of relapsing optic neuritis, the patient's previously normal visual acuity decreased to between 20/350 and 20/400 in the right eye and to 20/70 in the left eye. Significant visual field loss developed bilaterally. The patient underwent a right eye vitrectomy with injection of BMSCs into the optic nerve of the right eye and retrobulbar, subtenon, and intravitreal injection of BMSCs in the left eye. At 15 months after SCOTS treatment, the patient's visual acuity had improved to 20/150 in the right eye and 20/20 in the left eye. Bilateral visual fields improved markedly. Both macular thickness and fast retinal nerve fiber layer thickness were maximally improved at 3 and 6 months after SCOTS treatment. The patient also reduced her mycophenylate dose from 1500 to 500 mg per day and required no steroid pulse therapy during the 15-month follow-up.

- Weiss JN, Levy S, Benes SC. Stem Cell Ophthalmology Treatment Study (SCOTS): bone marrow-derived stem cells in the treatment of Leber's hereditary optic neuropathy. Neural Regen Res. 2016 Oct;11(10):1685–1694. http://www.nrronline.org/article.asp?issn=1673-5374;year=2016;volume=11;issue=10;spage=1685;epage=1694;aulast=Weiss

Abstract The Stem Cell Ophthalmology Treatment Study (SCOTS) is currently the largest-scale stem cell ophthalmology trial registered at ClinicalTrials.gov (identifier: NCT01920867). SCOTS utilizes autologous bone marrow-derived stem cells (BMSCs) to treat optic nerve and retinal diseases. Treatment approaches include a combination of retrobulbar, subtenon, intravitreal, intraoptic nerve, subretinal, and intravenous injection of autologous BMSCs according to the nature of the disease, the degree of visual loss, and any risk factors related to the treatments. Patients with Leber's hereditary optic neuropathy had visual acuity gains on the Early Treatment Diabetic Retinopathy Study (ETDRS) of up to 35 letters and Snellen acuity improvements from hand motion to 20/200 and from counting fingers to 20/100. Visual field improvements were noted. Macular and optic nerve head nerve fiber layer typically thickened. No serious complications were seen. The increases in visual acuity obtained in our study were encouraging and suggest that the use of autologous BMSCs as provided in SCOTS for ophthalmologic mitochondrial diseases including Leber's hereditary optic neuropathy may be a viable treatment option.

- Weiss JN, Levy S. Stem Cell Ophthalmology Treatment Study (SCOTS): bone marrow-derived stem cells in the treatment of Dominant Optic Atrophy. Stem Cell Investig 2019;6:41. http://sci.amegroups.com/article/view/32664

Abstract Background: We report the results of six patients with Dominant Optic Atrophy (DOA) who met inclusion criteria and were treated in the Stem Cell Ophthalmology Treatment Study (SCOTS). SCOTS/SCOTS 2 is an Institutional Review Board approved and NIH registered (NCT 03011541) clinical study that uses autologous bone marrow-derived stem cells (BMSC) in the treatment of optic nerve and retinal disease.

Methods: This is an open-label, nonrandomized clinical study using natural history of the disease as the comparator. BMSC were separated from aspirated autologous bone marrow with minimal manipulation using an FDA cleared Class II medical device. Patients were treated with combinations of retrobulbar, subtenons, intravitreal or subretinal placement of BMSC followed by intravenous injection of BMSC depending on the arm of the study chosen. There were no surgical complications.

Results: Of the patients treated, 83.3% (5 of 6 patients) experienced visual improvements and in all of these cases both eyes improved. Ten eyes or 83.3% experienced gains in visual acuity with a median improvement of 2.125 Snellen lines, or approximately 10.63 letters. Two eyes were considered unchanged compared to longstanding measurements. Using LogMAR, the average improvement in vision for all eyes was 29.5%. The average visual acuity increase in eyes that improved was 33.3%. Findings were statistically significant with $P < 0.001$.

Conclusions: Using autologous BMSC per protocols developed in the SCOTS/SCOTS 2 clinical studies resulted in statistically significant visual acuity improvements in patients with DOA or Kjers Optic Neuropathy. Improvements occurred in 83.3% of eyes and averaged 29.5%. Mitochondrial transfer and neuroprotective exosome secretions from the BMSC may have been keys to the improvements observed in this mitochondrial disease.

Recruiting

Autologous Stem Cell Transplant for Neurologic Autoimmune Diseases

ClinicalTrials.gov ID NCT00716066

Sponsor Fred Hutchinson Cancer Center
Information provided by Fred Hutchinson Cancer Center (Responsible Party)
Last Update Posted 2023-09-15
Study record dates

Brief Summary
This phase II trial studies the side effects and how well carmustine, etoposide, cytarabine, and melphalan together with antithymocyte globulin before a stem cell transplant works in treating patients with autoimmune neurologic disease that did not respond to previous therapy. In autoimmune neurological diseases, the patient's own immune system "attacks" the nervous system which might include the brain/spinal cord and/or the peripheral nerves. Giving high-dose chemotherapy, including carmustine, etoposide, cytarabine, melphalan, and antithymocyte globulin, before a stem cell transplant weakens the immune system and may help stop the

immune system from "attacking" a patient's nervous system. When the patient's own (autologous) stem cells are infused into the patient, they help the bone marrow make red blood cells, white blood cells, and platelets so the blood counts can improve.

Outline

Patients receive carmustine intravenously (IV) on day −6, etoposide IV and cytarabine IV twice daily (BID) on days −5 to −2, melphalan IV on day −1, and antithymocyte globulin IV on days −2 and −1. Patients then undergo autologous or syngeneic stem cell transplant on day 0. Patients also receive prednisone orally (PO) once daily (QD) on days 7–21, followed by 2 week taper.

After completion of study treatment, patients are followed up at 3 months, 1 year, and then annually thereafter for up to 5 years.

Official Title

High-Dose Immunosuppressive Therapy Using Carmustine, Etoposide, Cytarabine, and Melphalan (BEAM) + Thymoglobulin Followed by Syngeneic or Autologous Hematopoietic Cell Transplantation for Patients with Autoimmune Neurologic Diseases

Conditions

Autoimmune Disease
Neurologic Autoimmune Disease
Autologous Transplant Autoimmune
Multiple Sclerosis Transplant
MS Stem Cell Transplant
Multiple Sclerosis Stem Cell Transplant
Stiff Person Syndrome
HCT for Neurologic Autoimmune Disorders
CIDP Transplant
Myasthenia Gravis Transplant
Autoimmune Nervous System Disorder
Central Nervous System Vasculitis
Cerebellar Degeneration
Chronic Inflammatory Demyelinating Polyneuropathy
Lambert Eaton Myasthenic Syndrome
Myasthenia Gravis
Neuromyelitis Optica
Opsoclonus Myoclonus Syndrome
Rasmussen Subacute Encephalitis

Study Type

Interventional

Enrollment (Estimated)

80

Intervention/Treatment
Biological: Antithymocyte Globulin
Procedure: Autologous Hematopoietic Stem Cell Transplantation
Drug: Carmustine
Drug: Cytarabine
Drug: Etoposide
Other: Laboratory Biomarker Analysis
Drug: Melphalan
Procedure: Peripheral Blood Stem Cell Transplantation
Drug: Prednisone
Procedure: Syngeneic Bone Marrow Transplantation

Phase
Phase 2

Other Study ID Numbers
2260.00
NCI-2010-00403 (Registry Identifier) (Registry: CTRP (Clinical Trial Reporting Program))
2260.00 (Other Identifier) (Other: Fred Hutch/University of Washington Cancer Consortium)
RG9213030 (Other Identifier) (Other: Fred Hutch/University of Washington Cancer Consortium)

Study Start
2008-06

Primary Completion (Estimated)
2028-01-30

Study Completion (Estimated)
2033-06-30

Study Contact
Name: Bernie McLaughlin
Phone Number: 206.667-4916
Email: bmclaugh@fredhutch.org
United States
Colorado Locations

Denver, Colorado, United States, 80218
Recruiting
Colorado Blood Cancer Institute

Contact
Richard A. Nash
720-754-4800 Richard.Nash@Healthonecares.com

Contact
Sarah Wright
303-577-6488 sarah.wright@healthonecares.com

Principal Investigator
Richard A. Nash

Washington Locations

Seattle, Washington, United States, 98109
Recruiting
Fred Hutch/University of Washington Cancer Consortium

Contact
Bernie McLaughlin
206-667-4916 bmclaugh@fredhutch.org

Principal Investigator
Leona Holmberg

Seattle, Washington, United States, 98122-4307
Recruiting
Swedish Medical Center-First Hill

Contact
Bernie McLaughlin
206-667-4916 bmclaugh@fredhutch.org

Principal Investigator
James Bowen

Eligibility Criteria
Ages Eligible for Study
Up to 71 Years (Child, Adult, Older Adult)

Accepts Healthy Volunteer
No

Sexes Eligible for Study
All

Inclusion Criteria

- Patients with an autoimmune disorder of the central or peripheral nervous system will be eligible; this will include:
  - Primary Central Nervous System (CNS) vasculitis
  - Rasmussen's encephalitis
  - Autoimmune peripheral neuropathy (anti-Hu [Anna-1], anti-GM1 [GD1b], anti-MAG, antiganglioside, antisulfatide)
  - Autoimmune cerebellar degeneration
  - Gait Ataxia with Late age-Onset Polyneuropathy (GALOP)
  - Stiff Person Syndrome
  - Chronic Inflammatory Demyelinating Polyneuropathy
  - Myasthenia Gravis
  - Lambert-Eaton myasthenic syndrome
  - Human T-cell lymphotropic virus (HTLV)-1-associated myelopathy (HAM)/ tropical spastic paraparesis (TSP)
  - Opsoclonus/myoclonus (anti-Ri)
  - Neuromyelitis optica
  - Multiple sclerosis
  - Other central or peripheral nervous system autoimmune diseases as approved by study neurologists and the Fred Hutchinson Cancer Research Center (FHCRC) faculty at Patient Care Conference (PCC)
- Patients must satisfy the criteria for a diagnosis of one of the severe neurological autoimmune disorders outlined
- Patients age = <70 years
- Evidence of disease activity as outlined (e.g., gadolinium enhancement on magnetic resonance imaging of the brain or clinical progression)
- Patients must have failed at least two lines of standard therapy as outlined for the specific diseases
- DONOR: Sibling of any patient enrolled on this protocol proven by ABO typing, human leukocyte antigen (HLA) typing, and variable number tandem repeat (VNTR) analysis to be syngeneic with the patient (e.g., identical twin)
- DONOR: Willing to undergo multiple apheresis procedures (except donors <12 years who will undergo bone marrow harvests)

Exclusion Criteria

- Age ≥ 71 years.
- Pregnancy or expressed plans to become pregnant within 1 year of the procedure.
- Patients who are serologically positive for human immunodeficiency virus (HIV).

- Patients with pulmonary, cardiac, hepatic or renal impairment that would limit their ability to receive cytoreductive therapy and compromise their survival; this should include patients with any of the following:
  - Severe pulmonary dysfunction associated with a carbon monoxide diffusing capacity (DLCO) (corrected for hemoglobin) <60%, or requires supplemental oxygen; patients who are unable to perform pulmonary function test (because of underlying disease) will be excluded if the oxygen saturation is <92% on room air.
  - Uncontrolled malignant arrhythmias, or clinical evidence of congestive heart failure (New York class III–IV) or ejection fraction <50%.
  - Renal disease with estimated glomerular filtration rate (GFR) by creatinine clearance or iothalamate clearance <50 mL/min/1.73 m^2 body surface area.
  - Serum glutamate pyruvate transaminase (SGPT)/aspartate aminotransferase (AST) >3 times normal or direct bilirubin greater than 2.5 mg/dL on two repeated tests.
- Active uncontrolled infection.
- Demonstrated lack of compliance with prior medical care.
- Patients whose life expectancy is limited by illness other than their neurological condition.
- Patients with evidence of myelodysplasia.
- Active malignancy (excluding localized squamous cell or basal cell carcinoma of the skin).
- DONOR: Inadequate documentation that donor and recipient are syngeneic.
- DONOR: Donors who do not fulfill criteria as apheresis donors as established by institutional guidelines.
- DONOR: Concordant for autoimmune neurological disease(s) as determined by neurological evaluation.

Primary Purpose: Treatment
Allocation: N/A
Interventional Model: Single Group Assignment
Masking: None (Open Label)

Arms and interventions

Participant group/arm	Intervention/treatment
Experimental: treatment (immunosuppressive therapy followed by transplant) Patients receive carmustine IV on day −6, etoposide IV and cytarabine IV BID on days −5 to −2, melphalan IV on day −1 and antithymocyte globulin IV on days −2 and −1. Patients then undergo autologous or syngeneic stem cell transplant on day 0. Patients also receive prednisone PO QD on days 7–21, followed by a 2 week taper	Biological: antithymocyte globulin • Given IV • Other names: – Antithymocyte globulin – Antithymocyte serum – ATG – ATGAM – ATS – Thymoglobulin Procedure: autologous hematopoietic stem cell transplantation • Undergo autologous or syngeneic stem cell transplantation • Other names: – Autologous stem cell transplantation Drug: carmustine • Given IV • Other names: – BCNU – Becenum – Becenun – BiCNU – Bis(chloroethyl) nitrosourea – Bis-chloronitrosourea – Carmubris – Carmustin – Carmustinum – FDA 0345 – Gliadel – *N,N'*-bis(2-chloroethyl)-*N*-nitrosourea – Nitrourean – Nitrumon – SK 27702 – SRI 1720 – WR-139021 – 154-93-8 Drug: cytarabine • Given IV • Other names: –.beta.-cytosine arabinoside – 1-.beta.-D-arabinofuranosyl-4-amino-2(1H)pyrimidinone – 1-.beta.-D-arabinofuranosylcytosine – 1-Beta-D-arabinofuranosyl-4-amino-2(1H)pyrimidinone – 1-Beta-D-arabinofuranosylcytosine – 1-.beta.-D-arabinofuranosylcytosine – 2(1H)-pyrimidinone, 4-amino-1-beta-D-arabinofuranosyl- – 2(1H)-pyrimidinone, 4-amino-1.beta.-D-arabinofuranosyl- – Alexan – Ara-C – ARA-cell – Arabine – Arabinofuranosylcytosine – Arabinosylcytosine – Aracytidine – Aracytin – Aracytine

- Beta-cytosine arabinoside
- CHX-3311
- Cytarabinum
- Cytarbel
- Cytosar
- Cytosar-U
- Cytosine arabinoside
- Cytosine-.beta.-arabinoside
- Cytosine-beta-arabinoside
- Erpalfa
- Starasid
- Tarabine PFS
- U 19920
- U-19920
- Udicil
- WR-28453
- 147-94-4

Drug: etoposide
- Given IV
- Other names:
  - Demethyl epipodophyllotoxin ethylidine glucoside
  - EPEG
  - Lastet
  - Toposar
  - Vepesid
  - VP 16-213
  - VP-16
  - VP-16-213
  - 33419-42-0

Other: laboratory biomarker analysis
- Correlative studies

Drug: melphalan
- Given IV
- Other names:
  - Alanine nitrogen mustard
  - CB-3025
  - L-PAM
  - L-phenylalanine mustard
  - L-sarcolysin
  - L-sarcolysin phenylalanine mustard
  - L-sarcolysine
  - Melphalanum
  - Phenylalanine mustard
  - Phenylalanine nitrogen mustard
  - Sarcoclorin
  - Sarkolysin
  - WR-19813
  - 148-82-3

Procedure: peripheral blood stem cell transplantation
- Undergo autologous or syngeneic stem cell transplantation
- Other names:
  - PBPC transplantation
  - Peripheral blood progenitor cell transplantation
  - Peripheral stem cell support
  - Peripheral stem cell transplantation

Drug: prednisone
- Given PO
- Other names:
  - .delta.1-cortisone
  - 1,2-Dehydrocortisone
  - Adasone
  - Cortancyl
  - Dacortin
  - DeCortin
  - Decortisyl
  - Decorton
  - Delta 1-cortisone
  - Delta-dome
  - Deltacortene
  - Deltacortisone
  - Deltadehydrocortisone
  - Deltasone
  - Deltison
  - Deltra
  - Econosone
  - Lisacort
  - Meprosona-F
  - Metacortandracin
  - Meticorten
  - Ofisolona
  - Orasone
  - Panafcort
  - Panasol-S
  - Paracort
  - PRED
  - Predicor
  - Predicorten
  - Prednicen-M
  - Prednicort
  - Prednidib
  - Prednilonga
  - Predniment
  - Prednisonum
  - Prednitone
  - Promifen
  - Servisone
  - SK-Prednisone
  - 53-03-2

Procedure: syngeneic bone marrow transplantation
- Undergo syngeneic bone marrow transplantation

Primary outcome measures

Outcome measure	Measure description	Time frame
Incidence of grades 4–5 regimen-related toxicity	Assessed by the regimen-related toxicity scale. Using the National Cancer Institute Common Terminology Criteria for Adverse Events version 3.0. The development of grade 4–5 toxicity of any of the included major organ systems within the first 365 days after transplant will be defined as regimen-related toxicity	Up to 1 year posttransplant

Secondary outcome measures

Outcome measure	Measure description	Time frame
Transplant-related mortality	Defined as death within the first 100 days of transplant due to transplant-related complications	Within 100 days posttransplant
Disease responses	Assessed by clinical, laboratory, and radiologic evaluation	Up to 5 years
Engraftment kinetics	Monitored for engraftment kinetics of granulocytes, platelets, and red cells posttransplant	Over first 60 days posttransplant
Number of subjects achieving greater than or equal to 4.0×10^6 CD34+ cells/kg, after up to two peripheral blood stem cell mobilizations	Efficacy of peripheral blood stem cell mobilization as evaluated by total number of harvested CD34+ cells/kg, for autologous transplant	Baseline to postmobilization, assessed up to 20 days after starting final mobilization (up to two mobilizations)
Number of subjects with an exacerbation of autoimmune disease symptoms secondary to G-CSF (filgrastim) during peripheral blood stem cell mobilization	Subjects are evaluated by standardized clinical neurologic tests specific to autoimmune disease type	Baseline to postmobilization, assessed up to 20 days after starting final mobilization (up to two mobilizations)

Sponsor
Fred Hutchinson Cancer Center

Collaborators
No information provided

Investigators
Principal Investigator: Leona Holmberg, Fred Hutch/University of Washington Cancer Consortium

General Publications
No publications available

Recruiting

Neurologic Stem Cell Treatment Study (NEST)

ClinicalTrials.gov ID NCT02795052

Sponsor MD Stem Cells
Information provided by MD Stem Cells (Responsible Party)
Last Update Posted 2023-06-06

Brief Summary
This is a human clinical study involving the isolation of autologous bone marrow-derived stem cells (BMSC) and transfer to the vascular system and inferior 1/3 of the nasal passages in order to determine if such a treatment will provide improvement in neurologic function for patients with certain neurologic conditions. http://mdstemcells.com/nest/

Detailed Description
Various clinical studies have registered with the National Institutes of Health (NIH) to study neurologic diseases and damage. There have also been a number of journal reports on the benefits of treatment with BMSC for diseases and damage to nervous tissue. The investigators hope to add to the volume of literature regarding the use of BMSC in those neurologic diseases and conditions identified as likely to respond to this treatment.

Intravenous administration of BMSC is a well-established approach to neurologic disease and injury with much support for its effectiveness in the preclinical and clinical literature. BMSC and the associated bone marrow fraction are posited to have a number of different mechanisms by which they may potentially improve neurologic function. In regards to their ability to penetrate the blood–brain barrier for potential neuronal transdifferentiation and direct impact on the neurons and glial tissue within the brain, it should be remembered that within the diencephalon there are specific circumventricular organs which lie in the wall of the third ventricle. These are noteworthy for a significantly diminished blood–brain barrier and glial limitans which facilitates their function of coordinating homeostatic mechanisms of the endocrine and nervous systems.

Therefore, the investigators believe entry of BMSC may be facilitated in this area of the brain.

The NEST Study provides a treatment Arm 1 which combines intravenous BMSC with topical application of BMSC to the lower 1/3 of the nasal passages as a means of introducing BMSC to the Central Nervous System (CNS). This is applied bilaterally to the inferior nasal conchas and meatuses. The Trigeminal Nerve or fifth Cranial Nerve is a paired, large sensory and motor nerve with multiple branches. It provides sensation to the surface and interior structures of the face including the nasal mucosa that lines the nose. The nerves of the Trigeminal Nerve providing sensation to this area converge and enter the brain at the level of the pons.

There is documentation in the scientific literature that intranasal delivery of BMSC allows the BMSC to follow the pathways of the trigeminal nerve, facilitating entry into the parenchyma and cerebral spinal fluid (CSF) for effects on the CNS.

Official Title
Neurologic Bone Marrow-Derived Stem Cell Treatment Study

Conditions
Neurologic Disorders
Nervous System Diseases
Neurodegenerative Diseases
Neurological Disorders
Stroke
Traumatic Brain Injury
Cadasil
Chronic Traumatic Encephalopathy
Cerebral Infarction
Cerebral Ischemia
Cerebral Stroke
Cerebral Hemorrhage
Parkinson
Multisystem Degeneration
MSA—Multiple System Atrophy
Progressive Supranuclear Palsy
ALS
Amyotrophic Lateral Sclerosis
Neuropathy
Diabetic Neuropathies
Alzheimer Disease
Dementia
Frontotemporal Dementia
Lewy Body Disease
Cognitive Impairment
Lewy Body Variant of Alzheimer Disease

Study Type
Interventional

Enrollment (Estimated)
500

Intervention/Treatment
Procedure: Intravenous and Intranasal BMSC

Phase
Not Applicable

Other Study ID Numbers
MDSC-NEST

Study Start
2016-06

Primary Completion (Estimated)
2024-07

Study Completion (Estimated)
2025-07

Study Contact
Name: Steven Levy, MD
Phone Number: 203-423-9494
Email: stevenlevy@mdstemcells.com
United States
Connecticut Locations

Westport, Connecticut, United States, 06880
Recruiting
MD Stem Cells

Contact
Steven Levy, MD
203-423-9494 stevenlevy@mdstemcells.com

Contact
203-423-9494

Florida Locations

Coral Springs, Florida, United States, 33065
Recruiting
MD Stem Cells

Contact
Steven Levy, MD
203-423-9494 stevenlevy@mdstemcells.com
203-423-9494

Sub-Investigator
Steven Levy, MD

United Arab Emirates

Dubai, United Arab Emirates
Recruiting
Medcare Orthopaedics & Spine Hospital

Contact
Steven Levy, MD
(001) 2034239494 stevenlevy@mdstemcells.com

Ages Eligible for Study
18 Years and older (Adult, Older Adult)

Accepts Healthy Volunteer
No

Sexes Eligible for Study
All

Inclusion Criteria

- Have documented functional damage to the central or peripheral nervous system unlikely to improve with the present standard of care.
- Be at least 6 months postonset of the disease.
- If under current medical therapy (pharmacologic or surgical treatment), the condition be considered stable on that treatment and unlikely to have a reversal of the associated neurologic functional damage as a result of the ongoing pharmacologic or surgical treatment.
- In the estimation of Dr. Weiss, the neurologists have the potential for improvement with BMSC treatment and are at minimal risk of any potential harm from the procedure.
- Be over the age of 18 and capable of providing informed consent.
- Be medically stable and able to be medically cleared by their primary care physician or a licensed primary care practitioner for the procedure. Medical clearance means that in the estimation of the primary care practitioner, the patient can reasonably be expected to undergo the procedure without significant medical risk to health.

Exclusion Criteria

- All patients must be capable of an adequate neurologic examination and evaluation to document the pathology. This will include the ability to cooperate with the exam.
- Patients must be capable and willing to undergo follow-up neurologic exams with the sub-investigators or their own neurologists as outlined in the protocol.
- Patients must be capable of providing informed consent.
- In the estimation of Dr. Weiss, the BMSC collection and treatment will not present a significant risk of harm to the patient's general health or their neurologic function.
- Patients who are not medically stable or who may be at significant risk to their health undergoing the procedure will not be eligible.
- Women of childbearing age must not be pregnant at the time of treatment and should refrain from becoming pregnant for 3 months posttreatment.

Primary Purpose: Treatment.
Allocation: N/A.
Interventional Model: Single Group Assignment.
Interventional Model Description: Intravenous and intranasal bone marrow-derived stem cells.
Masking: None (Open Label).

Arms and interventions

Participant group/arm	Intervention/treatment
Other: arm 1—intravenous and intranasal BMSC Intervention—autologous bone marrow aspiration and separation of bone marrow-derived stem cell (BMSC) fraction then provided intravenously and intranasally (lower 1/3 of nasal passages)	Procedure: intravenous and intranasal BMSC • Autologous bone marrow-derived stem cells provided intravenous and intranasal (lower 1/3 of nose) • Other names: – IV and IN BMSC

Primary outcome measures

Outcome measure	Measure description	Time frame
Change in neurologic function	Neurologic function from prior to treatment (0 month) and the change in neurologic function at 1, 3, 6, and 12 months posttreatment will be compared to pretreatment using the neuro-QOL (neurology quality of life) questionnaire. The scales of the neuro-QOL assess the following outcome measures: communication, social roles and activities, anxiety, depression, emotional and behavioral dyscontrol, lower extremity function (mobility), positive affect and well-being, sleep disturbance, upper extremity function (fine motor, ADL/activities of daily living), stigma, satisfaction with social roles and activities, cognitive function. The scale for each question ranges from 1 to 5 with 1 being the most impairment and 5 being no impairment; higher numbers are better. The scale can range from 5 indicating no impairment to 45 for significant impairment. Each scale will be recorded and presented as separate outcome measurements	0, 1, 3, 6, and 12 months

Sponsor
MD Stem Cells

Collaborators
No information provided

Investigators
- Study Chair: Steven Levy, MD, MD Stem Cells
- Principal Investigator: Jeffrey Weiss, MD, Coral Springs

General Publications

- Chapman CD, Frey WH 2nd, Craft S, Danielyan L, Hallschmid M, Schioth HB, Benedict C. Intranasal treatment of central nervous system dysfunction in humans. Pharm Res. 2013 Oct;30(10):2475–84. https://doi.org/10.1007/s11095-012-0915-1. Epub 2012 Nov 8.
- Jiang Y, Zhu J, Xu G, Liu X. Intranasal delivery of stem cells to the brain. Expert Opin Drug Deliv. 2011 May;8(5):623–32. https://doi.org/10.1517/17425247.2011.566267. Epub 2011 Mar 19.

- Bhasin A, Srivastava M, Bhatia R, Mohanty S, Kumaran S, Bose S. Autologous intravenous mononuclear stem cell therapy in chronic ischemic stroke. J Stem Cells Regen Med. 2012 Nov 26;8(3):181–9. https://doi.org/10.46582/jsrm.0803011.eCollection2012.
- Teixeira FG, Carvalho MM, Sousa N, Salgado AJ. Mesenchymal stem cells secretome: a new paradigm for central nervous system regeneration? Cell Mol Life Sci. 2013 Oct;70(20):3871–82. https://doi.org/10.1007/s00018-013-1290-8. Epub 2013 Mar 1.
- Lescaudron L, Naveilhan P, Neveu I. The use of stem cells in regenerative medicine for Parkinson's and Huntington's Diseases. Curr Med Chem. 2012;19(35):6018–35.
- Laroni A, de Rosbo NK, Uccelli A. Mesenchymal stem cells for the treatment of neurological diseases: immunoregulation beyond neuroprotection. Immunol Lett. 2015 Dec;168(2):183–90. https://doi.org/10.1016/j.imlet.2015.08.007. Epub 2015 Aug 18.
- Anbari F, Khalili MA, Bahrami AR, Khoradmehr A, Sadeghian F, Fesahat F, Nabi A. Intravenous transplantation of bone marrow mesenchymal stem cells promotes neural regeneration after traumatic brain injury. Neural Regen Res. 2014 May 1;9(9):919–23. https://doi.org/10.4103/1673-5374.133133.
- Weiss JN, Levy S. Neurologic Stem Cell Treatment Study (NEST) using bone marrow-derived stem cells for the treatment of neurological disorders and injuries: study protocol for a nonrandomized efficacy trial. Clin Trials Degener Dis. 2016 [cited 2019 Jun 18];1:176–80.
- Cella D, Lai JS, Nowinski CJ, Victorson D, Peterman A, Miller D, Bethoux F, Heinemann A, Rubin S, Cavazos JE, Reder AT, Sufit R, Simuni T, Holmes GL, Siderowf A, Wojna V, Bode R, McKinney N, Podrabsky T, Wortman K, Choi S, Gershon R, Rothrock N, Moy C. Neuro-QOL: brief measures of health-related quality of life for clinical research in neurology. Neurology. 2012 Jun 5;78(23):1860–7. https://doi.org/10.1212/WNL.0b013e318258f744. Epub 2012 May 9.
- Cella D, Nowinski C, Peterman A, Victorson D, Miller D, Lai JS, Moy C. The neurology quality-of-life measurement initiative. Arch Phys Med Rehabil. 2011 Oct;92(10 Suppl): S28–36. https://doi.org/10.1016/j.apmr.2011.01.025.

Recruiting

Caribbean/South America

Safety of Cultured Allogeneic Adult Umbilical Cord-Derived Mesenchymal Stem Cells for Eye Diseases

ClinicalTrials.gov ID NCT05147701

Sponsor The Foundation for Orthopaedics and Regenerative Medicine
Information provided by The Foundation for Orthopaedics and Regenerative Medicine (Responsible Party)
Last Update Posted 2022-10-27

Brief Summary
This trial will study the safety and efficacy of intravenous and subtenon delivery of cultured allogeneic adult umbilical cord-derived mesenchymal stem cells for the treatment of eye diseases.

Detailed Description
This patient-funded trial aims to study the safety and efficacy of intravenous and subtenon delivery of cultured allogeneic adult umbilical cord-derived mesenchymal stem cells (UC-MSCs) for the treatment of eye diseases. The total dose will be 100 million cells. Patients will be evaluated within 1 month pretreatment and at 1, 6, 12, 24, 36, and 48 months posttreatment for safety and efficacy.

For patients with more severe disease, an autologous Effector cells (activated lymphocytes) treatment will be utilized created from the patient's own cells obtained by apheresis.

Official Title
Safety of Cultured Allogeneic Adult Umbilical Cord-Derived Mesenchymal Stem Cells for the Treatment of Eye Diseases

Conditions
Eye Diseases
Retinitis Pigmentosa
Glaucoma
Diabetic Retinopathy
Macular Degeneration
Traumatic Optic Neuropathy
Optic Atrophy

Study Type
Interventional

Enrollment (Estimated)
20

Intervention/Treatment
Biological: AlloRx

Phase
Phase 1

Other Study ID Numbers
ATG-1-MSC-014

Study Start (Actual)
2022-02-01

Primary Completion (Estimated)
2026-01

Study Completion (Estimated)
2026-01

Antigua and Barbuda

St. John's, Antigua and Barbuda
Recruiting
Medical Surgical Associates Center

Contact
Chadwick Prodromos, M.D.
8476996810 care@thepsci.com

Argentina

Buenos Aires, Argentina
Recruiting
Center for Investigation in Tissue Engineering and Cellular Therapy

Contact
Chadwick Prodromos, M.D.
8476996810 ext 202 Care@thepsci.com

Mexico

San Pedro Garza García, N.L, Mexico
Recruiting
Medyca Bosques

Contact
Chadwick Prodromos, M.D.
8476996810 ext. 202 Care@thepsci.com

Eligibility Criteria
Ages Eligible for Study
(Child, Adult, Older Adult)

Accepts Healthy Volunteer
No

Sexes Eligible for Study
All

Description

Inclusion Criteria
- Diagnosis of eye disease
- Understanding and willingness to sign a written informed consent document

Exclusion Criteria
- Active infection.
- Active cancer.
- Chronic multisystem organ failure.
- Pregnancy.
- Clinically significant abnormalities on pretreatment laboratory evaluation.
- Medical condition that would (based on the opinion of the investigator) compromise patient's safety.
- Continued drug abuse.
- Premenopausal women not using contraception.
- Previous organ transplant.
- Hypersensitivity to sulfur.

Design Details
Primary Purpose: Treatment
Allocation: N/A
Interventional Model: Single Group Assignment
Masking: None (Open Label)

Arms and interventions

Participant group/arm	Intervention/treatment
Experimental: treatment group (AlloRx) intravenous and subtenon delivery (total dose of 100 million cells)	Biological: AlloRx • Cultured allogeneic adult umbilical cord-derived mesenchymal stem cells

Primary outcome measures

Outcome measure	Measure description	Time frame
Safety (adverse events)	Clinical monitoring of possible adverse events or complications	4-year follow-up

Sponsor
The Foundation for Orthopaedics and Regenerative Medicine

Collaborators
No information provided

Investigators
Principal Investigator: Chadwick Prodromos, MD, The Foundation for Orthopaedics and Regenerative Medicine

General Publications

- Sung Y, Lee SM, Park M, Choi HJ, Kang S, Choi BI, Lew H. Treatment of traumatic optic neuropathy using human placenta-derived mesenchymal stem cells in Asian patients. Regen Med. 2020 Oct;15(10):2163–2179. https://doi.org/10.2217/rme-2020-0044. Epub 2020 Dec 14.
- Zhao T, Liang Q, Meng X, Duan P, Wang F, Li S, Liu Y, Yin ZQ. Intravenous Infusion of Umbilical Cord Mesenchymal Stem Cells Maintains and Partially Improves Visual Function in Patients with Advanced Retinitis Pigmentosa. Stem Cells Dev. 2020 Aug;29(16):1029–1037. https://doi.org/10.1089/scd.2020.0037. Epub 2020 Jul 15.
- Ozmert E, Arslan U. Management of retinitis pigmentosa by Wharton's jelly-derived mesenchymal stem cells: preliminary clinical results. Stem Cell Res Ther. 2020 Jan 13;11(1):25. https://doi.org/10.1186/s13287-020-1549-6.

Completed

United States

Hematopoietic Stem Cell Transplant in Devic's Disease

ClinicalTrials.gov ID NCT00787722

Sponsor Northwestern University
Information provided by Richard Burt, MD, Northwestern University (Responsible Party)
Last Update Posted 2020-02-28

Brief Summary
This study is designed to examine whether treating Devic's disease patients with high-dose cyclophosphamide together with rabbit antithymocyte globulin (rATG)/rituximab (drugs which reduce the function of the immune system), followed by return of previously collected patient's stem cells will result in improvement in Devic's disease. Stem cells are undeveloped cells that have the capacity to grow into mature blood cells, which normally circulate in the blood stream. The purpose of the intense chemotherapy is to destroy the cells in patient's immune system, which may be causing his/her disease. The purpose of the stem cell infusion is to produce a normal immune system that will no longer attack patient's body. The purpose of study is to examine the safety and efficacy of this treatment. The drugs used in this study treatment are drugs for commonly used for immune suppression.

Detailed Description

Neuromyelitis optica (NMO, Devic's disease) is an autoimmune, inflammatory, demyelinating central nervous system disorder in which a person's own immune system attacks the optic nerves and spinal cord and is characterized by the concurrence of optic neuritis and transverse myelitis, typically associated with a lesion in the spinal cord extending over three or more vertebral segments. Although it is most commonly relapsing, it is distinct from multiple sclerosis in that it is more severe, tends to spare the brain, and is associated with a longitudinally extensive lesion on spinal cord MRI. Furthermore, NMO is associated with a highly specific serum autoantibody marker, NMO-immunoglobulin G (IgG), which targets the water channel aquaporin-4. The disease follows a relapsing course in more than 90% of patients.

At present, parenteral corticosteroids are widely employed as first-line treatment of optic neuritis and myelitis attacks, whereas therapeutic plasmapheresis is applied in the case of corticosteroid failure. Various strategies for the prevention of NMO relapses have been employed in small case series with modest activity. Immune-based therapies, in order to be effective, need to be started early in the disease course while Devic's disease is predominantly an immune-mediated and inflammatory disease. Since 50% of patients with NMO are confined to a wheelchair within 5 years of onset, new therapies are needed in this disease.

We now propose, as a phase I study, complete immune ablation and subsequent reconstitution with autologous stem cells.

Based on the experience of the pilot studies, the current protocol will mobilize stem cells with granulocyte-colony-stimulating factor (G-CSF) and cyclophosphamide and collect stem cells by apheresis. A subsequent bone marrow harvest will be performed only if needed to supplement the peripheral blood stem cells (PBSC). Based on the experience of autoimmune flares in patients receiving G-CSF alone for mobilization, patients will be mobilized with cyclophosphamide 2.0 g/m^2 and G-CSF 5–10 μg/kg.

In order to avoid cumulative cardiac toxicity from cyclophosphamide and to allow culture of hematopoietic stem cell (HSC) product, 3 weeks must separate the administration of cyclophosphamide for mobilization and conditioning.

Cyclophosphamide 50 mg/kg/day will be given IV over 2 h in 500 cc of normal saline. If actual weight is < ideal weight, cyclophosphamide will be given based on actual weight. If actual weight is > ideal weight, cyclophosphamide will given as an adjusted weight. Adjusted weight = ideal weight + 25% (actual weight minus ideal weight).

Hydration-guidelines, normal saline (NS) at 150–200 mL/h should be given 2 h before cyclophosphamide and continued until 24 h after the last cyclophosphamide dose. The rate of hydration will be aggressively adjusted. Twice daily weights will be obtained. Amount of fluid can be modified based on patient's fluid status.

r ATG 0.5 mg/kg given on day −5, then 1.0 mg/kg given on day −4, then 1.5 mg/kg given on days −3 through −1. rATG is infused over 10 h. Premedicate with Acetaminophen 650 mg po and Diphenhydramine 25 mg po/IV 30 min before the infusion.

Rituxan (Rituximab)—The dose of 500 mg of Rituximab will be diluted in 500 mL 0.9% NS and infused per standard Rituximab infusion guidelines, given on days −6 and on day +1. Following the guidelines, Rituximab will be started at 50 mg/h. If no reaction occurs, the dose will be increased by 50 mg/h every 30 min to a maximum of 400 mg/h.

G-CSF-guidelines, 5–10 μg/kg/day will be started day +5 and continued until the absolute neutrophil counts reach at least 1000/μL.

Official Title
Trial of High-Dose Immunosuppressive Therapy with Hematopoietic Stem Cell Support in Devic's Disease

Conditions
Devic's Disease

Study Type
Interventional

Enrollment (Actual)
13

Intervention/Treatment
Procedure: Hematopoietic Stem Cell Transplantation
Drug: Cyclophosphamide
Drug: G-CSF
Drug: rATG
Drug: Mesna
Drug: Rituximab
Drug: Methylprednisolone

Phase
Phase 1 Phase 2

Other Study ID Numbers
DIAD Devic's Disease Auto 2008

Study Start (Actual)
2009-10-10

Primary Completion (Actual)
2018-11

Study Completion (Actual)
2018-11

United States
Illinois Locations

Chicago, Illinois, United States, 60611
Northwestern University, Feinberg School of Medicine

Ages Eligible for Study
16 Years to 65 Years (Child, Adult, Older Adult)

Accepts Healthy Volunteer
No

Sexes Eligible for Study
All

Inclusion Criteria
- Age between 16 and 65, at the time of pretransplant evaluation
- An established diagnosis of Devic's disease (more than one acute attack)
- NMO-IgG aquaporin-4 autoantibody-positive

Exclusion Criteria
- Paraplegia or quadriplegia and legal blindness (defined as visual acuity of 20/200 or less in the better eye with the best correction possible).
- Any illness that in the opinion of the investigators would jeopardize the ability of the patient to tolerate aggressive chemotherapy.
- Prior history of malignancy except localized basal cell, squamous skin cancer or carcinoma in situ of the cervix. Other malignancies for which the patient is judged to be cured, such as head and neck cancer, or breast cancer will be considered on an individual basis.
- Positive pregnancy test.
- Inability or unwillingness to pursue effective means of birth control. Effective birth control is defined as (1) refraining from all acts of vaginal intercourse (ABSTINENCE); (2) consistent use of birth control pills; (3) injectable birth control methods (Depo-provera, Norplant); (4) tubal sterilization or male partner who has undergone vasectomy; (5) placement of an intrauterine device (IUD); or (6) use, with every act of intercourse, of diaphragm with contraceptive jelly and/or condoms with contraceptive foam.
- Failure to willingly accept or comprehend irreversible sterility as a side effect of therapy.
- Forced expiratory volume at one (FEV1)/forced vital capacity (FVC) <60% of predicted after bronchodilator therapy (if necessary).
- Diffusing capacity of the lung for carbon monoxide (DLCO) <50% of predicted.
- Resting left ventricular ejection fraction (LVEF) <50%.
- Serum creatinine >2.0 mg/dL.
- Known hypersensitivity to mouse, rabbit, or *E. coli*-derived proteins.
- Presence of metallic objects implanted in the body that would preclude the ability of the patient to safely have MRI exams.
- Bilirubin >2.0 mg/dL.
- Platelet count <100,000/μL or absolute neutrophil count (ANC) <1000/μL.
- Psychiatric illness, mental deficiency or cognitive dysfunction making compliance with treatment or informed consent impossible.
- Active infection except for asymptomatic bacteriuria.
- Inability to give informed consent.

- HIV positive.
- Transaminases >3× of normal limits, liver cirrhosis.

Primary Purpose: Treatment
Allocation: N/A
Interventional Model: Single Group Assignment
Masking: None (Open Label)

Arms and interventions

Participant group/arm	Intervention/treatment
Experimental: hematopoietic stem cell transplantation Hematopoietic stem cell transplantation will be performed after a conditioning regimen of cyclophosphamide, G-CSF, Mesna, rATG, rituximab, and methylprednisolone	Procedure: hematopoietic stem cell transplantation • Infusion of participant's own stem cells Drug: cyclophosphamide • A medication used as chemotherapy and to suppress the immune system • Other names: – Cytoxan – Neosar Drug: G-CSF • A glycoprotein that stimulates the bone marrow to produce granulocytes and stem cells and release them into the bloodstream • Other names: – Neupogen – Filgrastim – Granix – Zarxio Drug: rATG • A rabbit polyclonal antibody to lymphocytes • Other names: – Thymoglobulin – Antithymocyte globulin Drug: mesna • A medication used in those taking cyclophosphamide or ifosfamide to decrease the risk of bleeding from the bladder • Other names: – Mesnex Drug: rituximab • Monoclonal antibody therapy used to treat certain autoimmune diseases and types of cancer • Other names: – Rituxan Drug: methylprednisolone • A corticosteroid medication used to suppress the immune system and decrease inflammation • Other names: – Solu-Medrol – Depo-Medrol

Primary outcome measures

Outcome measure	Measure description	Time frame
Survival	Survival rate will be evaluated at 6 months,1 year, 2 years, 3 years, 4 years, 5 years after the transplant	6 months, 1 year, 2 years, 3 years, 4 years, 5 years—after the transplant

Secondary outcome measures

Outcome measure	Measure description	Time frame
Quality of Life (QOL) Short Form-36 (SF-36)	SF-36 is a self-administered quality-of-life exam. The evaluation of the results was done by attributing scores to each question, which were then transformed into a scale ranging from 0 to 100, where 0 corresponds to the worst quality of life and 100 to the best	Pretransplant 12 months and 5 years
Post-HSCT immune-modulating medication and relapse	Number of immune-modulating medication and relapse evaluated at 5 years—after the transplant	Pretransplant and 6 months, 1 year, 2 years, 3 years, 4 years, and 5 years after transplant
Number of patients who require no device assistance for ambulation	No device assistance needed for ambulation evaluated at 6 months, 1 year, 2 years, 3 years, 4 years, 5 years—after the transplant	6 months, 1 year, 2 years, 3 years, 4 years, 5 years—after the transplant
Disability score: expanded disability status scale (EDSS)	Disability scores (disease improvement) defined by at least a 1 point increase in the Expanded Disability Status Scale (EDSS) on consecutive evaluations at least 3 months apart The EDSS scale ranges from 0 to 10 in 0.5 unit increments that represent higher levels of disability)	Pretransplant 6 month, 5 year
NMO-IgG aquaporin-4 autoantibody titer	NMO-IgG aquaporin-4 autoantibody titer will be tested pretransplant and posttransplant	Pretransplant and 5 year posttransplant

Sponsor

Northwestern University

Collaborators

No information provided

Investigators

- Principal Investigator: Richard Burt, MD, Northwestern University

General Publications

- Burt RK, Balabanov R, Han X, Burns C, Gastala J, Jovanovic B, Helenowski I, Jitprapaikulsan J, Fryer JP, Pittock SJ. Autologous nonmyeloablative hematopoietic stem cell transplantation for neuromyelitis optica. Neurology. 2019 Oct 29;93(18):e1732–e1741. https://doi.org/10.1212/WNL.0000000000008394. Epub 2019 Oct 2.

Completed

China

Autologous Mesenchymal Stem Cells for the Treatment of Neuromyelitis Optica Spectrum Disorders

ClinicalTrials.gov ID NCT02249676

Sponsor Tianjin Medical University General Hospital
Information provided by Fu-Dong Shi, Tianjin Medical University General Hospital (Responsible Party)
Last Update Posted 2018-10-17

Brief Summary
Neuromyelitis optica (NMO) is a demyelinating and degenerative disorder of the central nervous system affecting vision and brain and spinal cord function which leads to accumulating disability with a 5-year mortality of approximately 30%. Survivors are typically left with severe morbidity secondary to blindness, quadriparesis, and respiratory failure. No agent has been found to be highly effective in halting disease activity. Based on recent outcomes of Multipotent mesenchymal stromal cells in autoimmune diseases including multiple sclerosis, and based on the mechanisms of neuromyelitis optica, the investigators anticipate that mesenchymal stem cells transplantation may provide lasting disease stability for neuromyelitis optica patients.

Detailed Description
Primary objective was to assess feasibility and safety; the investigators compared adverse events from up to 3 months before treatment until up to 12 months after the infusion.

As a secondary objective, the investigators chose efficacy outcomes to assess the Expanded Disability Status (EDSS), annual relapse rate (ARR), and time to next relapse after transplant.

Third objective anterior visual pathway and pyramidal tract as a model of wider disease. Masked endpoint analyses were used for electrophysiological and selected imaging outcomes.

Official Title
Autologous Mesenchymal Stem Cells for the Treatment of Progressive and Refractory Neuromyelitis Optica Spectrum Disorders: An Open-Label Phase 2a Proof-of-Concept Study

Conditions
Devic's Syndrome
Devic's Neuromyelitis Optica
Devic Syndrome
Devic's Disease
Devic Disease

Study Type
Interventional

Enrollment (Actual)
15

Intervention/Treatment
Biological: Autologous mesenchymal stem cells

Phase
Phase 2

Other Study ID Numbers
IRB2013-055-02

Study Start (Actual)
2013-01

Primary Completion (Actual)
2014-12-31

Study Completion (Actual)
2014-12-31

China
Tianjin Locations

Tianjin, Tianjin, China, 300052
Tianjin Medical University General Hospital

Eligibility Criteria
Ages Eligible for Study
18 Years to 80 Years (Adult, Older Adult)

Accepts Healthy Volunteer
No

Sexes Eligible for Study
All

Inclusion Criteria
- Clinically definite neuromyelitis optica or neuromyelitis optica spectrum disorder
- Age >18 year
- EDSS >3
- Progression of continued relapses or worsening MRI after at least a year of attempted therapy as evidenced by one or more of the following:
  - Increase of 1 EDSS point (if baseline EDSS <5.0) or 0.5 EDSS points (if baseline EDSS >5.5)
  - Moderate-severe relapses in past 18 months
  - Gadolinium-enhancing lesions (double- or triple-dose Gd)
  - One new T2 lesion

- Evidence of recent inflammatory disease, as evidenced by any one of the following:
  - One moderate-severe relapse in the past 18 months
  - One Gd-enhancing lesion (single-, double- or triple-dose Gd)
  - One new T2 lesion

Exclusion Criteria

- Received immune inhibitors immunomodulator during the 3 months before the trial
- Significant cardiac, renal, or hepatic failure or any other disease that may affect the results of the study
- Allergies
- Pregnant or possibly pregnant
- Cognitive decline to understand or sign the informed consent
- Brain tumor, HIV (+) tumor marker (+), blood pressure (BP): 200/110 mmHg
- Judged not suitable by doctors

Primary Purpose: Treatment
Allocation: Randomized
Interventional Model: Parallel Assignment
Masking: None (Open Label)

Arms and interventions

Participant group/arm	Intervention/treatment
Experimental: autologous mesenchymal stem cells group Generated clinical-grade MSC 10 mg chlorpheniramine Po.; 100 mg hydrocortisone i.v.; 10 mg metoclopramide im.; 30 min before administration of the cells MSC a day-case 2.0 × 10^6 cells/kg i.v. 15 min infused normal saline 500 Ml over 4 h i.v.	Biological: autologous mesenchymal stem cells • Autologous mesenchymal stem cells • Other names: – MSC
Placebo comparator: control group Patients with progressive and refractory NMO treated with regular methods	Biological: autologous mesenchymal stem cells • Autologous mesenchymal stem cells • Other names: – MSC

Primary outcome measures

Outcome measure	Measure description	Time frame
EDSS	Compare EDSS change before and 1 year after mesenchymal stem cell (MSC) infusion	Change from baseline to 1 year

Secondary outcome measures

Outcome measure	Measure description	Time frame
Annual relapse rate	Compare annual relapse rate before and 1 year after MSC infusion	1 year after infusion
Lesion load	Compared lesion load before and 1 year after MSC infusion	1 year after infusion
Retinal nerve fiber layer (RNFL)	Compared RNFL before and 1 year after MSC infusion	1 year after infusion
Cognition	Compare cognition questionnaire scale before and 1 year after MSC infusion	1 year after infusion
Immunological assessments	Compare antiaquaporin4-ab before and 1 year after MSC infusion	1 year after infusion
Immunological assessments	Compare immune cell subpopulation before and 1 year after MSC infusion	1 year after infusion
Immunological assessments	Compare cytokine kinetics before and 1 year after MSC infusion	1 year after infusion
Cerebral volume	Compare cerebral volume before and 1 year after MSC infusion	1 year after infusion

Sponsor
Tianjin Medical University General Hospital

Collaborators
No information provided

Investigators
Principal Investigator: Fu-Dong Shi, MD, PhD, Tianjin Medical University General Hospital

General Publications
No publications available

Completed

Turkey

Therapy of Toxic Optic Neuropathy Via Combination of Stem Cells with Electromagnetic Stimulation (Magnovision)

ClinicalTrials.gov ID NCT04877067

Sponsor Ankara Universitesi Teknokent
Information provided by Umut Arslan, Ankara Universitesi Teknokent (Responsible Party)
Last Update Posted 2021-05-10

Brief Summary

The axons of the retinal ganglion cells combine to form the optic nerve. The optic nerve transmits electrical signals to the visual cortex by various synapses. Optic nerve axons are more sensitive to toxins than retina because they are outside the blood–retinal barrier. Methanol, various solvents and heavy metals, carbon dioxide, antiarrhythmic, antiepileptic, antibiotics, and some vasoactive drugs can cause toxic optic neuropathy. There is a different pathophysiology for each toxin. Methanol is easily accessible alcohol in all types of disinfectants. Methanol is converted into formaldehyde and formic acid while metabolized in the liver. Formaldehyde disrupts ATP synthesis by blocking mitochondrial function and oxidative phosphorylation. Formic acid causes demyelination as a result of metabolic acidosis. Neuroinflammation occurs when denatured proteins block axoplasmic flow. All these processes can lead to apoptosis and permanent vision loss. Sildenafil is a vasoactive drug used in erectile dysfunction. Sildenafil decreases optic nerve head blood flow. Neuroinflammation develops secondary to the cessation of axoplasmic flow after hypoxia. If hypoxia and neuroinflammation persist, apoptosis and permanent vision loss develop. Amiodarone is an ion channel blocker used in the treatment of cardiac arrhythmias. Long-term use may cause disruption of ion channel balance in the optic nerve. This condition leads to asymmetric neuroinflammation and apoptosis.

Wharton's jelly-derived mesenchymal stem cells (WJ-MSC) can increase mitochondrial ATP synthesis with paracrine effects and suppress neuroinflammation with immunomodulatory effects. Repetitive electromagnetic stimulation (rEMS) can rearrange ion channel balances and axoplasmic flow. The aim of this prospective phase-3 clinical study is to investigate the effect of WJ-MSC and rEMS combination in the therapy of toxic optic neuropathies. This combination is the first study in the literature for the therapy of toxic optic neuropathies.

Detailed Description

This prospective, open-label clinical phase-3 study was conducted at Ankara University Faculty of Medicine, Department of Ophthalmology between April 2019 and April 2021. Thirty-six eyes of 18 patients with toxic optic neuropathy were included in the study. The primary toxic optic neuropathy (TON) diagnosis was made in emergency or intensive care clinics. Patients who admitted within 3 months after the first intervention were included in the study. All patients enrolled underwent a complete routine ophthalmic examination, including the best-corrected visual acuity (BCVA) measurement with the early treatment of diabetic retinopathy study (ETDRS) chart (Topcon CC 100 XP, Japan). The patients were further evaluated with optical coherence tomography angiography (OCTA) from RTVue XR (Avanti, Optovue, Fremont, CA, USA) to analyze and measure the changes in the ganglion cell complex (GCC) layer that provided a typical co-registered en face and cross-sectional multimodal imaging platform. Functional evaluation of the optic nerve was followed by Compass 24/2 visual field (VF) test (Compass, CenterVue, Padova, Italy) and 120′ pattern visual evoked potential (pVEP) test (Mon 2018F, Metrovision, Perenchies, France).

Subjects Thirty-six eyes of 18 TON patients were included in the study. Inclusion criteria consisted of several parameters:

- Cases poisoned with a toxic agent within 3 months
- Patients with BCVA better than 35 letters
- Any degree of visual field loss
- Patients over 18 years old

Exclusion criteria consisted of several parameters:

- Cases poisoned with a toxic agent more than 3 months
- Patients with BCVA less than 35 letters: to perform the visual field test correctly
- Neurological sequelae that cannot be cooperated
- Smoking

The same treatment protocol was applied to all patients with methanol intoxication before admission to our clinic. Hemodialysis, bicarbonate, and ethanol were administered to all patients. The cases were divided into three groups according to similar demographic characteristics.

Group 1: Consists of 12 eyes of 12 patients treated with WJ-MSC and rEMS combination in one eye. WJ-MSC was applied only one time before rEMS applications. rEMS application was started 10 days after WJ-MSC application. The rEMS was applied with a custom-designed helmet for 30 min after the WJ-MSC application. rEMS applications were repeated 10 times with a 1-week interval. The course was evaluated by comparing the BCVA, FPDI, GCC thickness, pVEP-p100 latency, and amplitude parameters before and third month of applications.

Group 2: Consists of 12 eyes of 12 patients treated with only rEMS in one eye. The rEMS was applied with a custom-designed helmet for 30 min. rEMS applications were repeated 10 times with a 1-week interval. The course was evaluated by comparing the BCVA, FPDI, GCC thickness, pVEP-p100 latency, and amplitude parameters before and third month of applications.

Group 3: Consists of 12 eyes of six patients treated with only WJ-MSC in two eyes. WJ-MSC was applied only one time for both eyes. The course was evaluated by comparing the BCVA, FPDI, GCC thickness, pVEP-p100 latency, and amplitude parameters before and third month of applications.

Umbilical Cord Wharton's Jelly-Derived Mesenchymal Stem Cells Preparation: The mesenchymal stem cells used in this study were isolated from Wharton's jelly of the umbilical cord that was collected allogenicly from a single donor with the mother's consent. The umbilical cord sample was treated following several steps. Briefly, cord tissue was washed twice with phosphate-buffered saline (Lonza, Switzerland) and the Wharton's jelly part was minced using forceps and a scalpel. Minced pieces were cultivated in a cell culture dish (Greiner Bio-One, Germany) with Dulbecco's modified Eagle's medium F12 (DMEM)-low glucose with no L-glutamine (Biological Industries, Israel) and 10% human AB serum (Capricorn, Germany), 1% 10.000 U/mL penicillin, and 10.000 μg/mL streptomycin (Gibco, USA). All cell preparations and cultivation procedures were conducted in a current Good Manufacturing Practice (cGMP) accredited laboratory (Onkim Stem Cell

Technologies, Turkey). The culture-expanded cells were cryopreserved at P3 using standard cryopreservation protocols until used in the following experiment. CryoSure-DEX40 (WAK-Chemie Medical, Germany) containing 55% Dimethyl Sulfoxide and 5% Dextran 40 was used as cryopreservant. The cells were characterized at the time of cryopreservation using flow cytometric analysis to determine the expression of the positive cluster of differentiation (CD) surface markers, CD90, CD105, CD73, CD44, CD29, and negative for CD34, CD45, and CD11b. Using real-time polymerase chain reaction (qPCR), the expressions of several genes, such as tumor necrosis alpha (TNF alpha) and vimentin (VIM) were analyzed. Additionally, quality control analyses, such as mycoplasma and endotoxin analyses (using the PCR and LAL test combined with sterility analysis, respectively) were also completed. Cells were solubilized from cryopreservation before being prepared for injection. Average cell viability for each treatment was over 90.0%, and each patient received 2–6 × 10^6 cells in a 1.5 mL saline solution.

Injection of Umbilical Cord WJ-MSCs: The WJ-MSCs suspension from the culture was delivered to the operating room by cold chain and used within 24 h. A total of 1.5 mL of the WJ-MSC suspension was immediately injected into the subtenon space of each eye. The procedure was conducted under topical anesthesia with proparacaine hydrochloride drops (Alcaine, Alcon, USA) and sterile conditions. 5/0 atraumatic traction suture was applied to the limbus for easy access and manipulation to the application area. Postoperatively, loteprednol and tobramycin combination eye drops were given four times per day for 1 week, and oral amoxicillin clavulonate (1 g) was given twice a day for 5 days.

Retinal Repetitive Electromagnetic Stimulation (rEMS): The rEMS helmet (Magnovision™, Bioretina Biotechnology, Ankara, Turkey) stimulated the retina and visual pathways with an electromagnetic field strength of 2000 mG, frequency of 42 Hz, and duration 30 min. These values were previously determined to be effective for other clinical and preclinical studies.

Time Frame

The patients were evaluated at several study timepoints:

- T0 (baseline): immediately before the applications
- T1: first month of applications
- T2: third month of applications

Primary Outcome Measure

- ETDRS visual acuity: The visual acuity scores obtained from the T0 and T2 examinations were analyzed and compared using statistical tests to determine effectiveness.

Secondary Outcome Measures

- Visual Field Sensitivity: Fundus perimetry deviation index (FPDI, %) FPDI was examined in the 24/2 visual field of the computerized perimetry records. The FPDI offers data explaining how many of the 100 flashing points and what percentage of the visual field could be correctly seen by the patient. For VF analysis,

in order to avoid mistakes during the test, practice rounds were carried out three times before applications.
- Ganglion Cell Complex Thickness (GCC thickness, μm): GCC is the thickness from the internal limiting membrane to the inner plexiform layer in the 3 × 3 mm of foveal area. The measurement is done automatically by the OCTA device. GCC is the total thickness of the ganglion cells and retinal nerve fibers.
- Pattern Visual Evoked Potential (pVEP): pVEP is an objective test that measures the electrical activity of the optical pathway in response to a light stimulus. The 120′ pattern reveals responses from the all retinal quadrants. The measurements were taken according to the ISCEV standards for both eyes. We used the 120′ pattern VEP protocol, which combines p100 implicit time and amplitude, to create a numerical result.

Turkey

Ankara, Turkey, 06000
Umut Arslan

Türkiye Locations

Ankara, Türkiye, Turkey, 06312
Ankara University Biotechnology Institute

Sponsor
Ankara Universitesi Teknokent

Collaborators
- International Olympic Committee

Investigators
No information provided

General Publications

- Ozmert E, Arslan U. Management of retinitis pigmentosa by Wharton's jelly-derived mesenchymal stem cells: preliminary clinical results. Stem Cell Res Ther. 2020 Jan 13;11(1):25. https://doi.org/10.1186/s13287-020-1549-6.
- Ozmert E, Arslan U. Management of retinitis pigmentosa by Wharton's jelly-derived mesenchymal stem cells: prospective analysis of 1-year results. Stem Cell Res Ther. 2020 Aug 12;11(1):353. https://doi.org/10.1186/s13287-020-01870-w.
- Arslan U, Ozmert E. Treatment of resistant chronic central serous chorioretinopathy via platelet-rich plasma with electromagnetic stimulation. Regen Med. 2020 Aug;15(8):2001–2014. https://doi.org/10.2217/rme-2020-0056. Epub 2020 Oct 27.
- Ozmert E, Arslan U. Management of Deep Retinal Capillary Ischemia by Electromagnetic Stimulation and Platelet-Rich Plasma: Preliminary Clinical Results. Adv Ther. 2019 Sep;36(9):2273–2286. https://doi.org/10.1007/s12325-019-01040-2. Epub 2019 Aug 5.

- Arslan U, Ozmert E. Management of Retinitis Pigmentosa via Platelet-Rich Plasma or Combination with Electromagnetic Stimulation: Retrospective Analysis of 1-Year Results. Adv Ther. 2020 May;37(5):2390–2412. https://doi.org/10.1007/s12325-020-01308-y. Epub 2020 Apr 18.

Completed

United Kingdom

Mesenchymal Stem Cells in Multiple Sclerosis (MSCIMS)

ClinicalTrials.gov ID NCT00395200

Sponsor University of Cambridge
Information provided by Peter Connick, University of Cambridge (Responsible Party)
Last Update Posted 2011-10-25

Brief Summary
Hypothesis: Intravenous administration of bone marrow-derived autologous adult human mesenchymal stem cells is a safe novel therapeutic approach for patients with multiple sclerosis.

Mesenchymal Stem Cells in Multiple Sclerosis (MSCIMS) is a phase I/IIA trial designed to establish the safety of intravenous administration of bone marrow-derived autologous adult human mesenchymal stem cells to patients with multiple sclerosis.

Detailed Description

Disease under investigation: Multiple Sclerosis
Phase: I/IIA
Number of patients: 10
Design: 18 month cross over, single treatment at 6 months
Intervention: Administration of bone marrow-derived autologous mesenchymal stem cells
Route of administration: Intravenous
Dose: Up to 2,000,000 Mesenchymal Stem Cells per kilogram
Source of patients: Referrals accepted from Neurologists in East Anglia and North London, UK
Referral Criteria: (all three required)

1. Clinically definite multiple sclerosis
2. Expanded Kurtzke Disability Status Score 2.0–6.5 (inclusive)
3. Evidence of optic nerve damage by
    (a) History of optic neuritis, or
    (b) Relative afferent pupillary defect, or

(c) Optic atrophy on fundoscopy, or
(d) Abnormal visual evoked potential from either or both eyes suggestive of demyelination

Primary Objective: Establish the safety of intravenously administered bone marrow-derived autologous mesenchymal stem cells at a dose of up to 2,000,000 cells/kg over 12 months by monitoring adverse reactions.

Secondary Objectives: Explore the efficacy of intravenously administered bone marrow-derived autologous mesenchymal stem cells at a dose of up to 2,000,000 cells/kg over 12 months on visual function by clinical, neurophysiological, and imaging assessments.

Outcome Measures

1. Primary
   (a) Adverse events
2. Secondary
   (a) Visual function (acuity and color)
   (b) Visual evoked potential latency
   (c) Optic nerve Magnetization Transfer Ratio
   (d) Retinal nerve fiber layer thickness (by optical coherence tomography)
   (e) Brain lesion Magnetization Transfer Ratio
   (f) MRI brain T1 hypointensity load
   (g) T cell response suppression
3. Tertiary
   (a) Multiple Sclerosis Functional Composite Score
   (b) Expanded Kurtzke Disability Status Score

Official Title
Autologous Adult Human Mesenchymal Stem Cells: A Neuroprotective Therapy for Multiple Sclerosis

Conditions
Multiple Sclerosis

Study Type
Interventional

Enrollment (Actual)
10

Intervention/Treatment
Procedure: MSC Treatment

Phase
Phase 1 Phase 2

Other Study ID Numbers
MRCRG44871
REC Reference: 07/Q0108/104

Study Start
2008-07

Primary Completion (Actual)
2010-12

Study Completion (Actual)
2010-12

United Kingdom

London, United Kingdom, WC1N 3BG
University College London Institute of Neurology

Cambridgeshire Locations

Cambridge, Cambridgeshire, United Kingdom, CB2 0PY
University of Cambridge, Dept of Clinical Neurosciences

Participation Criteria
- Researchers look for people who fit a certain description, called eligibility criteria. Some examples of these criteria are a person's general health condition or prior treatments.

Ages Eligible for Study
18 Years to 65 Years (Adult, Older Adult)

Accepts Healthy Volunteer
No

Sexes Eligible for Study
All

Inclusion Criteria
- Clinically definite multiple sclerosis
- Expanded Kurtzke Disability Status Score 2.0–6.5 (inclusive)
- Evidence of optic nerve damage by:
- History of optic neuritis, or
- Relative afferent pupillary defect, or
- Optic atrophy on fundoscopy, or
- Abnormal visual evoked potential from either or both eyes suggestive of demyelination
- Prolonged visual evoked potential P100 latency with preserved waveform
- T2 lesion on MRI optic nerve
- Retinal nerve fiber layer thickness on optical coherence tomography >40 μm

Exclusion Criteria

- Age <18 years
- Age >65 years
- Patient lacks capacity to give informed consent
- Presence of a severe bleeding disorder
- Planning a pregnancy during the trial period
- Current MS disease-modifying therapy

Primary Purpose: Treatment
Allocation: Nonrandomized
Interventional Model: Single Group Assignment
Masking: None (Open Label)

Arms and interventions

Participant group/arm	Intervention/treatment
Experimental: MSC treatment	Procedure: MSC treatment • Intravenous administration of up to 2×10^6 autologous MSCs per kg • Other names: – Mesenchymal stem cells – Multipotent mesenchymal stem cells – Multipotent mesenchymal stromal cells

Primary outcome measures

Outcome measure	Measure description	Time frame
Adverse events		0, 1, 2, 3, 4, 12, and 52 weeks posttreatment

Secondary outcome measures

Outcome measure	Measure description	Time frame
Visual function (acuity and color)		12 and 52 weeks posttreatment
Visual evoked potential latency		12 and 52 weeks posttreatment
Optic nerve magnetization transfer ratio		12 and 52 weeks posttreatment
Retinal nerve fiber layer thickness (by optical coherence tomography)		12 and 52 weeks posttreatment
Brain lesion magnetization transfer ratio		12 and 52 weeks posttreatment
MRI brain T1 hypointensity load		12 and 52 weeks posttreatment
Multiple sclerosis functional composite score		12 and 52 weeks posttreatment
Expanded Kurtzke disability status score		12 and 52 weeks posttreatment

Sponsor

University of Cambridge

Collaborators

- Cambridge University Hospitals NHS Foundation Trust
- Medical Research Council

Investigators
- Principal Investigator: Siddharthan Chandran, MBChB, PhD, University of Cambridge

General Publications

- Connick P, Kolappan M, Patani R, Scott MA, Crawley C, He XL, Richardson K, Barber K, Webber DJ, Wheeler-Kingshott CA, Tozer DJ, Samson RS, Thomas DL, Du MQ, Luan SL, Michell AW, Altmann DR, Thompson AJ, Miller DH, Compston A, Chandran S. The mesenchymal stem cells in multiple sclerosis (MSCIMS) trial protocol and baseline cohort characteristics: an open-label pre-test: post-test study with blinded outcome assessments. Trials. 2011 Mar 2;12:62. https://doi.org/10.1186/1745-6215-12-62.

Terminated

Canada

Reason: Recruitment Failure

Autologous Hematopoietic Stem Cell Transplant in Neuromyelitis Optica (SCT-NMO)

ClinicalTrials.gov ID NCT01339455

Sponsor University of Calgary
Information provided by Jodie Burton MD, MSc, FRCPC, University of Calgary (Responsible Party)
Last Update Posted 2018-05-02

Brief Summary
Neuromyelitis Optica (NMO) is a demyelinating and degenerative disorder of the CNS affecting vision and spinal cord function. This disease is rare compared to Multiple Sclerosis (MS), but it is devastating and often leads to accumulating disability with a 5-year mortality of approximately 30%. Survivors are typically left with severe morbidity secondary to blindness, quadriparesis, and respiratory failure. No agent has been found to be highly effective in halting disease activity. Based on recent outcomes of stem cell transplant trials and reports in autoimmune diseases including MS, and based on the mechanisms of NMO, we anticipate that stem cell transplantation may provide lasting disease stability for NMO patients. The hypothesis of the present trial is that autologous hematopoetic stem cell transplantation in patients with NMO will provide lasting benefit in relapse prevention. Specifically, we anticipate a 50% reduction in the proportion of patients experiencing relapse over a 3-year period. We will be following patients for a total of 5 years after transplantation.

Detailed Description
Patients who are deemed eligible will be enrolled and undergo a two-stage transplant process followed by neurological assessments every 6 months for the following 5 years assessing EDSS, visual metrics, MRI, AQP-4 antibodies, MSFC, and SF36.

Official Title
Autologous Hematopoietic Stem Cell Transplant in Patients with Neuromyelitis Optica

Conditions
Neuromyelitis Optica

Intervention/Treatment
Procedure: AHSCT

Study Start
2011-03

Primary Completion (Actual)
2017-03

Study Completion (Actual)
2017-03

Enrollment (Actual)
3

Study Type
Interventional

Phase
Phase 1 Phase 2

Canada
Alberta Locations

Calgary, Alberta, Canada, T2N 2 T9
Foothills Medical Centre, University of Calgary

Eligibility Criteria
Inclusion Criteria
- Age between 18 and 65, inclusive.
- Diagnosis of NMO using Wingerchuk 2006 NMO Criteria.
- EDSS 0–6.5.
- Treatment with a minimum of one NMO therapy in past 12 months.
- One objective and documented relapse in the past 12 months and two relapse events in the past 24 months despite medical therapy.
- ECOG performance status 0–3.
- Platelets $\geq 100 \times 10^9$/L.
- ALT $\leq 3 \times$ ULN.
- Total bilirubin $\leq 2.0 \times$ ULN, except in patients with Gilbert syndrome or in patients in whom the bilirubin rise is of nonhepatic origin.

- Serum creatinine <1.5 × ULN or creatinine clearance ≥50 cc/min.
- Patients must reside in Alberta, Canada for the duration of the transplant period of the trial.

Exclusion Criteria

- Any illness that would jeopardize the ability of the patient to complete study protocol.
- Prior malignancy unless nonmelanoma skin cancer, carcinoma in situ of the cervix (CIN) or breast, or malignancy treated more than 5 years previously with no evidence of recurrent disease since initial treatment.
- Pregnant or lactating females. Women of childbearing potential must have a negative serum or urine β-hCG pregnancy test at screening.
- Inability or unwillingness to pursue effective means of birth control.
- FEV1/FVC <50% of predicted.
- DLCO <50% of predicted.
- Resting LVEF <50%.
- Known hypersensitivity to mouse, rabbit, or *E. coli*-derived proteins, or to iron compounds/medications.
- Presence of metallic objects implanted in the body that would preclude the ability of the patient to safely have MRI exams.
- Unable or unwilling to provide written informed consent for participation.
- Active infection except asymptomatic bacteriuria.
- Any use of investigational therapies within 4 weeks prior to initiation of study treatment.
- Patients dependent on prednisone who cannot be successfully tapered to a maximum of 0.5 mg/kg/day prior to mobilization therapy.

Ages Eligible for Study

18 Years to 65 Years (Adult, Older Adult)

Sexes Eligible for Study

All

Accepts Healthy Volunteers

No

Sponsor

University of Calgary

Collaborators

No information provided

Investigators

- Principal Investigator: Jodie M Burton, MD, MSc, FRCPC, Department of Clinical Neurosciences, Hotchkiss Brain Institute, University of Calgary
- Principal Investigator: Jan Storek, MD, PhD, Department of Medicine, University of Calgary

General Publications

No publications available

Withdrawn

United States

Reason: Discontinued by Investigator

Autologous Transplant to End NMO Spectrum Disorder (ATTEND)

ClinicalTrials.gov ID NCT03829566

Sponsor Northwestern University
Information provided by Richard Burt, MD, Northwestern University (Responsible Party)
Last Update Posted 2019-11-20

Brief Summary
This study is designed to treat your disease with an autologous stem cell transplant using a regimen of immune suppressant drugs and chemotherapy to reset your immune system and to determine if your disease will go into long-term remission.

Detailed Description
The autologous stem cell transplant used in this research study is an investigational procedure that uses cyclophosphamide (chemotherapy), rabbit antithymocyte globulin (rATG) (a protein that kills the immune cells that are thought to be causing your disease), rituximab (a biologic drug that targets B cells of your immune system), and intravenous immunoglobulin (IVIg) (pooled IgG antibodies from plasma donors with immunomodulatory and anti-inflammatory effects), followed by return of your own previously collected blood stem cells (autologous stem cell transplant). One day of plasmapheresis will also be performed the day prior to admission for stem cell transplant to remove disease-causing antibodies. The ability of this experimental treatment to stop relapses and progression (worsening) of your NMOSD will be assessed.

Official Title
Autologous Hematopoietic Stem Cell Transplant for Neuromyelitis Optica Spectrum Disorder (NMOSD)

Conditions
Neuromyelitis Optica
Devic's Disease
NMO Spectrum Disorder
Intervention/Treatment
Drug: Rituximab
Drug: Cyclophosphamide
Drug: Mesna
Drug: rATG
Drug: Methylprednisolone

Drug: G-CSF
Biological: IVIg
Biological: Autologous Stem Cells
Show fewer interventions/treatments

Study Start (Estimated)
2019-11

Primary Completion (Estimated)
2025-01

Study Completion (Estimated)
2025-11-28

Enrollment (Actual)
0

Study Type
Interventional

Phase
Phase 2 Phase 3

United States
Illinois Locations

Chicago, Illinois, United States, 60611
Northwestern University, Feinberg School of Medicine

Chicago, Illinois, United States, 60611
Northwestern University

Eligibility Criteria
Inclusion Criteria

- Age 18–65 years old at the time of pretransplant evaluation
- An established diagnosis of NMOSD (with or without aquaporin 4 (AQP4)-IgG antibody)

Exclusion Criteria

- Under age of 18 or over age of 65.
- Prisoners.
- Psychiatric illness or mental deficiency making compliance with treatment or informed consent impossible, or any adult who is unable to consent (for adults cognitively impaired due to disease, consent may be obtained from the closest living relative).
- Paraplegia or quadriplegia (must be able to use a walker if even for only a few feet).
- Extensive subcortical white matter lesions.
- Uncontrolled diabetes mellitus or any other illness that in the opinion of the investigators would jeopardize the ability of the patient to tolerate aggressive treatment.

- Myocardial infarction within the last 12 months. If longer than 12 months, must pass a dobutamine stress test and be cleared by cardiology.
- Active systemic lupus erythematous, Sjogren's, myasthenia gravis, or another autoimmune disease.
- Sickle cell disease, sickle cell disease, or coagulopathy
- Prior history of malignancy that required any radiotherapy, chemotherapy, or biological therapy.
- Positive pregnancy test, inability or unable to pursue effective means of birth control, or failure to willingly accept or comprehend irreversible sterility as a side effect of therapy.
- Women who are breastfeeding.
- Untreated life-threatening cardiac arrhythmia on electrocardiogram (EKG) or 24-h Holter.
- Left ventricular ejection fraction (LVEF) <50%.
- Tiffeneau-Pinelli index (FEV1/FVC) <70% of predicted after bronchodilator therapy (if necessary), or diffusing capacity of lung for carbon monoxide (DLCO) hemoglobin corrected <70% predicted.
- Serum creatinine >2.0 mg/dL.
- Liver cirrhosis, transaminases >2× of normal limits, or bilirubin >2.0 mg/dL unless due to Gilbert's disease.
- Major hematological abnormalities such as platelet count <100,000/μL or absolute neutrophil count (ANC) <1000/μL.
- Active infection except asymptomatic bacteriuria.
- Presence of metallic objects implanted in the body that would preclude the ability of the patient to safely have magnetic resonance imaging (MRI) exams.
- Known hypersensitivity to mouse, rabbit, or *E. coli*-derived proteins.
- Human immunodeficiency virus (HIV) positive.
- Hepatitis B or C positive.
- Use of natalizumab (Tysabri) within the previous 6 months.
- Use of fingolimod (Gilenya) within the previous 3 months.
- Use of dimethyl fumarate (Tecfidera) within the previous 3 months.
- Use of teriflunomide (Aubagio) unless cleared from the body (plasma concentration <0.02 μg/mL) following elimination from the body with cholestyramine 8 g three times a day for 11 days.
- Use of alemtuzumab (Lemtrada/Campath) within previous 12 months.
- Use of rituximab (Rituxan) or ocrelizumab (Ocrevus) within previous 6 months.
- Prior treatment with mitoxantrone (Novantrone).

Ages Eligible for Study
18 Years to 65 Years (Adult, Older Adult)

Sexes Eligible for Study
All

Accepts Healthy Volunteers
No

Design Details

Primary Purpose: Treatment
Allocation: N/A
Interventional Model: Single Group Assignment
Masking: None (Open Label)

Arms and interventions

Participant group/arm	Intervention/treatment
Experimental: hematopoietic stem cell transplantation Hematopoietic stem cell therapy will be performed as follows: autologous stem cells will be infused after conditioning with rituximab, cyclophosphamide, mesna, rATG (rabbit), and methylprednisolone. Granulocyte-colony-stimulating factor (G-CSF) and intravenous immunoglobulin (IVIg) will be administered posttransplant	Drug: rituximab • Monoclonal antibody therapy used to treat certain autoimmune diseases and types of cancer • Other names: – Rituxan Drug: cyclophosphamide • A medication used as chemotherapy and to suppress the immune system • Other names: – Cytoxan Drug: mesna • A medication used in those taking cyclophosphamide or ifosfamide to decrease the risk of bleeding from the bladder • Other names: – Mesnex Drug: rATG • A rabbit polyclonal antibody to lymphocytes • Other names: – Thymoglobulin – Antithymocyte globulin Drug: methylprednisolone • A corticosteroid medication used to suppress the immune system and decrease inflammation • Other names: – Solu-Medrol – Depo-Medrol Drug: G-CSF • A glycoprotein that stimulates the bone marrow to produce granulocytes and stem cells and release them into the bloodstream • Other names: – Neupogen – Filgrastim – Granix – Zarxio Biological: IVIg • Pooled immunoglobulin (IgG) from thousands of plasma donors that has immunomodulatory and anti-inflammatory effects • Other names: – Bivigam – Carimune nanofiltered (NF) – Gammagard – Privigen – Octagam Biological: autologous stem cells • Infusion of patient's own stem cells

Primary outcome measures

Outcome measure	Measure description	Time frame
Progression-free survival	Disease progression defined as: 1.0-point increase in the expanded disability status scale (EDSS) on consecutive evaluations at least 6 months apart and not due to a non-NMO disease process. The EDSS scale ranges from 0 to 10 in 0.5 increments that represent higher levels of disability	5 years

Secondary outcome measures

Outcome measure	Measure description	Time frame
Relapse-free survival	Relapse defined as: acute neurologic deterioration occurring after engraftment and lasting more than 24 h, accompanied by objective worsening on neurological examination that are documented by a neurologist and not explained by fever, infection, stress, heat, drugs or related pseudo-exacerbation. Supportive confirmation by enhancement on MRI is preferred but not mandatory	5 years
Expanded disability status scale (EDSS) improvement	The EDSS scale ranges from 0 to 10 in 0.5 increments that represent higher levels of disability. Improvement in EDSS is defined by both a 0.5 or 1.0 points sustained for more than 6 months	6 months, 1 year, 2 years, 3 years, 4 years, 5 years
Scripps neurological rating scale (NRS) improvement	The NRS scale ranges from 0 to 100 in 1 point increments that represent lower levels of disability	6 months, 1 year, 2 years, 3 years, 4 years, 5 years
Improvement in quality of life	Measured using the short form (SF)-36 health survey	6 months, 1 year, 2 years, 3 years, 4 years, 5 years
Paced auditory serial addition test (PASAT) improvement	The PASAT is a measure of cognitive function that specifically assesses auditory information processing speed and flexibility, as well as calculation ability. Improvement measured with the 2″ and 3″ versions	6 months, 1 year, 2 years, 3 years, 4 years, 5 years
Ambulation index improvement	The subject's walk of 25 ft is timed and a score from 0 to 10 is assigned based on their walk/gait and/or assistance required	6 months, 1 year, 2 years, 3 years, 4 years, 5 years
9-Hole peg test (9-HPT) improvement	The 9-HPT is a brief, standardized, quantitative test of upper extremity function. Both the dominant and nondominant hands are tested twice, with the total time to complete the task each time recorded and then averaged	6 months, 1 year, 2 years, 3 years, 4 years, 5 years
Change in NMO IgG (aquaporin-4) antibody titer	Evaluation of the antibody titer, looking for a change from positive to negative	6 months, 1 year, 2 years, 3 years, 4 years, 5 years
Improvement in visual acuity	A visual acuity test is an eye exam that checks how well one sees the details of a letter or symbol from a specific distance	6 months, 1 year, 2 years, 3 years, 4 years, 5 years

Sponsor
Northwestern University

Collaborators
No information provided

Investigators
- Principal Investigator: Richard Burt, MD, Northwestern University

General Publications
No publications available

Unknown Status

China

Safety and Efficacy of Umbilical Cord Mesenchymal Stem Cell Therapy for Patients with Progressive Multiple Sclerosis and Neuromyelitis Optica

ClinicalTrials.gov ID NCT01364246

Sponsor Shenzhen Beike Bio-Technology Co., Ltd.
Information provided by Shenzhen Beike Bio-Technology Co., Ltd. (Responsible Party)
Last Update Posted 2012-11-28

Brief Summary
Multiple sclerosis (MS) has been classically regarded as a chronic inflammatory autoimmune demyelinating disease of the central nervous system, along with a considerable pathological heterogeneity. Neuromyelitis optica (NMO) is a severe inflammatory, demyelinating disease, and its clinical characteristics include recurrent optic neuritis and longitudinally extensive transverse myelitis.

Current therapies provide only modest control of progressive Multiple Sclerosis and Neuromyelitis Optica. Stem cell therapy might open a light horizon in approaching to an efficient treatment in progressive MS and NMO. In this study, the safety and efficacy of Human Umbilical Cord Mesenchymal Stem Cells transplantation will be evaluated in patients with progressive MS and NMO.

Official Title
Phase I/II Study of Umbilical Cord Mesenchymal Stem Cell Therapy for Patients with Progressive Multiple Sclerosis and Neuromyelitis Optica

Conditions
Progressive Multiple Sclerosis
Neuromyelitis Optica.

Intervention/Treatment
Biological: human umbilical cord mesenchymal stem cells

Study Start
2010-01

Primary Completion (Estimated)
2013-03

Study Completion (Estimated)
2014-12

Enrollment (Estimated)
20

Study Type
Interventional

Phase
Phase 1 Phase 2

Study Contact
Name: Yun Yun Xu
Email: xuyun20042001@yahoo.com.cn
China
Jiangsu Locations

Nanjing, Jiangsu, China
Recruiting
Nanjing University Medical College Affiliated Drum Tower Hospital

Contact
Yun Xu
xuyun20042001@yahoo.com.cn

Eligibility Criteria
Inclusion Criteria
- McDonald Diagnosis of Multiple Sclerosis or 2006 Diagnosis of neuromyelitis optica.
- Aged 16–65 years.
- Disease duration ≥2 years
- Poor response to steroid therapy
- Written informed consent and follow the clinic trial procedure

Exclusion Criteria
- Cardiac insufficiency; Renal insufficiency; hepatic insufficiency; Total bilirubin higher than 1.5 times of upper limit of normal value; AST/ALT higher than 2.5 times of upper limit of normal value.
- Combined Pneumonia or other severe systemic bacteria infection.

- Severe drug allergic history or anaphylaxis to two or more food or medicine.
- Intracranial hypertension due to other brain lesions (e.g., Brain cancer).
- HIV+, TPPA +, patients diagnosed as HBV or HCV.
- Tumor Markers +.
- Severe psychotic patients, cognitive dysfunction, or cannot understand or sign the Consent Form.
- Coagulation disorders.
- Uncontrolled hypertension after treatment, blood pressure ≥180 mmHg/110 mmHg.
- Pregnancy.
- Enrollment in other trials in the last 3 months.
- Other criteria the investigator considers improper for inclusion.

Ages Eligible for Study
18 Years to 60 Years (Adult)

Sexes Eligible for Study
All

Accepts Healthy Volunteers
No

Primary Purpose: Treatment
Allocation: Nonrandomized
Interventional Model: Single Group Assignment
Masking: None (Open Label)

Arms and interventions

Participant group/arm	Intervention/treatment
Experimental: human umbilical cord mesenchymal stem cells transplantation Intervention group	Biological: human umbilical cord mesenchymal stem cells • Participants will be given hUC-MSCs transplantation

Primary outcome measures

Outcome measure	Measure description	Time frame
Score of expanded disability status scale (EDSS)		1 year after treatment

Secondary outcome measures

Outcome measure	Measure description	Time frame
Visual evoked potential (VEP)		1 year after treatment
Brainstem auditory evoked potential (BAEP)		1 year after treatment
Somatosensory evoked potential (SEP)		1 year after treatment
Brain magnetic resonance imaging (MRI) scan		1 year after treatment

Sponsor
Shenzhen Beike Bio-Technology Co., Ltd.

Collaborators
- The Affiliated Nanjing Drum Tower Hospital of Nanjing University Medical School
- The Affiliated Nanjing Brain Hospital of Nanjing University Medical School
- Nanjing University Medical College Affiliated Wuxi Second Hospital
- Xuzhou Medical University
- The Second Hospital of Nanjing Medical University

Investigators
- No information provided

General Publications
No publications available

Unknown Status

India

Study the Safety and Efficacy of Bone Marrow-Derived Autologous Cells for the Treatment of Optic Nerve Disease (OND)

ClinicalTrials.gov ID NCT01834079

Sponsor Chaitanya Hospital, Pune
Information provided by Dr. Sachin Jamadar, Chaitanya Hospital, Pune (Responsible Party)
Last Update Posted 2014-09-17

Brief Summary
This is a single-arm, single-center trial to check the safety and efficacy of bone marrow-derived autologous mono nuclear cell (100 million per dose) clinical trial to be conducted for 36 months in patients with optic nerve diseases.

Detailed Description
Optic Nerve Diseases: Conditions which produce injury or dysfunction of the second cranial or optic nerve, which is generally considered a component of the central nervous system. Damage to optic nerve fibers may occur at or near their origin in the retina, at the optic disk, or in the nerve, optic chiasm, optic tract, or lateral geniculate nuclei. Clinical manifestations may include decreased visual acuity and contrast sensitivity, impaired color vision, and an afferent papillary defect. Primary output of clinical study is to measure improvement in visual loss and improvement in idiopathic intracranial. This is a single-arm, single-center trial to check the safety and efficacy of bone marrow-derived autologous mono nuclear cell (100 million per dose) clinical trial to be conducted for 36 months.

Official Title
Study the Safety and Efficacy of Bone Marrow-Derived Autologous Cells for the Treatment of Optic Nerve Disease. It is Self-Funded (Patients' Own Funding) Clinical Trial

Conditions
Optic Atrophy

Intervention/Treatment
Biological: Stem Cell Therapy

Study Start
2014-09

Primary Completion (Estimated)
2016-07

Study Completion (Estimated)
2016-07

Enrollment (Estimated)
24

Study Type
Interventional

Phase
Phase 1 Phase 2

Other Study ID Numbers
00104

Study Contact
Name: Sachin P Jamadar, D. Ortho
Phone Number: +918888788880
Email: sac2751982@gmail.com

Study Contact Backup
Name: Smita S Bhoyar, B.A.M.S. PGCR
Phone Number: 9372620569
Email: drsmitabhoyar@rediff.com
India
Maharashtra Locations

Pune, Maharashtra, India, 4
Recruiting
Chaitanya Hospital

Contact
Sachin P Jamadar, D. Ortho
8888788880 sac2751982@gmail.com

Contact
Smita S Bhoyar, BAMS.PGCR
9372620569 drsmitabhoyar@rediffmail.com

Principal Investigator
Anant E Bagul, MS

Eligibility Criteria
Inclusion Criteria

- Patient should suffer from optic nerve diseases like diabetic retinopathy, retinal pigmentation.
- Age between 18 and 50.
- Willingness to undergo bone marrow-derived autologous cell therapy.
- Ability to comprehend the explained protocol and thereafter give an informed consent as well as sign the require Informed consent form (ICF) for the study.
- An ability and willingness to regular visit to hospital for protocol and follow-up.

Exclusion Criteria

- Patients with preexisting or current systemic disease such as lung, liver (exception; History of uncomplicated Hepatitis A), gastrointestinal, cardiac, immunodeficiency (including HIV), or laboratory investigation that could cause a neurological defect including syphilis, clinically relevant polyneuropathy, etc.
- History of life-threatening allergic or immune-mediated reaction.
- Hemodynamically unstable.

Ages Eligible for Study
18 Years to 50 Years (Adult)

Sexes Eligible for Study
All

Accepts Healthy Volunteers
Yes

Design Details
Primary Purpose: Treatment
Allocation: N/A
Interventional Model: Single Group Assignment
Masking: None (Open Label)

Arms and interventions

Participant group/arm	Intervention/treatment
Other: STEM CELL intrathecal injection of MNC stem cell therapy	Biological: STEM CELL THERAPY • Autologous stem cells (MNCs) intrathecal. Intrathecal transplantation of single-arm autologous MNCs 100 million per dose in three divided doses at interval of 7 days, intrathecal/intravenous. Follow-up will be taken to 3 months or as required • Other names: – Intrathecal transplantation of autologous stem cells

Primary outcome measures

Outcome measure	Measure description	Time frame
Reduction in degeneration of the optic nerve with improvement in vision		6 months

Secondary outcome measures

Outcome measure	Measure description	Time frame
Increase in visual function		6 months
Improvement in idiopathic intracranial hypertension		6 months

Sponsor
Chaitanya Hospital, Pune

Collaborators
No information provided

Investigators
- Principal Investigator: Anant E Bagul, M.S., Chaitanya Hospital

General Publications
No publications available

Unknown Status

Jordan

Treatment of Optic Neuropathies Using Autologous Bone Marrow-Derived Stem Cells

ClinicalTrials.gov ID NCT02638714

Sponsor Stem Cells Arabia
Information provided by Stem Cells Arabia (Responsible Party)
Last Update Posted 2020-03-17

Brief Summary
A single-arm, single-center trial to assess the safety and efficacy of restoring function in damaged optic nerves using autologous purified populations of bone marrow-derived stem cells (BM-SCs) through a 24-month follow-up period.

Detailed Description
Optic nerve atrophy (ONA) is a condition defined as a damage to the optic nerve that harmfully affects central and peripheral vision. ONA may occur as a result of optic neuritis, compression by tumors or aneurysms, toxic and nutritional neuropathies, trauma, or as a secondary complication to other systemic diseases such as

diabetes. Symptoms of ONA vary diversely, but mainly include blurred vision and a reduction in optic sharpness and color visualization. ONA is irreversible process, and current medical strategies focus on finding the underlying cause, and trying to prevent further vision loss and protect the other healthy eye. This is a single-arm, single-center trial to assess the safety and efficacy of purified adult autologous bone marrow-derived CD34+, CD133+, and CD271+ stem cells through a 24-month follow-up period. The combination of these three cell types was based on their diverse potentialities to differentiate into specific functional cell types to regenerate damaged optic nerves and supporting issues and vasculature, and the availability of clinical-grade purification system (CliniMACS) and Microbeads to purify the target cell populations in clinically approved methods. Anticipated outcomes of this study are defined as an overall improvement of vision, restoration of functions to damaged optic nerves, and improvement in the quality of life of patients.

Official Title

Treatment of Optic Neuropathies Using Autologous Bone Marrow-Derived Clusters of Differentiation (CD) 34+, 133+, and 271+ Stem Cells: A Pilot Study

Conditions

Optic Neuropathy

Intervention/Treatment

Biological: Stem Cells

Study Start

2013-04

Primary Completion (Estimated)

2021-09-01

Study Completion (Estimated)

2021-10-01

Enrollment (Estimated)

100

Study Type

Interventional

Phase

Phase 1 Phase 2

Jordan

Amman, Jordan, 11953
Recruiting
Stem Cells of Arabia

Contact

Adeeb AlZoubi, PhD
adeebalzoubi@stemcellsarabia.net

Principal Investigator
Adeeb AlZoubi, PhD

Eligibility Criteria
Inclusion Criteria
- Patient should suffer from Optic Nerve Atrophy diseases like diabetic retinopathy and retinal pigmentation.
- Age between 18 and 55 years old.
- Willingness to undergo bone marrow-derived autologous cell therapy.
- Ability to comprehend the explained protocol.
- Ability and willingness to regularly visit to hospital for protocol and follow-up.

Exclusion Criteria
- Patients with preexisting or current systemic disease such as lung, liver, gastrointestinal, cardiac, immunodeficiency, syphilis, or clinically relevant polyneuropathies.
- History of life-threatening allergic or immune-mediated reaction.

Ages Eligible for Study
18 Years to 55 Years (Adult)

Sexes Eligible for Study
All

Accepts Healthy Volunteers
No

Primary Purpose: Treatment
Allocation: N/A
Interventional Model: Single Group Assignment
Masking: None (Open Label)

Arms and interventions

Participant group/arm	Intervention/treatment
Experimental: stem cells Intervention: transplantation of autologous purified stem cells	Biological: stem cells • Intervention: transplantation of autologous purified stem cells

Primary outcome measures

Outcome measure	Measure description	Time frame
Reduction in degeneration of the optic nerve using the visual field assessment with the Humphrey automated and Goldmann manual perimeters		24 months

Secondary outcome measures

Outcome measure	Measure description	Time frame
Improvement in visual function using the documentation of visual acuity using the Snellen chart		24 months

Sponsor
Stem Cells Arabia

Collaborators
No information provided

Investigators

- Principal Investigator: Adeeb AlZoubi, PhD

General Publications
No publications available

Unknown Status

Russian Federation

Effectiveness and Safety of Adipose-Derived Regenerative Cells for Treatment of Glaucomatous Neurodegeneration

ClinicalTrials.gov ID NCT02144103

Sponsor Central Clinical Hospital w/Outpatient Health Center of Business Administration for the President of Russian Federation
Information provided by Central Clinical Hospital w/Outpatient Health Center of Business Administration for the President of Russian Federation (Responsible Party)
Last Update Posted 2017-07-21

Brief Summary
Autologous adipose-derived regenerative cells (ADRC) extracted using Celution 800/CRS System (Cytori Therapeutics Inc.) from a portion of the fat harvested from the patient's front abdominal wall. ADRC will be administered one time into sub-tenon space of patient's eyeball. This is a single-arm study with no control. All patients receive cell therapy.

Detailed Description
Fat Tissue Obtainment

Subjects will undergo liposuction under local anesthesia. In this procedure, Ringer's solution with the anesthetic lidocaine and vasoconstrictor adrenaline is infused into the adipose compartment to minimize blood loss and contamination of the tissue by peripheral blood cells. Fifteen minutes later, a hollow blunt-tipped 3 mm cannula is introduced into the subcutaneous space through small (0.5 cm) incision. The cannula is attached to a syringe and under gentle suction moves through the adipose compartment, mechanically disrupting the fat tissue. Aspirate volume—approximately 150–200 cc. Procedure time—30 min.

ADRC Isolation

Aspirated fat tissue is placed into sterile vessel which is inserted into Celution 800/CRS System (Cytori Therapeutics Inc.)—closed system for automated and standardized extraction and concentration of ADRC. Celution 800/CRS System drains excess fluid from fat tissue and estimates its volume After that lipoaspirate washed extensively with equal volumes of Ringer's solution to remove blood. At the end of this process, System indicates required volume of enzyme reagent (Celase®) which should be added immediately by operator. After enzyme treatment Celution 800/CRS System automatically transfers isolated ADRC into washing compartment where ADRC washed and concentrated in 5 mL suspension. Tissue processing time—approximately 60 min. ADRC suspension matches all requirements listed in technical documentation for Celution 800/CRS System. Obtained ADRC is divided into two portions. First portion (0.2–0.5 mL) is used for counting, viability, and sterility assessment. Second portion is placed into sterile syringe for injection.

Subtenon Injection of ADRC

Antiseptic and anesthetic solutions are instilled into conjunctival sac. After that blepharostat is installed. The patient is asked to look in opposite to the injection side direction. Doctor inserts a needle into inferior temporal quadrant between rectus muscles, 10–12 mm from the limbus. Needle should be moved slowly, as close as possible to the eyeball. After needle placement at the depth of 5–7 mm, doctor injects concentrated solution of ADRC (up to 0.5 mL per single injection). Injection is made by insulin syringe with a needle size 0.45 mm * 12 mm (26 G).

Official Title

Effectiveness and Safety of Subtenon Administration of Autologous Adipose-Derived Regenerative Cells for Treatment of Glaucomatous Neurodegeneration

Conditions

Retinal Degeneration
Primary Open-Angle Glaucoma

Intervention/Treatment

Other: Subtenon administration of autologous ADRC
Procedure: Liposuction
Device: ADRC isolation

Study Start (Actual)

2014-05

Primary Completion (Estimated)

2018-07

Study Completion (Estimated)

2019-01

Enrollment (Estimated)

16

Study Type
Interventional

Phase
Phase 1 Phase 2

Moscow, Russian Federation, 119002
Federal State Budgetary Institution "Outpatient Health Center №1" of the Business Administration for the President of the Russian Federation

Moscow, Russian Federation, 121359
Federal State Budgetary Institution "Central Clinical Hospital with Outpatient Health Center" of the Business Administration for the President of the Russian Federation; Center for Biomedical Technologies

Eligibility Criteria
Inclusion Criteria
- Patient suffers from primary open-angle glaucoma (II and III stages; single eye or both eyes) at least for 6 months.
- Intraocular pressure is stable for at least for 3 months.
- Visual acuity of each eye (measured by using visual acuity charts projector) is not less than 0.1.
- Patient is familiar with Participant information sheet.
- Patient signed informed consent form.

Noninclusion Criteria
- Contraindications to the local anesthesia or medical history of allergic reactions to local anesthetics.
- Any anomalies or conditions of at least one eye which can limit tonometry implementation.
- Inflammatory disease of at least one eye or auxiliary apparatus (both infectious and noninfectious etiology: conjunctivitis, keratitis, uveitis, dacryocystitis, etc.).
- Medical history of surgery on at least one eye during preceding 6 months.
- Medical history of heavy traumatic injury of eyes.
- Patient has a cataract with high degree of lens opacification which can limit planned eye examination.
- Patient prescribed for systemic corticosteroids or other medications treatment with proven effect leading on intraocular pressure increase.
- Medical history or present dry eye syndrome accompanied by corneal and conjunctival xerosis.
- Subcompensated or decompensated forms of chronic diseases of internal organs.
- Clinically significant abnormalities in results of laboratory tests.
- Any conditions limiting compliance (dementia, neuropsychiatric disease, drug and alcohol abuse etc.).
- Participation in other clinical trials (or administration of investigational drugs) during 3 months prior inclusion.
- Patients with malignant tumors including postoperative period, patients receiving chemotherapy and/or radiotherapy.

- Patient's activated partial thromboplastin time exceeds normal levels more than 1.8 times.
- Patients prescribed for anticoagulants treatment or patient received anticoagulants at least 1 h prior to lipoaspiration.
- Medical history of heterotopic ossifications.
- Patients prescribed for glycoprotein inhibitors treatment.
- Acute vascular pathology.
- Age-related macular degeneration.

Exclusion Criteria

- Patient's refusal from the further participation in trial.
- Patient's refusal from compliance with the requirements of contraception during the participation in research.
- Chronic kidney disease IV–V stages (creatinine clearance <30 mL/min estimated by Cockroft-Gault formula).
- Confirmed syphilis, HIV, hepatitis B or C infections.

Dropout Criteria

- Direct indications on immediate initiation of treatment with medications with proven effect leading to intraocular pressure increase.
- Pregnancy.
- Development of cataract with high degree of lens opacification which can limit planned eye examination.

Ages Eligible for Study

18 Years to 75 Years (Adult, Older Adult)

Sexes Eligible for Study

All

Accepts Healthy Volunteers

No

Design Details

Primary Purpose: Treatment
Allocation: N/A
Interventional Model: Single Group Assignment
Masking: None (Open Label)

Arms and interventions

Participant group/arm	Intervention/treatment
Experimental: ADRC injection Subjects will undergo liposuction under local anesthesia. Lipoaspirate will be processed to isolate and concentrate adipose-derived regenerative cells (ADRC). After ADRC isolation autologous cells suspension will be injected into subtenon space of patient's eye	Other: subtenon administration of autologous ADRC Procedure: liposuction Device: ADRC isolation • ADRC isolation performed using Celution 800/CRS System (Cytori Therapeutics Inc.) according to manufacturer's protocol

Primary outcome measures

Outcome measure	Measure description	Time frame
SAEs and SARs monitoring	Types, probability, and severity of treatment emergent serious adverse events (SAEs) and serious adverse reactions (SARs)	4 weeks after treatment

Secondary outcome measures

Outcome measure	Measure description	Time frame
Change in visual acuity	Change from baseline in visual acuity assessed by visual acuity test	Follow up to completion (up to 48 weeks after treatment)
Changes in structures of fundus of the eye-1	Changes in structures of fundus of the eye assessed by funduscopy: changes of configuration and size of optic disc, neuroretinal rim thinning, degree of optic disc pallor, hemorrhages on the optic nerve and retina, vascular changes, presence of degenerative changes of retina, optic disc drusen, edema, and retinal detachment	Follow up to completion (up to 48 weeks after treatment)
Changes in structures of fundus of the eye-2	Changes in structures of fundus of the eye assessed by optical coherence tomography: changes of optic disc, neuroretinal rim and macula, retinal nerve fiber layer thickness	Follow up to completion (up to 48 weeks after treatment)
Change in visual field	Change from baseline in visual field assessed by computer perimetry	Follow up to completion (up to 48 weeks after treatment)
Change in retinal flicker response	Change from baseline in critical flicker fusion threshold	Follow up to completion (up to 48 weeks after treatment)
Change in intraocular pressure	Change from baseline in intraocular pressure assessed by pneumotonometry and tonography	Follow up to completion (up to 48 weeks after treatment)
Quality-of-life monitoring	Quality of life estimated by validated questionnaires: the short form (36) health survey (SF-36), visual functioning-14 quality of life (VF-14 QOL), and glaucoma quality of life-15 (GQL-15)	Follow up to completion (up to 48 weeks after treatment)

Sponsor

Central Clinical Hospital w/Outpatient Health Center of Business Administration for the President of Russian Federation

Collaborators

No information provided

Investigators

- Study Director: Alina K Drakon, MD, Federal State Budgetary Institution "Central Clinical Hospital with Outpatient Health Center" of the Business Administration for the President of the Russian Federation

- Principal Investigator: Ilya I Eremin, MD, PhD, Federal State Budgetary Institution "Central Clinical Hospital with Outpatient Health Center" of the Business Administration for the President of the Russian Federation; Center for Biomedical Technologies
- Principal Investigator: Julia P Sotnikova, MD, Federal State Budgetary Institution "Outpatient Health Center №1" of the Business Administration for the President of the Russian Federation

General Publications

No publications available

Unknown Status

Spain

Safety Assessment of Intravitreal Mesenchymal Stem Cells for Acute Nonarteritic Anterior Ischemic Optic Neuropathy (NEUROSTEM)

ClinicalTrials.gov ID NCT03173638

Sponsor Instituto Universitario de Oftalmobiología Aplicada (Institute of Applied Ophthalmobiology)—IOBA

Information provided by Instituto Universitario de Oftalmobiología Aplicada (Institute of Applied Ophthalmobiology)—IOBA (Responsible Party)

Last Update Posted 2021-04-06

Brief Summary

In this study, the investigators propose to perform a Phase II Clinical Trial which seeks to evaluate the safety of cell therapy as a new treatment for patients who suffer from acute nonarteritic anterior ischemic optic neuropathy (NAION). If it is successful, a later study to assess efficacy will be performed.

This disease has an age-adjusted incidence rate of 10/100,000, and in many cases it results in blindness. Currently, there is no available treatment and second eye involvement occurs in approximately 15–25% of the cases.

All this background originates a particularly dramatic outcome for the patient. Therefore, it seems justified to evaluate new therapies that maintain or improve the visual function in these patients.

The Project includes a clinical trial whose purpose is the assessment of the safety of intravitreal administration of allogenic mesenchymal stem cells (MSC) in patients with NAION, a product in clinical research phase (PEI No. 15-007) already approved for other human clinical applications (PEI No. 15-007).

It can be considered that the therapy with intravitreal injection of MSC is a treatment option in patients with acute NAION, since through the paracrine properties of these cells (secretion of neurotrophic, immunomodulatory, and antiapoptotic factors), it may prevent or reduce the progression of axonal degeneration caused by this disease.

Official Title
Phase II Safety Assessment of Intravitreal Injection of Mesenchymal Stem Cells for Acute Nonarteritic Anterior Ischemic Optic Neuropathy (NAION)

Conditions
Nonarteritic Ischemic Optic Neuropathy

Intervention/Treatment
Procedure: intravitreal injection of MSV

Study Start (Actual)
2018-03-23

Primary Completion (Estimated)
2022-04

Study Completion (Estimated)
2022-12

Enrollment (Actual)
5

Study Type
Interventional

Phase
Phase 2

Spain

Valladolid, Spain, 47011
IOBA—Applied Ophthalmobiology Institute

Inclusion Criteria

- Patients with acute unilateral NAION (within 2 weeks after the first symptoms) with at least two of the following:
  - Sudden and unpainful monocular vision loss
  - Visual field defects
  - Dyschromatopsia
  - Ocular nerve head edema
  - Afferent relative pupil defect
- Patients ≥50 years old, able to freely give informed consent.
- Best-corrected visual acuity (BCVA) ≤0.1 in study eye.
- Pseudophakia in study eye.
- Preserved pupil sphincter muscle motility.
- Signed informed consent form before any study procedure.
- Signed data protection consent form before any study procedure.

Exclusion Criteria
- Giant cell arteritis evidence (clinical history, erythrocyte sedimentation rate (ESR), C-Reactive Protein).
- Evidence of any other etiology that may justify the optic neuropathy (even in the nonstudy eye).
- History of systemic vasculitis, multiple sclerosis, collagenopathies or previous cancer treatments.
- Hypersensitivity or allergy to any compound used in the study, including investigational medicinal product (IMP).
- Positive pregnancy test at baseline.
- Participation in any other research study within 2 months.

Ophthalmic Exclusion Criteria
- History of uveitis or active ocular inflammation.
- History or evidence of glaucoma or high intraocular pressure ($\geq$24 mmHg in either eye).
- Mean opacities or retinal pathologies in the study eye.
- Any previous vitreous or glaucoma surgery in the study eye.
- Cataract surgery within 3 months in the study eye.

Ages Eligible for Study
- 18 Years to 80 Years (Adult, Older Adult)

Sexes Eligible for Study
- All

Accepts Healthy Volunteers

Primary Purpose: Treatment
Allocation: N/A
Interventional Model: Single Group Assignment
Masking: None (Open Label)

Arms and interventions

Participant group/arm	Intervention/treatment
Experimental: mesenchymal stem from valladolid (MSV) Allogenic mesenchymal stem cells from bone marrow	Procedure: intravitreal injection of MSV • A unique intravitreal injection of MSV in acute phase of NAION

Primary outcome measures

Outcome measure	Measure description	Time frame
Absence of inflammatory reaction—slit lamp exploration—SUN (standardization of uveitis nomenclature) scale	Following the SUN scale, the parameters that will be taken into account in the slit lamp exploration will be: cells and flare in the anterior chamber, and vitreous flare	Changes compared to baseline in visits V1 (1 day), V2 (1 week), V3 (1 month), V4 (3 months), V5 (6 months), and V6 (12 months) and in any unscheduled visit any patient might need

Secondary outcome measures

Outcome measure	Measure description	Time frame
Adverse events procedure-related (intravitreal injection)	Conjunctival hemorrhages, anterior chamber inflammation, changes in intraocular pressure, infectious endophthalmitis, vitreous inflammation, retinal detachment, choroidal detachment, corneal opacities, lens opacities, neovascularization, macular edema, or any other adverse event that may appear	Throughout the study after treatment in visits V1 (1 day), V2 (1 week), V3 (1 month), V4 (3 months), V5 (6 months), and V6 (12 months) and in any unscheduled visit any patient might need

Sponsor

Instituto Universitario de Oftalmobiología Aplicada (Institute of Applied Ophthalmobiology)—IOBA

Collaborators

University of Valladolid

Investigators

- Principal Investigator: José C Pastor Jimeno, MD, PhD, IOBA-UVA

General Publications

No publications available

Chapter 3
Gene Therapy Studies in Optic Nerve Disease Treatment

Recruiting

China

Gene Therapy Clinical Trial for the Treatment of Leber's Hereditary Optic Neuropathy (GOLD)

ClinicalTrials.gov ID NCT04912843

Sponsor Wuhan Neurophth Biotechnology Limited Company
Information provided by Wuhan Neurophth Biotechnology Limited Company (Responsible Party)
Last Update Posted 2022-11-14

Brief Summary
The objective of this clinical study is to select the optimal dose and evaluate the safety and efficacy of NR082 in treatment of LHON caused by mitochondrial ND4 gene mutation. Part 1 (Phase 1/2) is a safety dose-finding study, which will enroll subjects aged ≥18 years old and ≤ 75 years old to receive a single unilateral intravitreal (IVT) injection of NR082 to observe its safety and efficacy. In Part 2 (Phase 3) of the clinical study, the dose recommended after the end of Part 1 is used to further verify the safety and efficacy of the study drug. Part 2 of the study is divided into the safety run-in phase and the randomized, double-blind, and control study. Subjects aged ≥12 and ≤75 years will be enrolled in the Part 2. The run-in phase will enroll six evaluable subjects. After monitoring for at least 6 weeks, if no new safety signals are observed, the clinical trial will enter the randomized, double-blind, and control study phase upon approval by the Safety Review Committee (SRC). The clinical manifestation of all subjects is reduced visual acuity caused by LHON associated with ND4 mutation, and central laboratory test showed G11778A

J. N. Weiss, *Clinical Trials in Optic Nerve Disease Treatment*,
https://doi.org/10.1007/978-3-031-58815-0_3

mutation (a CLIA-certified laboratory), while the reduced visual acuity lasted for >6 months and < 10 years.

Detailed Description

Part 1: Dose-Finding At the dose-finding part, the principle is that the Safety Review Committee (SRC) will determine whether to make dose adjustment based on the safety data of the starting dose in Part 1. The recommended dose (safe and effective dose) of the Part 2 study will be determined jointly by the SRC, IDMC, sponsor, and the drug regulatory authority after the interim analysis in Part 1 is completed.

The starting dose in Part 1 is 1.5 × 109 vg, 0.05 mL eye/dose. The safety of the starting dose will be reviewed by the SRC and the dose escalation or de-escalation will be recommended by the SRC.

The safety of the starting dose will first be performed in six evaluable subjects.

Part 2 (including the safety run-in phase and the randomized, double-blind, and sham-injection control study):

First Stage: safety run-in phase:

The safety run-in phase of Part 2 will enroll six evaluable subjects (including at least one minor subject aged ≥12 years and < 18 years) aged ≥12 years and ≤75 years at the dose determined in Part 1, namely 4.5 × 109 vg, 0.05 mL eye/dose (high dose) and monitor the safety for at least 6 weeks. If there is no new safety concern evaluated by the SRC, the randomized, double-blind, sham-injection control study can be initiated.

Sccond Stage: randomized, double-blind, sham-injection control study:

The randomized, double-blind, sham-injection control study of Part 2 is to verify the efficacy and safety of NR082 in LHON caused by mitochondrial gene ND4 mutation at the dose determined in Part 1 of the study, namely 4.5 × 109 vg, 0.05 mL eye/dose (high dose). This part is divided into the NR082 treatment group and the control group (sham-injection group).

Official Title

A Phase 1/2/3, Multicenter, Two-Part Clinical Trial to Evaluate the Safety and Efficacy of Gene Therapy for Leber's Hereditary Optic Neuropathy (LHON) Associated with ND4 Mutation

Conditions

Leber's Hereditary Optic Neuropathy (LHON)

Study type

Interventional

Enrollment (Estimated)

102

Intervention/Treatment

Drug: NR082 injection
Device: Sham Injection

Phase
Phase 2 Phase 3

Other Study ID Numbers
NFS-01-101

Study Start (Actual)
2021-06-18

Primary Completion (Estimated)
2024-02-29

Study Completion (Estimated)
2028-02-29

Study Contact
Name: Xiaoning Guo, PHD
Phone Number: +86–21-64172955
Email: info@neurophth.com
China

Beijing, China
Recruiting
Beijing Tongren Hospital, Capital Medical University

Eligibility Criteria
Ages Eligible for Study
12 to 75 Years (Child, Adult, Older Adult)

Accepts Healthy Volunteer
No

Sexes Eligible for Study
All

Inclusion Criteria Age
- Age at signing of informed consent form
  - In Part 1, the age of the subjects must be ≥18 years old and ≤ 75 years old.
  - In Part 2, the age of the subjects must be ≥12 years old and ≤ 75 years old, and the six evaluable subjects must be monitored for at least 6 weeks during the safety run-in phase. If SRC believes that there is no safety issue, the randomized double-blind control study will be initiated Subject Type and Disease Characteristics.
- The clinical manifestation caused by LHON is vision loss, with a visual acuity of ≥0.5 LogMAR in BCVA in either eye.
- The genotype test result is that there is G11778A mutation in ND4 gene, and there are no other primary LHON-associated mutations in the mitochondrial DNA (mtDNA) (ND1[G3460A] or ND6[T14484C]) (confirmed by a CLIA-certified international laboratory).

- The duration of vision loss in the eye with worse visual acuity lasted >6 months and < 10 years at screening.
- Pupils can be adequately dilated for a comprehensive eye examination and visual acuity test.
- Each eye of the subject must maintain the VA determined by manual visual acuity test (≤2.3 LogMAR) as defined in the ocular/vision examination manual (operating manual for optometry and VA examinations) in this study.
- Sign the written informed consent form and willing to comply with the clinical study protocol Sex.
- Male or female.
  - Male Subjects:
    A male subject must agree to take contraceptive measures at least 6 months after the treatment visit.
  - Female Subjects:
    A female subject is eligible to participate if she is not pregnant, not breastfeeding, and at least one of the following conditions applies:
      Not a woman of childbearing potential (WOCBP). A WOCBP who agrees to follow the contraception guidance for at least 6 months after the treatment visit Informed Consent.
- Written informed consent form must be obtained from the subject or his/her parent/legal guardian (if the subject is under 18 years of age) (Part 2) before any study-related procedures are performed. If the subject is legally identified as blind (>1.0 LogMAR or decimal acuity meter reading <0.1), an impartial witness must be present throughout the informed consent process and discussion process.

Exclusion Criteria

Subjects who meet any of the following criteria will be excluded from the study:

- Any known allergy and/or hypersensitivity to the study drug or its constituents.
- Contraindication to IVT injection in any eye.
- IVT drug delivery to any eye within 30 days prior to the screening visit.
- History of vitrectomy in either eye.
- Narrow anterior chamber angle in any eye contraindicating pupillary dilation.
- Presence of disorders or diseases of the eye or adnexa, excluding LHON, which may interfere with visual or ocular assessments, including spectral-domain optical coherence tomography (FD-OCT), during the study.
- Presence of known/documented mutations, other than the LHON-related mutation, which are known to cause pathology of the optic nerve, retina or afferent visual system.
- Presence of systemic or ocular/vision diseases, disorders or pathologies, other than LHON, known to cause or be associated with vision loss, or whose associated treatment(s) or therapy(ies) is/are known to cause or be associated with vision loss.

- Presence of optic neuropathy from any cause other than LHON.
- Presence of illness or disease that, in the opinion of the investigator, includes symptoms and/or the associated treatments that can alter visual function, for instance cancers or pathology of the CNS, including multiple sclerosis (diagnosis of multiple sclerosis must be based on the 2010 Revisions to the McDonald Criteria) (Polman et al., 2011), and/or diseases or conditions that affect the safety of subjects participating in the study.
- History of recurrent uveitis (idiopathic or immune-related) or active ocular inflammation.
- Participated in another clinical study and received IP within 90 days prior to the screening visit.

(a) Exceptions: Subjects who have completed the clinical study of idebenone as IP within 90 days prior to the screening visit, and have completely discontinued idebenone at least 7 days prior to dosing are still eligible to participate in the study.

- Any eye has previously received ocular gene therapy.
- Subjects who refused to stop using idebenone.
- Have undergone ocular surgery of clinical relevance (per investigator's assessment) within 90 days prior to the screening visit.
- Female subjects who are breastfeeding or plan to breastfeed within the first 6 months after the administration of NR082 Injection.
- History of drug or alcohol abuse (including heavy smoking, i.e., >20 cigarettes per day or >20 pack-years [equivalent to one pack a day for 20 years or 2 packs a day for 10 years]).
- Subjects with positive human immunodeficiency virus (HIV), syphilis, and HCV antibodies are excluded; subjects who have clinically significant active infection requiring treatment as shown by hepatitis B test (defined as positive hepatitis B core antibody [HBcAb] or hepatitis B surface antigen [HBsAg], hepatitis B virus deoxyribonucleic acid (HBV-DNA) >1000 copies /mL or > lower limit of quantitative detection with the local laboratory method) will be excluded.
- Unable to tolerate or unable or unwilling to comply with all the protocol requirements.
- Subjects from the study site fail to comply with or do not agree to comply with local and institutional guidelines for suspected 2019 novel coronavirus (COVID-19) infection/testing.
- Any other exclusions determined by the investigator.

Primary Purpose: Treatment
Allocation: Randomized
Interventional Model: Sequential Assignment

Interventional Model Description
Part 1:

Dose-Finding at the dose-finding part, the principle is that the Safety Review Committee (SRC) will determine whether to make dose adjustment based on the safety data of the starting dose in Part 1. The recommended dose (safe and effective dose) of the Part 2 study will be determined jointly by the SRC, IDMC, sponsor, and the drug regulatory authority after the interim analysis in Part 1 is completed.

Part 2:

First Stage: safety run-in phase:

The safety run-in phase of Part 2 will enroll six evaluable subjects (including at least one minor subject aged ≥12 years and <18 years) aged ≥12 years and ≤75 years at the dose determined in Part 1, namely 4.5 × 109 vg, 0.05 mL eye/dose (high dose) and monitor the safety for at least 6 weeks. If there is no new safety concern evaluated by the SRC, the randomized, double-blind, sham-injection control study can be initiated.

Second Stage: randomized, double-blind, sham-injection control study:

Masking: Quadruple (Participant Care Provider Investigator Outcomes Assessor)
Masking Description: Part 1: Dose-Finding: open label; 12 subjects Part 2: First Stage: safety run-in phase: open label; six subjects Part 2: Second Stage: randomized, doublc-blind, sham-injection; 90 subjects.

Arms and interventions

Participant group/arm	Intervention/treatment
Experimental: NR082 injection 0.5E9 viral genomes (vg), 0.05 mL eye/dose, single-dose, only one eye per subject; 1.5E9 viral genomes (vg), 0.05 mL eye/dose single-dose, only one eye per subject; 4.5E9 viral genomes (vg), 0.05 mL eye/dose single-dose, only one eye per subject part 1: Dose-finding: The recommended dose (safe and effective dose) of the part 2 study will be determined jointly by the SRC, IDMC, sponsor, and the drug regulatory authority after the interim analysis in part 1 is completed.	Drug: NR082 injection • Intravitreal injection (IVT)
Sham comparator: sham-injection Part2. Second stage: randomized, double-blind, sham-injection control study one eye of each participant will undergo sham injection. Sham intravitreal injection will be performed by applying pressure to the eye at the location of a typical intravitreal injection procedure using the blunt end of a syringe without a needle	Device: Sham injection • Sham intravitreal injection

Primary outcome measures

Outcome measure	Measure description	Time frame
Safety and tolerability of NR082 at different doses	Incidence rates of AEs, SAEs, and DLTs within 12 weeks after injection of NR082 at different doses	Part 1 (phase1/2): 12 weeks
Safety after NR082 treatment among subjects 12≤ aged ≤75 years	Incidence rates of AEs and SAEs within 6 weeks after NR082 treatment	Part 2 (stage 1): 6 weeks
Efficacy of NR082 in study eye	Proportion of ≥0.3 logMAR from baseline in BCVA in the study eye in the NR082 treatment and the sham injection at week 52 after treatment	Part 2 (stage 2): 52 weeks

Secondary outcome measures

Outcome measure	Measure description	Time frame
The efficacy and safety following intravitreal injection of NR082 at different doses	Improvement and mean change from baseline in BCVA; change from baseline in visual field, contrast sensitivity, and visual evoked potential	Part 1 (phase1/2), part 2 (sStage 1 and stage 2): week 2, 6, 12, 26, 40, and 52
Further assess the efficacy and safety following intravitreal injection of NR082 at different doses	Descriptions of safety evaluation at weeks 26, 40, and 52	Part 1 (phase1/2) and part 2 (stage 1): at weeks 26, 40, and 52
Immunogenicity and vector shedding/biodistribution	Assessment of cell immunity, humoral immunity, vector DNA shedding in tears (both eyes), and biodistribution in whole blood	Part 1 (phase1/2), part 2 (stage 1 and stage 2): week 2, 6, 12, 26, 40, and 52
The change in quality of life from baseline	Change from baseline in VFQ-25 and SF-36	Part 1 (phase1/2), part 2 (stage 1 and stage 2): week 2, 26, and 52
Morphological improvement after NR082 treatment	Change from baseline in RNFL, GCL, and IPL thickness in the study eye	Part 1 (phase1/2), part 2 (stage 1 and stage 2): week 2, 6, 12, 26, 40, and 52
Safety and efficacy of NR082 caused by mitochondrial gene ND4 mutation	Incidence rates of AEs and SAEs between the NR082 treatment group and the sham-injection group (ocular and nonocular)	Part 2 (stage 2): week 2, 6, 12, 26, 40, and 52

Sponsor

Wuhan Neurophth Biotechnology Limited Company

Collaborators
No information provided

Investigators

- Study Chair: Bin Li, MD, Wuhan Neurophth Biotechnology Limited Company.

General Publications
No publications available

Recruiting

Gene Therapy Clinical Trial for the Treatment of Leber's Hereditary Optic Neuropathy Associated with ND1 Mutations

ClinicalTrials.gov ID NCT05820152

Sponsor Neurophth Therapeutics Inc.
Information provided by Neurophth Therapeutics Inc. (Responsible Party)
Last Update Posted 2023-09-13.

Brief Summary
The objective of this clinical study is to evaluate the safety, tolerability, and preliminary efficacy of NFS-02 in the treatment of LHON caused by mitochondrial ND1 gene mutation. This study will enroll subjects aged ≥18 years old and ≤75 years old to receive a single unilateral intravitreal (IVT) injection of NFS-02 to evaluate its safety, tolerability, and preliminary efficacy.

The clinical manifestations of all subjects are to be reduced visual acuity caused by LHON associated with ND1 mutation, with laboratory tests showing G3460A mutation (a CLIA-certified laboratory) and reduced visual acuity lasting for >6 months and <10 years.

Detailed Description
At the dose-finding stage, the principle is that the Safety Review Committee (SRC) will decide whether to make dose adjustment based on the safety data of the starting dose. The starting dose is 1.5 × 108 vg, 0.05 mL eye/dose. The safety of the starting dose will be reviewed by the SRC, and dose escalation or de-escalation is by recommendation of the SRC. The safety of the starting dose will first be performed in six evaluable subjects.

Criteria for Dose Modification
Dose Escalation:

If drug-related dose-limiting toxicity (DLT) events are observed in <2 of the six evaluable subjects within 6 weeks after the dosing of NFS-02 at the starting dose, the dose can be escalated to 5.0 × 108 vg, 0.05 mL eye/dose after the approval by SRC.

If drug-related dose-limiting toxicity (DLT) events are observed in <2 of the six evaluable subjects within 6 weeks after the dosing of NFS-02 at the 5.0 × 108 vg, 0.05 mL eye/dose, the dose can be escalated to 1.5 × 109 vg, 0.05 mL eye/dose after the approval by SRC.

Dose De-Escalation:

If drug-related dose-limiting toxicity (DLT) events are observed in ≥2 of the six evaluable subjects within 6 weeks after the dosing of NFS-02 at the starting dose, the dose can be de-escalated to 5.0 × 107 vg, 0.05 mL eye/dose after the approval by SRC.

Enrollment Sequence

- The enrollment sequence of any dose group (six subjects) is that the second subject and the third subject will be enrolled at least 7 days after the enrollment of the first subject.
- The fourth, fifth, and sixth subjects will be enrolled at least 7 days after the enrollment of the second and the third subjects.

The 7-day interval is to avoid acute safety events to the greatest possible extent.

Official Title

A Phase 1/2, Multiregional, Single-Arm, Open-Label, Dose-Finding Clinical Trial to Evaluate the Safety, Tolerability, and Efficacy of Gene Therapy for Leber's Hereditary Optic Neuropathy (LHON) Associated with ND1 Mutation

Conditions

Leber Hereditary Optic Neuropathy (LHON)

Study Type

Interventional

Enrollment (Estimated)

18

Intervention/Treatment

Drug: NFS-02 Injection

Phase

Phase 1 Phase 2

Other Study ID Numbers

NFS-02-101

Study Start (Actual)

2023-08-15

Primary Completion (Estimated)

2024-12-30

Study Completion (Estimated)

2029-12-30

Study Contact
Name: Bin LI
Phone Number: +8602765524119
Email: info@neurophth.com

China
Beijing Locations

Beijing, Beijing, China
Recruiting
The First Medical Center of the General Hospital of the Chinese People's Liberation Army

Contact
Shihui Wei, Doctor
+8613910079431 weishihui706@hotmail.com

Zhejiang Locations
Wenzhou, Zhejiang, China
Recruiting
Optometry Affiliated to Wenzhou Medical University

Contact
Jia Qu, Doctor
+8613806898805 13806898805@163.com

Eligibility Criteria
Ages Eligible for Study
18 to 75 Years (Adult, Older Adult)

Accepts Healthy Volunteer
No

Sexes Eligible for Study
All

Inclusion Criteria
Age

- Age at the time of signing the informed consent form: the age of the subjects must be ≥18 years old and ≤ 75 years old Type of Subject and Disease Characteristics.
- The clinical manifested vision loss due to LHON, and any eye BCVA ≥0.5 LogMAR.
- The genotype testing result shows the presence of G3460A mutation in the ND1 gene, and the absence of the other primary LHON-associated mutations in the mitochondrial DNA (mtDNA) (ND4 [G11778A] or ND6 [T14484C]) (confirmed by a CLIA-certified international laboratory).
- The vision loss in the eye with worse visual acuity lasted >6 months and < 10 years at screening.

- Pupils can be adequately dilated for a thorough ocular examination and visual acuity test.
- Each eye of the subject must maintain at least Hand Motion visual acuity (VA) ($\leq$ 2.3 LogMAR) as defined in the ocular/vision examination manual (operating manual for refraction and VA examinations) in this study.
- Willingness to comply with the clinical study protocol and 5 years of long-term follow-up after administration Sex.
- Male or female.
  - Male Subjects:

    A male subject must agree to take contraceptive measures at least 6 months after the treatment visit.
  - Female Subjects:

    A female subject is eligible to participate if she is not pregnant not breast-feeding, and at least one of the following conditions applies:
    Not a woman of childbearing potential (WOCBP). A WOCBP who agrees to follow the contraception guidance for at least 6 months after the treatment visit Informed Consent.
- Written informed consent form must be obtained from the subject or his/her parent/legal guardian before any study-related procedure is performed.
- If the subject is legally blind (> 1.0 LogMAR or the readings of decimal visual acuity chart <0.1), an impartial witness must be present throughout the informed consent process and discussion process.

Exclusion Criteria

- Any known allergy and/or hypersensitivity to the study drug or its constituents.
- Contraindication to IVT injection in any eye.
- IVT drug delivery to any eye within 30 days prior to the screening visit.
- History of vitrectomy in either eye.
- Narrow anterior chamber angle in any eye contraindicating pupillary dilation.
- Presence of disorders or diseases of the eye or adnexa, excluding LHON, which may interfere with visual or ocular assessments, including spectral-domain optical coherence tomography (SD-OCT), during the study.
- Presence of known/documented mutations, other than the LHON-related mutation, which are known to cause pathology of the optic nerve, retina, or afferent visual system.
- Presence of systemic or ocular/vision diseases, disorders, or pathologies, other than LHON, known to cause or be associated with vision loss, or whose associated treatment(s) or therapy(ies) is/are known to cause or be associated with vision loss.
- Presence of optic neuropathy from any cause other than LHON.
- Presence of illness or disease that, in the opinion of the investigator, includes symptoms and/or the associated treatments that can alter visual function, for instance cancers or pathology of the central nervous system (CNS), including multiple sclerosis (diagnosis of multiple sclerosis must be based on the 2010

Revisions to the McDonald Criteria) (Polman C H et al., 2011), and/or diseases or conditions that affect the safety of subjects participating in the study.
- History of recurrent uveitis (idiopathic or immune-related) or active ocular inflammation.
- Participated in another clinical study and receive an IMP within 90 days prior to the screening visit.

  (a) Exceptions: Subjects who have completed the clinical study of idebenone as IMP >90 days prior to the screening visit and has completely discontinued idebenone at least 7 days prior to dosing are still eligible to participate in the study.

- Any eye has previously received ocular gene therapy.
- Subjects who refused to stop using idebenone.
- Have undergone clinical-related ocular surgery (per investigator's assessment) within 90 days prior to the screening visit.
- Female subjects who are breastfeeding or plan to breastfeed within the first 6 months after the administration of NFS-02 Injection.
- History of drug or alcohol abuse (including heavy smoking, i.e., > 20 cigarettes per day or > 20 pack-years [equivalent to one pack a day for 20 years or 2 packs a day for 10 years]).
- Human immunodeficiency virus (HIV) antibody, syphilis antibody, and HCV antibody positive are excluded; hepatitis B test that shows a clinically significant active infection requiring treatment (defined as the presence of hepatitis B core antibody [HBcAb] positive or hepatitis B surface antigen [HBsAg] positive, and hepatitis B virus deoxyribonucleic acid [HBV-DNA] > 1000 copies/mL or according to local laboratory method above lower limit of quantitative detection) is excluded.
- Unable to tolerate or unable or unwilling to comply with all the protocol requirements.
- Subjects from the study site fail to comply with or do not agree to comply with local and institutional guidelines for suspected 2019 novel coronavirus (COVID-19) infection/testing.
- Any other exclusions determined by the investigator.

Design Details

Primary Purpose: Treatment.

Allocation: N/A

Interventional Model: Sequential Assignment

Interventional Model Description: 5.0 × 107 vg, 0.05 mL eye/dose (low dose); 1.5 × 108 vg, 0.05 mL eye/dose (starting dose); 5.0 × 108 vg, 0.05 mL eye/dose (intermediate dose); 1.5 × 109 vg, 0.05 mL eye/dose (high dose)

Masking: None (Open Label)

Arms and interventions

Participant group/arm	Intervention/treatment
Experimental: NFS-02 injection Potential doses at the dose-finding stage: 5.0 × 107 vg, 0.05 mL/eye/dose (low dose); 1.5 × 108 vg, 0.05 mL/eye/dose (starting dose); 5.0 × 108 vg, 0.05 mL/eye/dose (intermediate dose); 1.5 × 109 vg, 0.05 mL/eye/dose (high dose)	Drug: NFS-02 injection • The starting dose is 1.5 × 108 vg, 0.05 mL eye/dose. If drug-related dose-limiting toxicity (DLT) events are observed in <2 of the six evaluable subjects within 6 weeks after the dosing of NFS-02 at the starting dose, the dose can be escalated to 5.0 × 108 vg, 0.05 mL eye/dose after the approval by SRC. If drug-related dose-limiting toxicity (DLT) events are observed in <2 of the six evaluable subjects within 6 weeks after the dosing of NFS-02 at the 5.0 × 108 vg, 0.05 mL eye/dose, the dose can be escalated to 1.5 × 109 vg, 0.05 mL eye/dose after the approval by SRC. If drug-related dose-limiting toxicity (DLT) events are observed in ≥2 of the six evaluable subjects within 6 weeks after the dosing of NFS-02 at the starting dose, the dose can be de-escalated to 5.0 × 107 vg, 0.05 mL eye/dose after the approval by SRC

Primary outcome measures

Outcome measure	Measure description	Time frame
Incidence of adverse events (AEs)	Incidence of adverse events (AEs) within 52 weeks of NFS-02 intravitreal injection at different doses	52 weeks
Incidence of serious adverse events (SAEs)	Incidence of serious adverse events (SAEs)within 52 weeks of NFS-02 intravitreal injection at different doses	52 weeks
Incidence of dose-limiting toxicities (DLT)	Incidence of dose-limiting toxicities (DLT) (ocular and nonocular) within 52 weeks of NFS-02 intravitreal injection at different doses	52 weeks

Secondary outcome measures

Outcome measure	Measure description	Time frame
Proportion (%) of subjects with an improvement of ≥0.3 logMAR from baseline in BCVA in the injected eye and noninjected eye	ETDRS visual acuity charts will used to assess proportion (percent) of subjects with an improvement of ≥0.3 logMAR from baseline in best-corrected visual acuity (BCVA)	At weeks 2, 6,12, 26, 40, 52, 78, 104, 130, 156, 182, 208, 234, and 260
Mean change from baseline in BCVA (logMAR) in the injected eye and noninjected eye	ETDRS visual acuity charts will used to assess mean change from baseline in BCVA (logMAR)	At weeks 2, 6,12, 26, 40, 52, 78, 104, 130, 156, 182, 208, 234, and 260
Mean change in BCVA (logMAR) compared to nadir in the injected eye and noninjected eye	ETDRS visual acuity charts will used to assess mean change in BCVA (logMAR) compared to nadir	At weeks 2, 6,12, 26, 40, 52, 78, 104, 130, 156, 182, 208, 234, and 260

Change from baseline in the parameter of microperimetry in the injected eye and noninjected eye	Microperimetry parameters will evaluate alterations in function of different regions of the retina. The major parameter to be documented is mean sensitivity	At weeks 2, 6,12, 26, 40, 52, 78, 104, 130, 156, 182, 208, 234, and 260
Proportion (%) of subjects with a clinically meaningful improvement of injected eye from baseline in microperimetry in the injected eye and noninjected eye	Microperimetry parameters will evaluate alterations in function of different regions of the retina. The major parameter to be documented is mean sensitivity. A clinically meaningful improvement is defined as an improvement of 7 decibels (dB) or more posttreatment from a baseline in a predefined area consisting of five or more points in central 20° vision on microperimetry (a predefined area is set as central 36 loci among 68 loci of the whole grid)	At weeks 2, 6,12, 26, 40, 52, 78, 104, 130, 156, 182, 208, 234, and 260
Change from baseline in contrast sensitivity in the injected eye and noninjected eye	The contrast sensitivity examination measures the subject's ability to discern targets presented at varying spatial frequencies or sizes under different contrast levels. The contrast sensitivity examination measures the full range of visual sensitivity, including brightness and contrast, and it may be used as a comprehensive assessment of visual function	At weeks 2, 6,12, 26, 40, 52, 78, 104, 130, 156, 182, 208, 234, and 260
Change from baseline in visual evoked potential (VEP) parameters in the injected eye and noninjected eye	VEP is a visual electrophysiological examination used to identify possible ischemic optic neuropathy, including the P100 latency, P100 amplitude, P2 latency, P2 amplitude	At weeks 2, 6,12, 26, 40, 52, 78, 104, 130, 156, 182, 208, 234, and 260
To evaluate immunogenicity	A central laboratory will be used to evaluate anti-AAV2 neutralizing antibodies in the serum samples of all subjects. These samples will be tested by the sponsor or its designee to detect anti-AAV2 neutralizing antibodies in the samples and report the titer of confirmed positive samples. Samples confirmed positive for anti-AAV2 neutralizing antibodies will also be evaluated for the presence of neutralizing antibodies	At weeks 1, 2, 6, 12, 26, 40, and 52
To evaluate immunogenicity	The interferon gamma enzyme-linked immunospot (ELISpot) assay will be performed to measure the proliferative response of lymphocytes to AAV2 antigen and ND1 peptide. The number of activated cells in the sample were calculated	At weeks 1, 2, 6, 12, 26, 40, and 52
To evaluate vector shedding	Assessment of vector DNA shedding in tears (both eyes). Samples were analyzed to determine the presence of viral DNA in tears	At weeks 1, 2, 6, 12, 26, 40, and 52
To evaluate biodistribution	Assessment of biodistribution in whole blood. Samples were analyzed to determine the presence of viral DNA in whole blood	At weeks 1, 2, 6, 12, 26, 40, and 52

To evaluate the improvement in BCVA in the injected eye and noninjected eye (<0.3 logMAR)	ETDRS visual acuity charts will be used to assess proportion (percent) of subjects with an improvement of ≥0.2 logMAR and ≥0.1 logMAR from baseline in BCVA proportion (percent) of subjects with visual acuity of >1.0 logMAR before and after treatment	At weeks 52, 78, 104, 130, 156, 182, 208, 234, and 260
Change from baseline in retinal nerve fiber layer (RNFL) thickness in the injected eye and noninjected eye	OCT is an imaging technology to investigate the ocular fundus by using of the basic principle of low-coherence light interferometry. It detects the reflection or diffusion signals of biological tissue layers of different depths by inputting low-coherence light and obtains the images and quantitative results of the microscopic structure of the retina	At weeks 2, 6,12, 26, 52, 78, 104, 130, 156, 182, 208, 234, and 260
Change from baseline in retinal ganglion cell complex thickness in the injected eye and noninjected eye	OCT is an imaging technology to investigate the ocular fundus by using of the basic principle of low-coherence light interferometry. It detects the reflection or diffusion signals of biological tissue layers of different depths by inputting low-coherence light and obtains the images and quantitative results of the microscopic structure of the retina	At weeks 2, 6,12, 26, 52, 78, 104, 130, 156, 182, 208, 234, and 260
To evaluate the change from baseline in VFQ-25	VFQ-25 is a 25-item short form version of the 51-item National Eye Institute Visual Function Questionnaire (NEI VFQ), which can effectively measure patient-reported outcomes (including quality of life, QoL). All items are scored so that a high score represents better functioning. Each item is then converted to a 0 to 100 scale so that the lowest and highest possible scores are set at 0 and 100 points, respectively	At weeks 12, 26, 52, 78, 104, 130, 156, 182, 208, 234, and 260
To evaluate the change from baseline in quality of SF-36	The SF-36 questionnaire is a universal tool for evaluating patient-reported QoL outcome. SF-36 comprises 36 questions which cover eight domains of health: (1) limitations in physical activities because of health problems; (2) limitations in social activities because of physical or emotional problems; (3) limitations in usual role activities because of physical health problems; (4) bodily pain; (5) general mental health (psychological distress and well-being); (6) limitations in usual role activities because of emotional problems; (7) vitality (energy and fatigue); and (8) general health perceptions. The scale score of each domain will be calculated based on the total score of the items included in the said domain and readjusted to 0–100, higher scores mean a worse outcome	At weeks 12, 26, 52, 78, 104, 130, 156, 182, 208, 234, and 260

Sponsor
Neurophth Therapeutics Inc.

Collaborators
No information provided

Investigators
No information provided

General Publications
No publications available

Completed

United States/Europe

RESCUE and REVERSE Long-Term Follow-Up (RESTORE)

ClinicalTrials.gov ID NCT03406104

Sponsor GenSight Biologics
Information provided by GenSight Biologics (Responsible Party)
Last Update Posted 2022-07-27

Brief Summary
The goal of this clinical trial is to assess the long-term safety and efficacy of GS010, a gene therapy, and assess the quality of life in subjects with LHON due to the G11778A ND4 mitochondrial mutation and who were treated in the Rescue or Reverse studies.

Official Title
Long-Term Follow-Up of ND4 LHON Subjects Treated with GS010 Ocular Gene Therapy in the RESCUE or REVERSE Phase III Clinical Trials (RESTORE)

Conditions
Leber Hereditary Optic Neuropathy

Study Type
Interventional

Enrollment (Actual)
61

Intervention/Treatment
Genetic: GS010
Other: Sham

Phase
Phase 3

Study Start (Actual)
2018-01-09

Primary Completion (Actual)
2022-07-04

Study Completion (Actual)
2022-07-04

United States
California Locations

Pasadena, California, United States, 91,105
Doheny Eye Center UCLA

Georgia Locations
Atlanta, Georgia, United States, 30,322
Emory University Hospital

Pennsylvania Locations
Philadelphia, Pennsylvania, United States, 19,107
Wills Eye Institute

France
Paris, France, 75,012
CHNO Les Quinze Vingts

Germany
Munich, Germany, 80,336
LMU Klinikum der Universität München / Friedrich-Baur-Institut

Italy
Bologna, Italy, 40,139
Ospedale Bellaria

United Kingdom
Greater London Locations

London, Greater London, United Kingdom, EC1V 2PD
Moorfields Eye Hospital

Eligibility Criteria
Ages Eligible for Study
15 Years and older (Child, Adult, Older Adult)

Accepts Healthy Volunteer
No

Sexes Eligible for Study
All

Inclusion Criteria

- Subject was treated with GS010 IVT injection in either of the RESCUE or REVERSE Phase III clinical studies.
- Subject of legal consent age has provided informed consent; subjects who are not of legal consent age have undergone their country-approved clinical trial enrollment consent process.

Noninclusion Criteria

- Subject is unwilling or unable to comply with the protocol requirements.
- Subject has any medical or psychological condition that, in the opinion of the Investigator, may compromise his or her safe participation in the study.
- Subject is taking or intending to take idebenone during the long-term follow-up study period.

Design Details

Primary Purpose: Treatment
Allocation: Randomized
Interventional Model: Parallel Assignment
Interventional Model Description: intrapatient comparison
Masking: None (Open Label)

Arms and interventions

Participant group/arm	Intervention/treatment
Experimental: GS010 Lenadogene nolparvovec intravitreal ocular unilateral injection	Genetic: GS010 • Lenadogene nolparvovec intravitreal ocular unilateral injection
Sham comparator: Sham Sham intravitreal ocular unilateral injection	Other: Sham • Lenadogene nolparvovec intravitreal ocular unilateral injection

Primary outcome measures

Outcome measure	Measure description	Time frame
Adverse events (AEs) or serious adverse events (SAEs) (ocular or systemic)	AEs or SAEs (ocular or systemic) related to IMP or administration procedure, as judged by the investigator, reported during the long-term follow-up visits (2, 2.5, 3, 4, and 5 years) from the period of 96 weeks up to 5 years posttreatment and summarized descriptively by type, frequency (number, percentage), severity, causal relationship, and seriousness	Up to five-year posttreatment

Secondary outcome measures

Outcome measure	Measure description	Time frame
Best-corrected visual acuity (BCVA) reported with logMAR	Change in best BCVA reported with logMAR	Up to five-year posttreatment
HumphreyTM visual field (HVF) 30–2 parameters	Change of parameters measured with HVF 30-2	Up to five-year posttreatment
Spectral domain-optical coherence tomography (SD-OCT) parameters	Change of parameters measured with SD-OCT	Up to five-year posttreatment
Responder analysis	Response status of eyes treated with GS010 IVT injection compared to eyes treated with sham IVT injection (an improvement of at least 15 ETDRS letters/eyes that lose less than the 15 ETDRS letters)	Up to five-year posttreatment
Time course of the response	Time course of the response in eyes treated with GS010 IVT injection compared to eyes treated with sham IVT injection, for the BCVA reported with logMAR, for parameters measured with HVF 30–2 and SD-OCT	Up to five-year posttreatment
Visual improvement	Visual improvement as measured by logMAR by analysis of covariance (ANCOVA)	Up to five-year posttreatment
Change of ganglion cell layer (GCL) thickness/ volume and topographical map and other parameters measured by SD-OCT	Change of GCL thickness/volume and topographical map and other parameters measured by SD-OCT using a mixed model of ANCOVA	Up to five-year posttreatment
Quality of life: visual functioning questionnaire 25 (VFQ-25)	QOL as measured with VFQ-25 subject-rated instrument	Up to five-year posttreatment
Quality of life: 36-item short form health survey, version 2 (SF-36-v2)	QOL as measured with SF-36v2 subject-rated instrument	Up to five-year posttreatment

Sponsor
GenSight Biologics

Collaborators
No information provided

Investigators
- Principal Investigator: Nancy Newman, MD, Emory University Hospital Atlanta, Georgia, United States, 30322

General Publications
No publications available

Completed

Efficacy Study of GS010 for Treatment of Vision Loss from 7 Months to 1 Year from Onset in LHON Due to the ND4 Mutation (REVERSE) (REVERSE)

ClinicalTrials.gov ID NCT02652780

Sponsor GenSight Biologics
Information provided by GenSight Biologics (Responsible Party)
Last Update Posted 2020-01-23

Brief Summary
The goal of this clinical trial is to assess the effectiveness of GS010, a gene therapy, in improving the visual outcome in participants with Leber Hereditary Optic Neuropathy (LHON) due to the G11778A ND4 mitochondrial mutation when vision loss is present for more than 6 months and up to 1 year.

Official Title
Randomized, Double-Masked, Sham-Controlled Clinical Trial to Evaluate the Efficacy of a Single Intravitreal Injection of GS010 in Subjects Affected for More Than 6 Months and to 12 Months by LHON Due to the G11778A Mutation in the ND4 Gene

Conditions
Optic, Atrophy, Hereditary, Leber

Study Type
Interventional

Enrollment (Actual)
37

Intervention/Treatment
Biological: GS010
Device: Sham Intravitreal Injection

Phase
Phase 3

Other Study ID Numbers
GS-LHON-CLIN-03B
2015–001266-26 (EudraCT Number)

Study Start (Actual)
2016–01

Primary Completion (Actual)
2018–01

Study Completion (Actual)
2018–12

United States
California Locations

Los Angeles, California, United States
Doheny Eye Center, University of California, Los Angeles

Georgia Locations

Atlanta, Georgia, United States, 30,322
Department of Ophthalmology, Emory University School of Medicine

Pennsylvania Locations

Philadelphia, Pennsylvania, United States, 19,107
Neuro Ophthalmologic Associates, Wills Eye Hospital, Thomas Jefferson University

France
Paris, France
Centre National Hospitalier d'Ophtalmologie des Quinze-Vingt

Germany

Munich, Germany, 80336
Department of Neurology, University of Munich, Friedrich-Baur-Institute

Italy

Bologna, Italy
IRCCS Istituto delle Scienze Neurologiche di Bologna, UOC Clinica Neurologica, Ospedale Bellaria

United Kingdom

London, United Kingdom, EC1V 2PD
Moorfields Eye Hospital NHS Foundation Trust

Eligibility Criteria
Ages Eligible for Study
15 years and older (Child, Adult, Older Adult)

Accepts Healthy Volunteer
No

Sexes Eligible for Study
All

Inclusion Criteria

Selection Criteria
Participants must meet all the following criteria at the Screening Visit (Visit 1) in order to be included into the study.

- Age 15 years or older.
- Onset of vision loss based on medically documented history or participants testimony, in both eyes for 181 and ≤365 days in duration.
- Each eye of the participant maintaining visual ability to allow at least for counting of the examiner's fingers at any distance.
- Female participants (if of childbearing potential) must agree to use effective methods of birth control up to 6 months after IVT injection and male participants must agree to use condoms for up to 6 months after IVT injection.
- Ability to obtain adequate pupillary dilation to permit thorough ocular examination and testing.
- Signed written informed consent.

Inclusion Criteria
Participants included in the study must satisfy all the following criteria at the Inclusion Visit (Visit 2).

- Documented results of genotyping showing the presence of the G11778A mutation in the ND4 gene and the absence of the other primary LHON-associated mutations (ND1 or ND6) in the participant's mitochondrial DNA.
- Review of all selection criteria to ensure continued compliance.
- Have a negative test for infection with human immunodeficiency virus (HIV).
- Have a negative pregnancy test for women of childbearing potential (a woman who is 2 years postmenopausal or surgically sterile is not considered to be of childbearing potential).

Exclusion Criteria

Nonselection Criteria
Participants who meet at least one of the following criteria at the Screening Visit (Visit 1) will not be included into the study.

- Any known allergy or hypersensitivity to GS010 or its constituents.
- Contraindication to IVT injection.
- IVT drug delivery to either eye within 30 days prior to the Screening Visit (Visit 1).
- Previous vitrectomy in either eye.
- Narrow angle in either eye contraindicating pupillary dilation.

- Presence of disorders of the ocular media, such as the cornea and lens, which may interfere with visual acuity and other ocular assessments during the study period.
- Vision disorders, other than LHON, involving visual disability or with the potential to cause further vision loss during the trial period.
- Causes of optic neuropathy other than LHON and glaucoma.
- Participants with known mutations of other genes involved in pathological retinal or optic nerve conditions.
- Presence of ocular or systemic disease, other than LHON, whose pathology or associated treatments might affect the retina or the optic nerve.
- History of amblyopia associated with a Snellen visual acuity equivalent of worse than 20/80 (equivalent to 6/24 at 6 m, decimal acuity 0.25, logMAR +0.6) in the affected eye.
- Presence of ocular conditions, which in the opinion of the investigator will prevent good quality SD-OCT imaging from being obtained.
- Presence, in either eye, of uncontrolled glaucoma, defined as an IOP greater than 25 mmHg, despite maximal medical therapy with intraocular pressure (IOP)-lowering agents.
- Active ocular inflammation or history of idiopathic or autoimmune-associated uveitis.
- Participants participating in another clinical trial and receiving an IMP within 90 days prior to the Screening Visit (Visit 1).
- Previous treatment with an ocular gene therapy product.
- Participants who have undergone ocular surgery of clinical relevance (per Investigator opinion) within 90 days preceding the Screening Visit (Visit 1).
- Female participants who are or who intend to breastfeed during the trial period.

Exclusion Criteria

Participants who meet at least one of the following criteria at the Inclusion Visit (Visit 2) will not be included in the study.

- Any nonselection criteria which may have appeared after the screening visit.
- Participants taking idebenone who have not completely discontinued the idebenone at least 7 days prior to Visit 2. If the participant has not discontinued idebenone at least 7 days prior to Visit 2, the visit may be delayed until the seven-day period is complete.
- Presence, at the time of study inclusion, of infectious conjunctivitis, keratitis, scleritis or endophthalmitis in either eye.
- Presence of systemic illness, including alcohol and drug abuse (except nicotine), or medically significant abnormal laboratory values that are deemed by the Investigator to preclude the participant's safe participation in the study.

- Presence of illness or disease that, in the opinion of the Investigator, includes symptoms and/or the associated treatments that can alter visual function, for instance cancers or pathology of the central nervous system.
- Any medical or psychological condition that, in the opinion of the Investigator, may compromise the safe participation of the participant in the study or would preclude compliance with the study protocol or ability of the participant to successfully complete the study.
- Participants unable or unwilling to comply with the protocol requirements.

Design Details
Primary Purpose: Treatment
Allocation: Randomized
Interventional Model: Parallel Assignment
Masking: Quadruple (Participant Care Provider Investigator Outcomes Assessor)

Arms and interventions

Participant group/arm	Intervention/treatment
Experimental: GS010-treated Eyes Each participant will have one eye randomly selected to receive a single injection of GS010 and the other eye will receive a sham injection. GS010-treated eyes: GS010 is a recombinant adeno-associated viral vector serotype 2 (rAAV2/2) containing the wild-type ND4 gene (rAAV2/2-ND4). Participants will receive a single dose of GS010 in one of their randomly selected eyes, via intravitreal injection containing 9E10 viral genomes in 90 µL balanced salt solution (BSS) plus 0.001% Pluronic F68®.	Biological: GS010 • Both eyes of each participant will receive standard antiseptic preparation, administration of topical local ocular anesthetic agents and will undergo pupillary dilation. Administration of an intraocular pressure lowering agent will precede treatment for every participant. GS010-treated eyes: GS010 is a recombinant adeno-associated viral vector serotype 2 (rAAV2/2) containing the wild-type ND4 gene (rAAV2/2-ND4). Participants will receive a single dose of GS010 in one of their randomly selected eyes, via intravitreal injection containing 9E10 viral genomes in 90 µL balanced salt solution (BSS) plus 0.001% Pluronic F68®. • Other names: – Lenadogene olparvovec – rAAV2/2-ND4
Sham Comparator: Sham-treated Eyes Each participant will have one eye randomly selected to receive GS010 and the other eye will receive a sham injection. Eyes receiving sham injection will undergo the same preparatory procedures as eyes receiving GS010 injection, including pupillary dilation, topical antiinfection, and topical anesthetic procedures. Sham Intravitreal injection will be performed by applying pressure to the eye at the location of a typical intravitreal injection procedure using the blunt end of a syringe without a needle	Device: Sham Intravitreal Injection • Both eyes of each participant will receive standard antiseptic preparation, administration of topical local ocular anesthetic agents and will undergo pupillary dilation. Administration of an intraocular pressure lowering agent will precede treatment for every participant Sham-treated Eyes: One eye of each participant will undergo sham injection. Sham Intravitreal injection will be performed by applying pressure to the eye at the location of a typical intravitreal injection procedure using the blunt end of a syringe without a needle

Primary outcome measures

Outcome measure	Measure description	Time frame
Change from baseline in ETDRS visual acuity (quantitative score) at week 48	Visual acuity was derived from the early treatment diabetic retinopathy study (ETDRS) chart. The visual acuity logarithm of the minimal angle of resolution (logMAR) score was derived from the number of letters participants could read on the ETDRS chart 1 ETDRS line = 5 letters 1 ETDRS line = 0.1 logMAR A lower logMAR score denotes better visual acuity and a negative change from baseline indicates an improvement in visual acuity Change = (week 48 score–baseline score)	Baseline and week 48

Secondary outcome measures

Outcome measure	Measure description	Time frame
Change from baseline in ETDRS visual acuity (quantitative score) at week 96	Visual acuity was derived from the early treatment diabetic retinopathy study (ETDRS) chart. The visual acuity logarithm of the minimal angle of resolution (logMAR) score was derived from the number of letters participants could read on the ETDRS chart 1 ETDRS line = 5 letters 1 ETDRS line = 0.1 logMAR A lower logMAR score denotes better visual acuity and a negative change from baseline indicates an improvement in visual acuity Change = (week 96 score–baseline score)	Baseline and week 96
Number of eye responders to treatment at week 48 and week 96	An eye was determined as a responder to treatment based on 2 different definitions Definition 1: An eye responder was defined by an improvement of the early treatment diabetic retinopathy study (ETDRS) visual acuity score of at least 15 letters compared to baseline, or a final visual acuity greater than a Snellen acuity equivalent of 20/200 (a score of at least one letter) Definition 2: An eye responder was defined by an improvement of the ETDRS score of at least 20 letters compared to baseline	Baseline; week 48 and week 96
Number of subject responders to treatment at week 48 and week 96	A subject responder was defined as a participant whose early treatment diabetic retinopathy study (ETDRS) score of the treated eye (that received GS010), was at least 15 letters better than the sham eye, or whose treated eye had a logarithm of the minimal angle of resolution (logMAR) acuity score of at least 0.3 logMAR better than the sham eye	Week 48 and week 96

Change from baseline in GCL macular volume at week 48 and week 96	Ganglion cell layer (GCL) macular volume was measured as a parameter of spectral domain-optical coherence tomography (SD-OCT). SD-OCT was obtained with the Spectralis® OCT (Heidelberg Engineering)	Baseline and week 48; baseline and week 96
Change from baseline in RNFL temporal quadrant thickness at week 48 and week 96	Retinal nerve fiber layer (RNFL) temporal quadrant thickness was measured as a parameter of spectral domain-optical coherence tomography (SD-OCT). SD-OCT was obtained with the Spectralis® OCT (Heidelberg Engineering)	Baseline and week 48; baseline and week 96
Change from baseline in papillomacular bundle thickness at week 48 and week 96	Papillomacular bundle thickness was measured as a parameter of spectral domain-optical coherence tomography (SD-OCT). SD-OCT was obtained with the Spectralis® OCT (Heidelberg Engineering)	Baseline and week 48; baseline and week 96
Change from baseline in ETDRS total macular volume at week 48 and week 96	Early treatment diabetic retinopathy study (ETDRS) total macular volume was measured as a parameter of spectral domain-optical coherence tomography (SD-OCT). SD-OCT was obtained with the Spectralis® OCT (Heidelberg Engineering)	Baseline and week 48; baseline and week 96
Change from baseline in the foveal threshold sensitivities obtained with HVF analyzer II at week 48 and week 96	The assessment of standardized automated visual fields was measured using the Humphrey visual field (HVF) analyzer II. Automated visual fields included the assessment of foveal threshold sensitivities. Foveal threshold sensitivity is measured in decibels (dB), which ranges from 0 dB to 50 dB. A sensitivity threshold of 0 dB indicates not being able to see the most intense perimetric stimulus, while higher dB indicates better/normal foveal vision. A positive change from baseline indicates an improvement of symptoms	Baseline and week 48; baseline and week 96
Visual field mean deviation in decibels of sensitivity obtained with HVF analyzer II at week 48 and week 96	The assessment of standardized automated visual fields was measured using the Humphrey visual field (HVF) analyzer II. Automated visual fields included the assessment of the mean deviation (MD) in decibels (dB) of sensitivity	Baseline, week 48 and week 96

Change from baseline in contrast sensitivity at week 48 and week 96	The assessment of contrast sensitivity was measured using the Pelli-Robson chart. The chart uses letters arranged in groups whose contrast varies from high to low. Participants read the letters, starting with the highest contrast, until they are unable to read 2 or 3 letters in a single group. Each eye is assigned a score based on the contrast of the last group in which 2 or 3 letters were correctly read, ranging from 0 to 2.2 "log of contrast sensitivity" (LogCS) units. A score of 2.0 LogCS, represents a normal sensitivity contrast, and indicates the eye was able to detect two of the three letters with a contrast of 1 percent (contrast sensitivity = 100 percent or log 2). Scores less than 2.0 signify poorer contrast sensitivity. Pelli-Robson contrast sensitivity score of less than 1.5 is consistent with visual impairment and a score of less than 1.0 represents in visual disability. A positive change from baseline indicates improvement in symptoms	Baseline and week 48; baseline and week 96
Change from baseline in color vision	The assessment of color vision was measured using the Farnsworth-Munsell 100-Hue color test. Each of the four trays consisted of 21 caps. Participants were asked to sort the randomly arranged caps following the hue order from the first to the last fixed caps. The total error score (TES) was derived by the frequency, the caps were misplaced, and the severity, or distance of the misplacement Errors were made whenever caps were misplaced from the correct order. Error scores were calculated according to the distance between any two caps. The error score for each individual cap was the sum of the difference between the number of that cap and the numbers of the cap adjacent to it, minus 2. TES was the total sum of the error scores of the entire set of caps The best possible score was 0 and there is no defined upper limit to the total error score range. A lower score indicates improved color discrimination ability. A negative change from baseline indicates an improvement in symptoms	Baseline and week 48; baseline and week 96

Sponsor
GenSight Biologics

Collaborators
No information provided

Investigators

- Principal Investigator: Patrick Yu Wai Man, MD PhD FRCOpht, Moorfields Eye Hospital NHS Foundation Trust.

General Publications
No publications available

Results
Outcome Measures

1. Change from Baseline in ETDRS Visual Acuity (Quantitative Score) at Week 48
 Type: Primary | Time Frame: Baseline and Week 48

Description	Visual acuity was derived from the Early Treatment Diabetic Retinopathy Study (ETDRS) chart. The visual acuity logarithm of the minimal angle of resolution (logMAR) score was derived from the number of letters participants could read on the ETDRS chart 1 ETDRS line = 5 letters 1 ETDRS line = 0.1 logMAR A lower logMAR score denotes better visual acuity and a negative change from baseline indicates an improvement in visual acuity Change = (week 48 score–baseline score)
Time frame	Baseline and week 48
Analysis population description	All participants and all eyes that received study treatments, with data at both baseline and the applicable postdose visit (week 48). All participants received both GS010 and Sham simultaneously

Arm/group title	GS010-treated eyes	Sham-treated eyes
Arm/group description	All eyes that received the study treatment, GS010. Each participant was randomly assigned GS010 in either the right or left eye. The eye assigned to GS010 received one single dose of GS010 (9E10 vg/eye) via an intravitreal (IVT) injection. The volume of the injected formula was 90 μL. The injection was performed in the vitreous humor under local anesthesia The same participants also received the sham procedure in the right or left eye, which was not assigned to receive GS010, at the same study visit Show less	All eyes that received the Sham. Each participant was randomly assigned GS010 in either the right or left eye, the eye not assigned GS010 received the sham procedure. The eye assigned to the Sham received one single sham intravitreal (IVT) injection, which was performed by applying pressure to the eye at the location of a typical IVT injection procedure, using the blunt end of a syringe without a needle The same participants also received GS010 in the right or left eye, which did not receive the Sham, at the same study visit Show less

Overall number of participants analyzed	37	37
Overall number of units analyzed Type of units analyzed: eyes	37	37
Least squares mean (standard error) ǀ unit of measure: logMAR	−0.219 (0.055)	−0.211 (0.055)
Statistical Analysis 1: GS010-Treated Eyes, Sham-Treated Eyes ǀ Superiority ǀ ANCOVA		

2. Change from Baseline in ETDRS Visual Acuity (Quantitative Score) at Week 96
   Type: Secondary ǀ Time Frame: Baseline and Week 96

Description	Visual acuity was derived from the early treatment diabetic retinopathy study (ETDRS) chart. The visual acuity logarithm of the minimal angle of resolution (logMAR) score was derived from the number of letters participants could read on the ETDRS chart 1 ETDRS line = 5 letters 1 ETDRS line = 0.1 logMAR A lower logMAR score denotes better visual acuity and a negative change from baseline indicates an improvement in visual acuity Change = (week 96 score–baseline score)
Time frame	Baseline and week 96
Analysis population description	All participants and all eyes that received study treatments, with data at both baseline and the applicable postdose visit (week 96). All participants received both GS010 and Sham simultaneously

Arm/group title	GS010-treated eyes	Sham-treated eyes
Arm/group description	All eyes that received the study treatment, GS010. Each participant was randomly assigned GS010 in either the right or left eye. The eye assigned to GS010 received one single dose of GS010 (9E10 vg/eye) via an intravitreal (IVT) injection. The volume of the injected formula was 90 μL. The injection was performed in the vitreous humor under local anesthesia The same participants also received the sham procedure in the right or left eye, which was not assigned to receive GS010, at the same study visit Show less	All eyes that received the Sham. Each participant was randomly assigned GS010 in either the right or left eye, the eye not assigned GS010 received the sham procedure. The eye assigned to the Sham received one single sham intravitreal (IVT) injection, which was performed by applying pressure to the eye at the location of a typical IVT injection procedure, using the blunt end of a syringe without a needle The same participants also received GS010 in the right or left eye, which did not receive the sham procedure, at the same study visit Show less

Overall number of participants analyzed	37	37
Least squares mean (standard error) ǀ unit of measure: logMAR	−0.308 (0.068)	−0.259 (0.068)

3. Number of Eye Responders to Treatment at Week 48 and Week 96
   Type: Secondary ǀ Time Frame: Baseline; Week 48 and Week 96

Description	An eye was determined as a responder to treatment based on two different definitions Definition 1: An eye responder was defined by an improvement of the early treatment diabetic retinopathy study (ETDRS) visual acuity score of at least 15 letters compared to baseline, or a final visual acuity greater than a Snellen acuity equivalent of 20/200 (a score of at least one letter) Definition 2: An eye responder was defined by an improvement of the ETDRS score of at least 20 letters compared to baseline
Time frame	Baseline; week 48 and week 96
Analysis population description	All participants and all eyes that received study treatments, with data at both baseline and the applicable postdose visit (week 48 or week 96). All participants received both GS010 and Sham simultaneously

Arm/group title	GS010-treated eyes	Sham-treated eyes
Arm/group description	All eyes that received the study treatment, GS010. Each participant was randomly assigned GS010 in either the right or left eye. The eye assigned to GS010 received one single dose of GS010 (9E10 vg/eye) via an intravitreal (IVT) injection. The volume of the injected formula was 90 μL. The injection was performed in the vitreous humor under local anesthesia The same participants also received the sham procedure in the right or left eye, which was not assigned to receive GS010, at the same study visit Show less	All eyes that received the Sham. Each participant was randomly assigned GS010 in either the right or left eye, the eye not assigned GS010 received the sham procedure. The eye assigned to the Sham received one single sham intravitreal (IVT) injection, which was performed by applying pressure to the eye at the location of a typical IVT injection procedure, using the blunt end of a syringe without a needle The same participants also received GS010 in the right or left eye, which did not receive the sham procedure, at the same study visit Show less
Overall number of participants analyzed	37	37

Overall number of units analyzed Type of units analyzed: eyes	37	37
Definition 1: week 48 [a]unit of measure: eyes	718.9%	513.5%
Definition 1: week 96[a]	1232.4%	616.2%
Definition 2: week 48[a]	1027.0%	1335.1%
Definition 2: week 96[a]	1745.9%	1951.4%

[a]Unit of measure: eyes

4. Number of Subject Responders to Treatment at Week 48 and Week 96
   Type: Secondary | Time Frame: Week 48 and Week 96.

Description	A subject responder was defined as a participant whose early treatment diabetic retinopathy study (ETDRS) score of the treated eye (that received GS010) was at least 15 letters better than the sham eye, or whose treated eye had a logarithm of the minimal angle of resolution (logMAR) acuity score of at least 0.3 logMAR better than the sham eye
Time frame	Week 48 and week 96
Analysis population description	All participants that received study treatments, with data at the applicable postdose visit (week 48 or week 96). All participants received both GS010 and Sham simultaneously

Arm/group title	All participants
Arm/group description	All participants who were enrolled and received both study treatments, GS010 and Sham. Participants were randomly assigned to receive GS010 in either the right or left eye. The same participants also received the sham comparator in the eye not assigned to GS010 at the same visit GS010: Either the right or left eye received one single dose of GS010 (9E10 vg/eye) via an intravitreal (IVT) injection. The volume of the injected formula was 90 μL. The injection was performed in the vitreous humor under local anesthesia Sham procedure: Either the right or left eye (the eye not randomly assigned to GS010) received the sham procedure. One single sham IVT injection was performed by applying pressure to the eye at the location of a typical IVT injection procedure, using the blunt end of a syringe without a needle Show less
Overall number of participants analyzed	37

Week 48 [a]Measure type: count of participants ǀ unit of measure: participants	37100.0%
Week 96[a]	37100.0%

[a]Measure type: count of participants ǀ unit of measure: participants

5. Change from Baseline in GCL Macular Volume at Week 48 and Week 96
   Type: Secondary ǀ Time Frame: Baseline and Week 48; Baseline and Week 96

Description	Ganglion cell layer (GCL) macular volume was measured as a parameter of spectral domain-optical coherence tomography (SD-OCT). SD-OCT was obtained with the Spectralis® OCT (Heidelberg Engineering)
Time frame	Baseline and week 48; baseline and week 96
Analysis population description	All participants and all eyes that received study treatments, with data at both baseline and the applicable postdose visit (week 48 or week 96). All participants received both GS010 and Sham simultaneously

Arm/group title	GS010-treated eyes	Sham-treated eyes
Arm/group description	All eyes that received the study treatment, GS010. Each participant was randomly assigned GS010 in either the right or left eye. The eye assigned to GS010 received one single dose of GS010 (9E10 vg/eye) via an intravitreal (IVT) injection. The volume of the injected formula was 90 μL. The injection was performed in the vitreous humor under local anesthesia The same participants also received the sham procedure in the right or left eye, which was not assigned to receive GS010, at the same study visit Show less	All eyes that received the Sham. Each participant was randomly assigned GS010 in either the right or left eye, the eye not assigned GS010 received the sham procedure. The eye assigned to the Sham received one single sham intravitreal (IVT) injection, which was performed by applying pressure to the eye at the location of a typical IVT injection procedure, using the blunt end of a syringe without a needle The same participants also received GS010 in the right or left eye, which did not receive the sham procedure, at the same study visit Show less
Overall number of participants analyzed	36	36
Overall number of units analyzed Type of units analyzed: eyes	36	36
Week 48 [a]Least squares mean (standard error) ǀ unit of measure: mm^3	−0.003 (0.012)	−0.038 (0.012)
Week 96[a]	−0.018 (0.012)	−0.031 (0.012)

[a]Least squares mean (standard error) ǀ unit of measure: mm^3

6. Change from Baseline in RNFL Temporal Quadrant Thickness at Week 48 and Week 96

Type: Secondary | Time Frame: Baseline and Week 48; Baseline and Week 96

Description	Retinal nerve fiber layer (RNFL) temporal quadrant thickness was measured as a parameter of spectral domain-optical coherence tomography (SD-OCT). SD-OCT was obtained with the Spectralis® OCT (Heidelberg Engineering)
Time frame	Baseline and week 48; baseline and week 96
Analysis population description	All participants and all eyes that received study treatments, with data at both baseline and the applicable postdose visit (week 48 or week 96). All participants received both GS010 and Sham simultaneously

Arm/group title	GS010-treated eyes	Sham-treated eyes
Arm/group description	All eyes that received the study treatment, GS010. Each participant was randomly assigned GS010 in either the right or left eye. The eye assigned to GS010 received one single dose of GS010 (9E10 vg/eye) via an intravitreal (IVT) injection. The volume of the injected formula was 90 μL. The injection was performed in the vitreous humor under local anesthesia The same participants also received the sham procedure in the right or left eye, which was not assigned to receive GS010, at the same study visit Show more	All eyes that received the Sham. Each participant was randomly assigned GS010 in either the right or left eye, the eye not assigned GS010 received the sham procedure. The eye assigned to the Sham received one single sham intravitreal (IVT) injection, which was performed by applying pressure to the eye at the location of a typical IVT injection procedure, using the blunt end of a syringe without a needle The same participants also received GS010 in the right or left eye, which did not receive the sham procedure, at the same study visit Show more
Overall number of participants analyzed	37	36
Overall number of units analyzed Type of units analyzed: eyes	37	36
Week 48		
Number analyzed	37 eyes	35 eyes[a]
[b]Least squares mean (standard error) | unit of measure: μm	−0.562 (0.988)	−3.354 (1.017)
Week 96		
Number analyzed	35 eyes[a]	36 eyes
[b]	−1.791 (0.974)	−2.042 (0.951)

[a]35 participants

[b]Least squares mean (standard error) | unit of measure: μm

7. Change from Baseline in Papillomacular Bundle Thickness at Week 48 and Week 96

Type: Secondary | Time Frame: Baseline and Week 48; Baseline and Week 96

Description	Papillomacular bundle thickness was measured as a parameter of spectral domain-optical coherence tomography (SD-OCT). SD-OCT was obtained with the Spectralis® OCT (Heidelberg Engineering)
Time frame	Baseline and week 48; baseline and week 96
Analysis population description	All participants and all eyes that received study treatments, with data at both baseline and the applicable postdose visit (week 48 or week 96). All participants received both GS010 and Sham simultaneously

Arm/group title	GS010-treated eyes	Sham-treated eyes
Arm/group description	All eyes that received the study treatment, GS010. Each participant was randomly assigned GS010 in either the right or left eye. The eye assigned to GS010 received one single dose of GS010 (9E10 vg/eye) via an intravitreal (IVT) injection. The volume of the injected formula was 90 μL. The injection was performed in the vitreous humor under local anesthesia The same participants also received the sham procedure in the right or left eye, which was not assigned to receive GS010, at the same study visit Show more	All eyes that received the Sham. Each participant was randomly assigned GS010 in either the right or left eye, the eye not assigned GS010 received the sham procedure. The eye assigned to the Sham received one single sham intravitreal (IVT) injection, which was performed by applying pressure to the eye at the location of a typical IVT injection procedure, using the blunt end of a syringe without a needle The same participants also received GS010 in the right or left eye, which did not receive the sham procedure, at the same study visit Show more
Overall number of participants analyzed	37	36
Overall number of units analyzed Type of units analyzed: eyes	37	36
Week 48		
Number analyzed	37 eyes	35 eyes[a]
[b]Least squares mean (standard error) | unit of measure: μm	1.6 (1.3)	−1.0 (1.4)
Week 96		
Number analyzed	35 eyes[a]	36 eyes
[b]	1.2 (1.3)	0.7 (1.3)

[a]35 participants

[b]Least squares mean (standard error) | unit of measure: μm

8. Change from Baseline in ETDRS Total Macular Volume at Week 48 and Week 96
Type: Secondary | Time Frame: Baseline and Week 48; Baseline and Week 96

Description	Early treatment diabetic retinopathy study (ETDRS) total macular volume was measured as a parameter of spectral domain-optical coherence tomography (SD-OCT). SD-OCT was obtained with the Spectralis® OCT (Heidelberg Engineering)
Time frame	Baseline and week 48; baseline and week 96
Analysis population description	All participants and all eyes that received study treatments, with data at both baseline and the applicable postdose visit (week 48 or week 96). All participants received both GS010 and Sham simultaneously

Arm/group title	GS010-treated eyes	Sham-treated eyes
Arm/group description	All eyes that received the study treatment, GS010. Each participant was randomly assigned GS010 in either the right or left eye. The eye assigned to GS010 received one single dose of GS010 (9E10 vg/eye) via an intravitreal (IVT) injection. The volume of the injected formula was 90 μL. The injection was performed in the vitreous humor under local anesthesia The same participants also received the sham procedure in the right or left eye, which was not assigned to receive GS010, at the same study visit Show less	All eyes that received the Sham. Each participant was randomly assigned GS010 in either the right or left eye, the eye not assigned GS010 received the sham procedure. The eye assigned to the Sham received one single sham intravitreal (IVT) injection, which was performed by applying pressure to the eye at the location of a typical IVT injection procedure, using the blunt end of a syringe without a needle The same participants also received GS010 in the right or left eye, which did not receive the sham procedure, at the same study visit Show less
Overall number of participants analyzed	36	36
Overall number of units analyzed Type of units analyzed: eyes	36	36
Week 48 [a]Least squares mean (standard error) | unit of measure: mm^3	−0.104 (0.046)	−0.224 (0.046)
Week 96[a]	−0.200 (0.037)	−0.265 (0.037)

[a]Least squares mean (standard error) | unit of measure: mm^3

9. Change from Baseline in the Foveal Threshold Sensitivities Obtained with HVF Analyzer II at Week 48 and Week 96

Type: Secondary | Time Frame: Baseline and Week 48; Baseline and Week 96

Description	The assessment of standardized automated visual fields was measured using the Humphrey visual field (HVF) analyzer II. Automated visual fields included the assessment of foveal threshold sensitivities. Foveal threshold sensitivity is measured in decibels (dB), which ranges from 0 dB to 50 dB. A sensitivity threshold of 0 dB indicates not being able to see the most intense perimetric stimulus, while higher dB indicates better/normal foveal vision. A positive change from baseline indicates an improvement of symptoms
Time frame	Baseline and week 48; baseline and week 96
Analysis population description	All participants and all eyes that received study treatments, with data at both baseline and the applicable postdose visit (week 48 or week 96). All participants received both GS010 and Sham simultaneously

Arm/group title	GS010-treated eyes	Sham-treated eyes
Arm/group description	All eyes that received the study treatment, GS010. Each participant was randomly assigned GS010 in either the right or left eye. The eye assigned to GS010 received one single dose of GS010 (9E10 vg/eye) via an intravitreal (IVT) injection. The volume of the injected formula was 90 μL. The injection was performed in the vitreous humor under local anesthesia The same participants also received the sham procedure in the right or left eye, which was not assigned to receive GS010, at the same study visit Show more	All eyes that received the Sham. Each participant was randomly assigned GS010 in either the right or left eye, the eye not assigned GS010 received the sham procedure. The eye assigned to the Sham received one single sham intravitreal (IVT) injection, which was performed by applying pressure to the eye at the location of a typical IVT injection procedure, using the blunt end of a syringe without a needle The same participants also received GS010 in the right or left eye, which did not receive the sham procedure, at the same study visit Show more
Overall number of participants analyzed	9	11
Overall number of units analyzed Type of units analyzed: eyes	9	11
Week 48		
Number analyzed	9 eyes	11 eyes
[a]Mean (standard deviation) | unit of measure: decibels (dB)	0.7 (8.9)	−0.5 (11.9)
Week 96		

Number analyzed	8 eyes[b]	9 eyes[c]
[a]	1.3 (8.0)	2.4 (10.8)

[a]Mean (standard deviation) | unit of measure: decibels (dB)
[b]8 participants
[c]9 participants

10. Visual Field Mean Deviation in Decibels of Sensitivity Obtained with HVF Analyzer II at Week 48 and Week 96
    Type: Secondary | Time Frame: Baseline, Week 48 and Week 96

Description	The assessment of standardized automated visual fields was measured using the Humphrey visual field (HVF) analyzer II. Automated visual fields included the assessment of the mean deviation (MD) in decibels (dB) of sensitivity
Time frame	Baseline; week 48 and week 96
Analysis population description	All participants and all eyes that received study treatments, with data at both baseline and the applicable postdose visit (week 48 or week 96). All participants received both GS010 and Sham simultaneously

Arm/group title	GS010-treated eyes	Sham-treated eyes
Arm/group description	All eyes that received the study treatment, GS010. Each participant was randomly assigned GS010 in either the right or left eye. The eye assigned to GS010 received one single dose of GS010 (9E10 vg/eye) via an intravitreal (IVT) injection. The volume of the injected formula was 90 μL. The injection was performed in the vitreous humor under local anesthesia The same participants also received the sham procedure in the right or left eye, which was not assigned to receive GS010, at the same study visit Show less	All eyes that received the Sham. Each participant was randomly assigned GS010 in either the right or left eye, the eye not assigned GS010 received the sham procedure. The eye assigned to the Sham received one single sham intravitreal (IVT) injection, which was performed by applying pressure to the eye at the location of a typical IVT injection procedure, using the blunt end of a syringe without a needle The same participants also received GS010 in the right or left eye, which did not receive the sham procedure, at the same study visit Show less
Overall number of participants analyzed	37	37
Overall number of units analyzed Type of units analyzed: eyes	37	37
Baseline MD [a]Mean (standard deviation)	unit of measure: decibels (dB)	−25.99 (8.37)	−24.94 (9.70)

Week 48 MD[a]	−22.83 (9.43)	−22.94 (9.80)
Week 96 MD[a]	−23.22 (8.98)	−22.43 (9.39)

[a]Mean (standard deviation) | unit of measure: decibels (dB)

11. Change from Baseline in Contrast Sensitivity at Week 48 and Week 96
Type: Secondary | Time Frame: Baseline and Week 48; Baseline and Week 96

Description	The assessment of contrast sensitivity was measured using the Pelli-Robson chart. The chart uses letters arranged in groups whose contrast varies from high to low. Participants read the letters, starting with the highest contrast, until they are unable to read two or three letters in a single group. Each eye is assigned a score based on the contrast of the last group in which two or three letters were correctly read, ranging from 0 to 2.2 "log of contrast sensitivity" (LogCS) units. A score of 2.0 LogCS, represents a normal sensitivity contrast, and indicates the eye was able to detect two of the three letters with a contrast of 1 percent (contrast sensitivity = 100 percent or log 2). Scores less than 2.0 signify poorer contrast sensitivity. Pelli-Robson contrast sensitivity score of less than 1.5 is consistent with visual impairment and a score of less than 1.0 represents in visual disability. A positive change from baseline indicates improvement in symptoms
Time frame	Baseline and week 48; baseline and week 96
Analysis population description	All participants and all eyes that received study treatments, with data at both baseline and the applicable postdose visit (week 48 or week 96). All participants received both GS010 and Sham simultaneously

Arm/group title	GS010-treated eyes	Sham-treated eyes
Arm/group description	All eyes that received the study treatment, GS010. Each participant was randomly assigned GS010 in either the right or left eye. The eye assigned to GS010 received one single dose of GS010 (9E10 vg/eye) via an intravitreal (IVT) injection. The volume of the injected formula was 90 μL. The injection was performed in the vitreous humor under local anesthesia The same participants also received the sham procedure in the right or left eye, which was not assigned to receive GS010, at the same study visit Show less	All eyes that received the Sham. Each participant was randomly assigned GS010 in either the right or left eye, the eye not assigned GS010 received the sham procedure. The eye assigned to the Sham received one single sham intravitreal (IVT) injection, which was performed by applying pressure to the eye at the location of a typical IVT injection procedure, using the blunt end of a syringe without a needle The same participants also received GS010 in the right or left eye, which did not receive the sham procedure, at the same study visit Show less
Overall number of participants analyzed	37	37
Overall number of units analyzed Type of units analyzed: eyes	37	37

Week 48 [a]Least squares mean (standard error) I unit of measure: LogCS	0.19 (0.05)	0.09 (0.05)
Week 96[a]	0.22 (0.06)	0.12 (0.06)

[a]Least squares mean (standard error) I unit of measure: LogCS

12. Change from Baseline in Color Vision

Type: Secondary I Time Frame: Baseline and Week 48; Baseline and Week 96

Description	The assessment of color vision was measured using the Farnsworth-Munsell 100-Hue Color Test. Each of the four trays consisted of 21 caps. Participants were asked to sort the randomly arranged caps following the hue order from the first to the last fixed caps. The total error score (TES) was derived by the frequency, the caps were misplaced and the severity, or distance of the misplacement Errors were made whenever caps were misplaced from the correct order. Error scores were calculated according to the distance between any two caps. The error score for each individual cap was the sum of the difference between the number of that cap and the numbers of the cap adjacent to it, minus 2. TES was the total sum of the error scores of the entire set of caps The best possible score was 0 and there is no defined upper limit to the total error score range. A lower score indicates improved color discrimination ability. A negative change from baseline indicates an improvement in symptoms
Time frame	Baseline and week 48; baseline and week 96
Analysis population description	All participants and all eyes that received study treatments, with data at both baseline and the applicable postdose visit (week 48 or week 96). All participants received both GS010 and Sham simultaneously

Arm/group title	GS010-treated eyes	Sham-treated eyes
Arm/group description	All eyes that received the study treatment, GS010. Each participant was randomly assigned GS010 in either the right or left eye. The eye assigned to GS010 received one single dose of GS010 (9E10 vg/eye) via an intravitreal (IVT) injection. The volume of the injected formula was 90 μL. The injection was performed in the vitreous humor under local anesthesia The same participants also received the sham procedure in the right or left eye, which was not assigned to receive GS010, at the same study visit Show more	All eyes that received the Sham. Each participant was randomly assigned GS010 in either the right or left eye, the eye not assigned GS010 received the sham procedure. The eye assigned to the Sham received one single sham intravitreal (IVT) injection, which was performed by applying pressure to the eye at the location of a typical IVT injection procedure, using the blunt end of a syringe without a needle The same participants also received GS010 in the right or left eye, which did not receive the sham procedure, at the same study visit Show more
Overall number of participants analyzed	24	25

Overall number of units analyzed Type of units analyzed: eyes	24	25
Week 48		
Number analyzed	24 eyes	25 eyes
[a]Mean (standard deviation) ǀ unit of measure: score on a scale	−30.0 (255.0)	−44.3 (182.2)
Week 96		
Number analyzed	23 eyes[b]	24 eyes[c]
[a]	−10.3 (247.3)	−61.0 (188.9)

[a]Mean (standard deviation) ǀ unit of measure: score on a scale
[b]23 participants
[c]24 participants

Adverse Events

Time Frame

From first dose to end of study (a maximum of 96 weeks)

Adverse Event Reporting Description

Because participants received both treatment and sham procedure simultaneously, adverse events (AEs) are reported overall for systemic and ocular AEs. Reported events include AEs associated with sham procedure.

Arm/group title	All participants	
Arm/group description	All participants who were enrolled and received both study treatments, GS010 and Sham. Participants were randomly assigned to receive GS010 in either the right or left eye. The same participants also received the sham comparator in the eye not assigned to GS010 at the same visit GS010: Either the right or left eye received one single dose of GS010 (9E10 vg/eye) via an intravitreal (IVT) injection. The volume of the injected formula was 90 μL. The injection was performed in the vitreous humor under local anesthesia Sham procedure: Either the right or left eye (the eye not randomly assigned to GS010) received the sham procedure. One single sham IVT injection was performed by applying pressure to the eye at the location of a typical IVT injection procedure, using the blunt end of a syringe without a needle Show less	
All-cause mortality		
Arm/group title	All participants	
	Affected/at risk (%)	
Total	0/37 (0.00%)	
Serious adverse events		

Arm/group title	All participants	
	Affected/at risk (%)	# Events
Total	3/37 (8.11%)	
Cardiac disorders		
Acute myocardial infarction[a,b]	1/37 (2.70%)	1
Eye disorders		
Retinal tear[a,b,c]	1/37 (2.70%)	1
Gastrointestinal disorders		
Intestinal perforation[a,b]	1/37 (2.70%)	1
Infections and infestations		
Diverticulitis[a,b]	1/37 (2.70%)	1
[a]Indicates events were collected by systematic assessment b Term from vocabulary, MedDRA 20.1 c This event occurred only in an eye receiving the sham procedure.		
Other (not including serious) adverse events .		
5% Frequency threshold for reporting other adverse events		

Arm/group title	All participants	
	Affected / at risk (%)	# Events
Total	37/37 (100.00%)	
Eye disorders		
Anterior chamber cell[a,b]	9/37 (24.32%)	11
Autoimmune uveitis[a,b,c]	14/37 (37.84%)	15
Cataract[a,b,d]	4/37 (10.81%)	4
Conjunctival hemorrhage[a,b,e]	6/37 (16.22%)	7
Conjunctival hyperemia[a,b]	6/37 (16.22%)	7
Dry eye[a,b,f]	2/37 (5.41%)	3
Iridocyclitis[a,b,g]	15/37 (40.54%)	17
Iritis[a,b]	2/37 (5.41%)	2
Keratic precipitates[a,b]	13/37 (35.14%)	16
Eye pain[a,b,h]	3/37 (8.11%)	4
Intraocular pressure increased[a,b,i]	11/37 (29.73%)	13
Vitritis[a,b]	6/37 (16.22%)	6
Vitreous floaters[a,b]	2/37 (5.41%)	3
Vitreous detachment[a,b]	2/37 (5.41%)	2
Vitreal cells[a,b,j]	7/37 (18.92%)	7

Visual impairment[a,b]	3/37 (8.11%)	3
Punctate keratitis[a,b,k]	15/37 (40.54%)	17
Gastrointestinal disorders		
Abdominal pain upper[a,b]	2/37 (5.41%)	2
Immune system disorders		
Drug hypersensitivity[a,b]	2/37 (5.41%)	2
Infections and infestations		
Nasopharyngitis[a,b]	6/37 (16.22%)	9
Injury, poisoning, and procedural complications		
Arthropod bite[a,b]	2/37 (5.41%)	2
Investigations		
Gamma-glutamyl transferase increased[a,b]	8/37 (21.62%)	11
Alanine aminotransferase increased[a,b]	4/37 (10.81%)	4
Aspartate aminotransferase increased[a,b]	2/37 (5.41%)	2
Musculoskeletal and connective tissue disorders		
Arthralgia[a,b]	2/37 (5.41%)	2
Nervous system disorders		
Headache[a,b]	4/37 (10.81%)	8
Paresthesia[a,b]	2/37 (5.41%)	2
Psychiatric disorders		
Depression[a,b]	2/37 (5.41%)	2
Social circumstances		
Alcohol use[a,b]	2/37 (5.41%)	2
Vascular disorders		
Hypertension[a,b]	2/37 (5.41%)	2

[a]Indicates events were collected by systematic assessment
[b]Term from vocabulary, MedDRA 20.1
[c]The verbatim AE term is "intermediate uveitis." 1/14 affected participants experienced this event only in sham-treated eyes
[d]1/4 affected participants experienced this event only in sham-treated eyes
[e]3/6 affected participants experienced this event only in sham-treated eyes
[f]1/2 affected participants experienced this event only in sham-treated eyes
[g]1/15 affected participants experienced this event only in sham-treated eyes
[h]1/3 affected participants experienced this event only in sham-treated eyes
[i]1/11 affected participants experienced this event only in sham-treated eyes
[j]1/7 affected participants experienced this event only in sham-treated eyes
[k]4/15 affected participants experienced this event only in sham-treated eyes

Completed

Efficacy Study of GS010 for the Treatment of Vision Loss up to 6 Months from Onset in LHON Due to the ND4 Mutation (RESCUE)

ClinicalTrials.gov ID NCT02652767

Sponsor GenSight Biologics
Information provided by GenSight Biologics (Responsible Party)
Last Update Posted 2022-07-29

Brief Summary
The goal of this clinical trial is to assess the effectiveness of GS010, a gene therapy, in improving the visual outcome in participants with Leber Hereditary Optic Neuropathy (LHON) due to the G11778A ND4 mitochondrial mutation when vision loss is present for 6 months or less.

Official Title
A Randomized, Double-Masked, Sham-Controlled Clinical Trial to Evaluate the Efficacy of a Single Intravitreal Injection of GS010 in Subjects Affected for 6 Months or Less by LHON Due to the G11778A Mutation in the Mitochondrial ND4 Gene

Conditions
Optic, Atrophy, Hereditary, Leber

Intervention/Treatment
Biological: GS010
Device: Sham Intravitreal Injection

Study Start (Actual)
2016-02-23

Primary Completion (Actual)
2018-08-07

Study Completion (Actual)
2019-07-04

Enrollment (Actual)
39

Study Type
Interventional

Phase
Phase 3

United States
California Locations

Los Angeles, California, United States, 91,105
Doheny Eye Center, University of California, Los Angeles

Georgia Locations

Atlanta, Georgia, United States, 30322
Department of Ophthalmology, Emory University School of Medicine

Pennsylvania Locations

Philadelphia, Pennsylvania, United States, 19,107
Neuro Ophthalmologic Associates, Wills Eye Hospital, Thomas Jefferson University

France

Paris, France
Centre National Hospitalier d'Ophtalmologie des Quinze-VingtCentre National Hospitalier d'Ophtalmologie des Quinze-Vingt

Germany

Munich, Germany, 80,336
Department of Neurology, University of Munich, Friedrich-Baur-Institute

Italy

Bologna, Italy
IRCCS Istituto delle Scienze Neurologiche di Bologna, UOC Clinica Neurologica, Ospedale Bellaria

United Kingdom

London, United Kingdom, EC1V 2PD
Moorfields Eye Hospital NHS Foundation Trust

Inclusion Criteria

Selection Criteria

Participants must meet all the following criteria at the Screening Visit (Visit 1) in order to be included into the study.

- Age 15 years or older.
- Onset of vision loss based on medically documented history or participant testimony, in at least one eye for ≤180 days in duration and if both eyes are affected, the duration of vision loss in both eyes must be ≤180 days in duration.
- Each eye of the participant maintaining visual ability to allow at least for counting of the examiner's fingers at any distance.
- Female participants (if of childbearing potential) must agree to use effective methods of birth control up to 6 months after intravitreal (IVT) injection and

male participants must agree to use condoms for up to 6 months after IVT injection.
- Ability to obtain adequate pupillary dilation to permit thorough ocular examination and testing.
- Signed written informed consent.

Inclusion Criteria

Participants included in the study must satisfy all the following criteria at the Inclusion Visit (Visit 2).

- Documented results of genotyping showing the presence of the G11778A mutation in the ND4 gene and the absence of the other primary Leber Hereditary Optical Neuropathy (LHON) -associated mutations (ND1 or ND6) in the participant's mitochondrial DNA.
- Review of all selection criteria to ensure continued compliance.
- Have a negative test for infection with human immunodeficiency virus.
- Have a negative pregnancy test for women of childbearing potential (a woman who is 2 years postmenopausal or surgically sterile is not considered to be of childbearing potential).

Exclusion Criteria

Nonselection Criteria

Participants who meet at least one of the following criteria at the Screening Visit (Visit 1) will not be included into the study.

- Any known allergy or hypersensitivity to GS010 or its constituents.
- Contraindication to IVT injection.
- IVT drug delivery to either eye within 30 days prior to the Screening Visit (Visit 1).
- Previous vitrectomy in either eye.
- Narrow angle in either eye contraindicating pupillary dilation.
- Presence of disorders of the ocular media, such as the cornea and lens, which may interfere with visual acuity and other ocular assessments during the study period.
- Vision disorders, other than LHON, involving visual disability or with the potential to cause further vision loss during the trial period.
- Causes of optic neuropathy other than LHON and glaucoma.
- Participants with known mutations of other genes involved in pathological retinal or optic nerve conditions.
- Presence of ocular or systemic disease, other than LHON, whose pathology or associated treatments might affect the retina or the optic nerve.
- History of amblyopia associated with a Snellen visual acuity equivalent of worse than 20/80 (equivalent to 6/24 at 6 m, decimal acuity 0.25, logMAR +0.6) in the affected eye.
- Presence of ocular conditions, which in the opinion of the Investigator will prevent good quality SD-OCT imaging from being obtained.

- Presence, in either eye, of uncontrolled glaucoma, defined as an intraocular pressure (IOP) greater than 25 mmHg, despite maximal medical therapy with IOP-lowering agents.
- Active ocular inflammation or history of idiopathic or autoimmune-associated uveitis.
- Participants participating in another clinical trial and receiving an investigational medicinal product within 90 days prior to the Screening Visit (Visit 1).
- Previous treatment with an ocular gene therapy product.
- Participants who have undergone ocular surgery of clinical relevance (per investigator opinion) within 90 days preceding the Screening Visit (Visit 1).
- Female participants who are or who intend to breastfeed during the trial period.

Exclusion Criteria
Participants who meet at least one of the following criteria at the Inclusion Visit (Visit 2) will not be included in the study.

- Any nonselection criteria which may have appeared after the Screening visit.
- Participants taking idebenone who have not completely discontinued the idebenone at least 7 days prior to Visit 2. If the participant has not discontinued idebenone at least 7 days prior to Visit 2, the visit may be delayed until the 7-day period is complete.
- Presence, at the time of study inclusion, of infectious conjunctivitis, keratitis, scleritis or endophthalmitis in either eye.
- Presence of systemic illness, including alcohol and drug abuse (except nicotine), or medically significant abnormal laboratory values that are deemed by the investigator to preclude the participant's safe participation in the study.
- Presence of illness or disease that, in the opinion of the investigator, includes symptoms and/or the associated treatments that can alter visual function, for instance cancers or pathology of the central nervous system.
- Any medical or psychological condition that, in the opinion of the investigator, may compromise the safe participation of the participant in the study or would preclude compliance with the study protocol or ability of the participant to successfully complete the study.
- Participants unable or unwilling to comply with the protocol requirements.

Ages Eligible for Study
15 years and older (Child, Adult, Older Adult)

Sexes Eligible for Study
All

Accepts Healthy Volunteers
No

Design Details
Primary Purpose: Treatment
Allocation: Randomized
Interventional Model: Parallel Assignment
Masking: Quadruple (Participant Care Provider Investigator Outcomes Assessor)

Arms and interventions

Participant group/arm	Intervention/treatment
Experimental: GS010-treated eyes Each participant will have one eye randomly selected to receive a single injection of GS010 and the other eye will receive a sham injection. GS010-treated eyes: GS010 is a recombinant adeno-associated viral vector serotype 2 (rAAV2/2) containing the wild-type ND4 gene (rAAV2/2-ND4). Participants will receive a single dose of GS010 in one of their randomly selected eyes, via intravitreal injection containing 9E10 viral genomes in 90 μL balanced salt solution (BSS) plus 0.001% Pluronic F68®	Biological: GS010 • Both eyes of each participant will receive standard antiseptic preparation, administration of topical local ocular anesthetic agents, and will undergo pupillary dilation. Administration of an intraocular pressure lowering agent will precede treatment for every participant. GS010-treated eyes: GS010 is a recombinant adeno-associated viral vector serotype 2 (rAAV2/2) containing the wild-type ND4 gene (rAAV2/2-ND4). Participants will receive a single dose of GS010 in one of their randomly selected eyes, via intravitreal injection containing 9E10 viral genomes in 90 μL balanced salt solution (BSS) plus 0.001% Pluronic F68®. • Other names: – Lenadogene nolparvovec – rAAV2/2-ND4
Sham comparator: Sham-treated eyes Each participant will have one eye randomly selected to receive GS010 and the other eye will receive a sham injection. Eyes receiving sham injection will undergo the same preparatory procedures as eyes receiving GS010 injection, including pupillary dilation, topical antiinfection, and topical anesthetic procedures. Sham intravitreal injection will be performed by applying pressure to the eye at the location of a typical intravitreal injection procedure using the blunt end of a syringe without a needle	Device: Sham intravitreal injection • Both eyes of each participant will receive standard antiseptic preparation, administration of topical local ocular anesthetic agents, and will undergo pupillary dilation. Administration of an intraocular pressure lowering agent will precede treatment for every participant Sham-treated eyes: One eye of each participant will undergo sham injection. Sham intravitreal injection will be performed by applying pressure to the eye at the location of a typical intravitreal injection procedure using the blunt end of a syringe without a needle

Primary outcome measures

Outcome measure	Measure description	Time frame
Change from baseline in ETDRS visual acuity (quantitative score) at week 48	Visual acuity was derived from the early treatment diabetic retinopathy study (ETDRS) chart. Visual acuity is measured in "logarithm of the minimal angle of resolution" (logMAR), which was derived from the number of letters participants could read on the ETDRS chart 1 ETDRS line = 5 letters 1 ETDRS line = 0.1 logMAR A lower logMAR score denotes better visual acuity. A positive change from baseline indicates a worsening in symptoms. Change = (week 48 score–baseline score)	Baseline and week 48

Secondary outcome measures

Outcome measure	Measure description	Time frame
Change from baseline in ETDRS visual acuity (quantitative score)	Visual acuity was derived from the Early Treatment Diabetic Retinopathy Study (ETDRS) chart. Visual acuity is measured in "logarithm of the minimal angle of resolution" (logMAR), which was derived from the number of letters participants could read on the ETDRS chart 1 ETDRS line = 5 letters 1 ETDRS line = 0.1 logMAR A lower logMAR score denotes better visual acuity. A positive change from baseline indicates a worsening in symptoms Change = (week 72 score–baseline score) or (week 96 score–baseline score). Missing data was imputed by the linear interpolation method	Baseline; week 72 and week 96
Number of eye responders to treatment	An eye was determined as a responder to treatment based on two different definitions Definition 1: An eye responder was defined by an improvement of the early treatment diabetic retinopathy study (ETDRS) visual acuity score of at least 15 letters compared to baseline, or a final visual acuity greater than a Snellen acuity equivalent of 20/200 (a score of at least one letter) Definition 2: An eye responder was defined by an improvement of the ETDRS score of at least 20 letters compared to baseline	Baseline; week 48; week 72; and week 96
Number of subject responders to treatment	A subject responder was defined as a participant whose early treatment diabetic retinopathy study (ETDRS) score of the treated eye (that received GS010), was at least 15 letters better than the sham eye, or whose treated eye had a "logarithm of the minimal angle of resolution" (logMAR) acuity score of at least 0.3 logMAR better than the sham eye For the week 96 analysis, if no score was available for week 96, the score from the previous visit was used	Week 48; week 72; and week 96
Change from baseline in GCL macular volume	Ganglion cell layer (GCL) macular volume was measured as a parameter of spectral domain-optical coherence tomography (SD-OCT). SD-OCT was obtained with the Spectralis® OCT (Heidelberg Engineering)	Baseline; week 48; week 72; and week 96
Change from baseline in RNFL temporal quadrant thickness	Retinal nerve fiber layer (RNFL) temporal quadrant thickness was measured as a parameter of spectral domain-optical coherence tomography (SD-OCT). SD-OCT was obtained with the Spectralis® OCT (Heidelberg Engineering)	Baseline; week 48; week 72; and week 96
Change from baseline in RNFL papillomacular bundle thickness	Papillomacular bundle thickness was measured as a parameter of spectral domain-optical coherence tomography (SD-OCT). SD-OCT was obtained with the Spectralis® OCT (Heidelberg Engineering)	Baseline; week 48; week 72; and week 96
Change from baseline in ETDRS total macular volume	Early treatment diabetic retinopathy study (ETDRS) total macular volume was measured as a parameter of spectral domain-optical coherence tomography (SD-OCT). SD-OCT was obtained with the Spectralis® OCT (Heidelberg Engineering)	Baseline; week 48; week 72; and week 96

Change from baseline in the foveal threshold sensitivities obtained with HVF Analyzer II	The assessment of standardized automated visual fields was measured using the Humphrey visual field (HVF) analyzer II. Automated visual fields included the assessment of foveal threshold sensitivities. Foveal threshold sensitivity is measured in decibels (dB), which ranges from 0 dB to 50 dB. A sensitivity threshold of 0 dB indicates not being able to see the most intense perimetric stimulus, while higher dB indicates better/normal foveal vision. A positive change from baseline indicates an improvement of symptoms	Baseline; week 48; week 72; and week 96
Visual field mean deviation in decibels of sensitivity obtained with HVF analyzer II	The assessment of standardized automated visual fields was measured using the Humphrey visual field (HVF) analyzer II. Automated visual fields included the assessment of the mean deviation (MD) in decibels (dB) of sensitivity	Baseline; week 48; week 72; and week 96
Change from baseline in contrast sensitivity	The assessment of contrast sensitivity was measured using the Pelli-Robson chart. The chart uses letters arranged in groups whose contrast varies from high to low. Participants read the letters, starting with the highest contrast, until they are unable to read two or three letters in a single group. Each eye is assigned a score based on the contrast of the last group in which two or three letters were correctly read, ranging from 0 to 2.2 "log of contrast sensitivity" (LogCS) units. A score of 2.0 LogCS, represents a normal sensitivity contrast, and indicates the eye was able to detect two of the three letters with a contrast of 1 percent (contrast sensitivity = 100 percent or log 2). Scores less than 2.0 signify poorer contrast sensitivity. Pelli-Robson contrast sensitivity score of less than 1.5 is consistent with visual impairment and a score of less than 1.0 represents in visual disability. A negative change from baseline indicates worsening in symptoms	Baseline; week 48; week 72; and week 96
Change from baseline in color vision	The assessment of color vision was measured using the Farnsworth-Munsell 100-Hue color test. Each of the four trays consisted of 21 caps. Participants were asked to sort the randomly arranged caps following the hue order from the first to the last fixed caps. The total error score (TES) was derived by the frequency, the caps were misplaced and the severity, or distance of the misplacement Errors were made whenever caps were misplaced from the correct order. Error scores were calculated according to the distance between any two caps. The error score for each individual cap was the sum of the difference between the number of that cap and the numbers of the cap adjacent to it, minus 2. TES was the total sum of the error scores of the entire set of caps The best possible score was 0 and there is no defined upper limit to the total error score range. A lower score indicates improved color discrimination ability. A positive change from baseline indicates a worsening in symptoms	Baseline; week 48 and week 96

Sponsor
GenSight Biologics

Collaborators
No information provided

Investigators

- Principal Investigator: Nancy J. Newman, MD, Department of Ophthalmology, Emory University School of Medicine

General Publications
No publications available

Results
Outcome Measures

1. Change from Baseline in ETDRS Visual Acuity (Quantitative Score) at Week 48
   Type: Primary | Time Frame: Baseline and Week 48

Description	Visual acuity was derived from the early treatment diabetic retinopathy study (ETDRS) chart. Visual acuity is measured in "logarithm of the minimal angle of resolution" (logMAR), which was derived from the number of letters participants could read on the ETDRS chart 1 ETDRS line = 5 letters 1 ETDRS line = 0.1 logMAR A lower logMAR score denotes better visual acuity. A positive change from baseline indicates a worsening in symptoms Change = (week 48 score–baseline score)
Time frame	Baseline and week 48
Analysis population description	Intent-to-treat (ITT) population: All participants and all eyes that received study treatments, with data at both baseline and the applicable postdose visit. One participant was excluded from the ITT population due to receiving a smaller volume of study treatment than specified in the protocol. Participants received GS010 and Sham simultaneously

Arm/group title	GS010-treated eyes	Sham-treated eyes
Arm/group description	All eyes that received the study treatment, GS010. Each participant was randomly assigned GS010 in either the right or left eye. The eye assigned to GS010 received one single dose of GS010 (9E10 vg/eye) via an intravitreal (IVT) injection. The volume of the injected formula was 90 μL. The injection was performed in the vitreous humor under local anesthesia The same participants also received the sham procedure in the right or left eye, which was not assigned to receive GS010, at the same study visit Show less	All eyes that received the Sham. Each participant was randomly assigned GS010 in either the right or left eye, the eye not assigned GS010 received the sham procedure. The eye assigned to the Sham received one single sham intravitreal (IVT) injection, which was performed by applying pressure to the eye at the location of a typical IVT injection procedure, using the blunt end of a syringe without a needle The same participants also received GS010 in the right or left eye, which did not receive the sham procedure, at the same study visit Show less

Overall number of participants analyzed	38	38
Overall number of units analyzed Type of units analyzed: eyes	38	38
Least squares mean (standard error) ǀ unit of measure: logMAR	0.380 (0.129)	0.392 (0.129)
Statistical analysis 1: GS010-treated eyes, Sham-treated eyes ǀ Superiority ǀ ANCOVA		

2. Change from Baseline in ETDRS Visual Acuity (Quantitative Score)
   Type: Secondary ǀ Time Frame: Baseline; Week 72 and Week 96

Description	Visual acuity was derived from the early treatment diabetic retinopathy study (ETDRS) chart. Visual acuity is measured in "logarithm of the minimal angle of resolution" (logMAR), which was derived from the number of letters participants could read on the ETDRS chart 1 ETDRS line = 5 letters 1 ETDRS line = 0.1 logMAR A lower logMAR score denotes better visual acuity. A positive change from baseline indicates a worsening in symptoms Change = (week 72 score–baseline score) or (week 96 score–baseline score). Missing data was imputed by the linear interpolation method
Time frame	Baseline; week 72 and week 96
Analysis population description	Intent-to-treat (ITT) population: All participants and all eyes that received study treatments, with data at both baseline and the applicable postdose visit. One participant was excluded from the ITT population due to receiving a smaller volume of study treatment than specified in the protocol. Participants received GS010 and Sham simultaneously

Arm/group title	GS010-treated eyes	Sham-treated eyes
Arm/group description	All eyes that received the study treatment, GS010. Each participant was randomly assigned GS010 in either the right or left eye. The eye assigned to GS010 received one single dose of GS010 (9E10 vg/eye) via an intravitreal (IVT) injection. The volume of the injected formula was 90 μL. The injection was performed in the vitreous humor under local anesthesia The same participants also received the sham procedure in the right or left eye, which was not assigned to receive GS010, at the same study visit Show less	All eyes that received the Sham. Each participant was randomly assigned GS010 in either the right or left eye, the eye not assigned GS010 received the sham procedure. The eye assigned to the Sham received one single sham intravitreal (IVT) injection, which was performed by applying pressure to the eye at the location of a typical IVT injection procedure, using the blunt end of a syringe without a needle The same participants also received GS010 in the right or left eye, which did not receive the sham procedure, at the same study visit Show less

Overall number of participants analyzed	38	38
Overall number of units analyzed Type of units analyzed: eyes	38	38
Week 72 [a]Least squares mean (standard error) ǀ unit of measure: logMAR	0.192 (0.104)	0.216 (0.104)
Week 96[a]	0.178 (0.120)	0.207 (0.120)

[a]Least squares mean (standard error) ǀ unit of measure: logMAR

3. Number of Eye Responders to Treatment
   Type: Secondary ǀ Time Frame: Baseline; Week 48; Week 72; and Week 96

Description	An eye was determined as a responder to treatment based on two different definitions Definition 1: An eye responder was defined by an improvement of the early treatment diabetic retinopathy study (ETDRS) visual acuity score of at least 15 letters compared to baseline, or a final visual acuity greater than a Snellen acuity equivalent of 20/200 (a score of at least one letter) Definition 2: An eye responder was defined by an improvement of the ETDRS score of at least 20 letters compared to baseline
Time frame	Baseline; week 48; week 72; and week 96
Analysis population description	Intent-to-treat (ITT) population: All participants and all eyes that received study treatments, with data at both baseline and the applicable postdose visit. One participant was excluded from the ITT population due to receiving a smaller volume of study treatment than specified in the protocol. Participants received GS010 and Sham simultaneously

Arm/group title	GS010-treated eyes	Sham-treated eyes
Arm/group description	All eyes that received the study treatment, GS010. Each participant was randomly assigned GS010 in either the right or left eye. The eye assigned to GS010 received one single dose of GS010 (9E10 vg/eye) via an intravitreal (IVT) injection. The volume of the injected formula was 90 μL. The injection was performed in the vitreous humor under local anesthesia The same participants also received the sham procedure in the right or left eye, which was not assigned to receive GS010, at the same study visit Show more	All eyes that received the Sham. Each participant was randomly assigned GS010 in either the right or left eye, the eye not assigned GS010 received the sham procedure. The eye assigned to the Sham received one single sham intravitreal (IVT) injection, which was performed by applying pressure to the eye at the location of a typical IVT injection procedure, using the blunt end of a syringe without a needle The same participants also received GS010 in the right or left eye, which did not receive the sham procedure, at the same study visit Show more

Overall number of participants analyzed	38	38
Overall number of units analyzed Type of units analyzed: eyes	38	38
Week 48 definition 1 [a]Unit of measure: eyes	410.5%	37.9%
Week 48 definition 2[a]	923.7%	1026.3%
Week 72 definition 1[a]	615.8%	513.2%
Week 72 definition 2[a]	1128.9%	923.7%
Week 96 definition 1[a]	718.4%	513.2%
Week 96 definition 2[a]	1334.2%	1128.9%

[a]Unit of measure: eyes

4. Number of Subject Responders to Treatment
   Type: Secondary | Time Frame: Week 48; Week 72; and Week 96

Description	A subject responder was defined as a participant whose early treatment diabetic retinopathy study (ETDRS) score of the treated eye (that received GS010), was at least 15 letters better than the sham eye, or whose treated eye had a "logarithm of the minimal angle of resolution" (logMAR) acuity score of at least 0.3 logMAR better than the sham eye For the week 96 analysis, if no score was available for week 96, the score from the previous visit was used
Time frame	Week 48; week 72; and week 96
Analysis population description	Intent-to-treat (ITT) population: All participants who received study treatments, with data at the applicable postdose visit. One participant was excluded from the ITT population due to receiving a smaller volume of study treatment than specified in the protocol. Participants received GS010 and Sham simultaneously

Arm/group title	All participants
Arm/group description	All participants who were enrolled and received both study treatments, GS010 and Sham. All participants in the study received both GS010 and the sham procedure. Participants were randomly assigned to receive GS010 in either the right or left eye. The same participants also received the sham procedure in the eye not assigned to receive GS010, at the same study visit GS010: Either the right or left eye received one single dose of GS010 (9E10 vg/eye) via an intravitreal (IVT) injection. The volume of the injected formula was 90 μL. The injection was performed in the vitreous humor under local anesthesia Sham: Either the right or left eye (the eye not randomly assigned to GS010) received the sham procedure. One single sham IVT injection was performed by applying pressure to the eye at the location of a typical IVT injection procedure, using the blunt end of a syringe without a needle Show less
Overall number of participants analyzed	38
Week 48 [a]Measure type: count of participants I unit of measure: participants	410.5%
Week 72[a]	25.3%
Week 96[a]	513.2%

[a]Measure type: count of participants I unit of measure: participants

5. Change from Baseline in GCL Macular Volume
   Type: Secondary I Time Frame: Baseline; Week 48; Week 72; and Week 96

Description	Ganglion cell layer (GCL) macular volume was measured as a parameter of spectral domain-optical coherence tomography (SD-OCT). SD-OCT was obtained with the Spectralis® OCT (Heidelberg Engineering)
Time frame	Baseline; Week 48; Week 72; and Week 96
Analysis population description	Intent-to-treat (ITT) population: All participants and all eyes that received study treatments, with data at both baseline and the applicable postdose visit. One participant was excluded from the ITT population due to receiving a smaller volume of study treatment than specified in the protocol. Participants received GS010 and Sham simultaneously

Arm/group title	GS010-treated eyes	Sham-treated eyes
Arm/group description	All eyes that received the study treatment, GS010. Each participant was randomly assigned GS010 in either the right or left eye. The eye assigned to GS010 received one single dose of GS010 (9E10 vg/eye) via an intravitreal (IVT) injection. The volume of the injected formula was 90 μL. The injection was performed in the vitreous humor under local anesthesia The same participants also received the sham procedure in the right or left eye, which was not assigned to receive GS010, at the same study visit Show more	All eyes that received the Sham. Each participant was randomly assigned GS010 in either the right or left eye, the eye not assigned GS010 received the sham procedure. The eye assigned to the Sham received one single sham intravitreal (IVT) injection, which was performed by applying pressure to the eye at the location of a typical IVT injection procedure, using the blunt end of a syringe without a needle The same participants also received GS010 in the right or left eye, which did not receive the sham procedure, at the same study visit Show more
Overall number of participants analyzed	36	37
Overall number of units analyzed Type of units analyzed: eyes	36	37
Week 48		
Number analyzed	36 eyes	37 eyes
[a]Least squares mean (standard error) ǀ unit of measure: mm^3	−0.184 (0.014)	−0.207 (0.014)
Week 72		
Number analyzed	33 eyes[b]	34 eyes[c]
[a]	−0.204 (0.015)	−0.226 (0.015)
Week 96		
Number analyzed	33 eyes[b]	33 eyes[b]
[a]	−0.208 (0.015)	−0.221 (0.015)

[a]Least squares mean (standard error) ǀ unit of measure: mm^3
[b]33 participants
[c]34 participants

6. Change from Baseline in RNFL Temporal Quadrant Thickness
Type: Secondary | Time Frame: Baseline; Week 48; Week 72; and Week 96

Description	Retinal nerve fiber layer (RNFL) temporal quadrant thickness was measured as a parameter of spectral domain-optical coherence tomography (SD-OCT). SD-OCT was obtained with the Spectralis® OCT (Heidelberg Engineering)
Time frame	Baseline; week 48; week 72; and week 96
Analysis population description	Intent-to-treat (ITT) population: All participants and all eyes that received study treatments, with data at both baseline and the applicable postdose visit. One participant was excluded from the ITT population due to receiving a smaller volume of study treatment than specified in the protocol. Participants received GS010 and Sham simultaneously

Arm/group title	GS010-treated eyes	Sham-treated eyes
Arm/group description	All eyes that received the study treatment, GS010. Each participant was randomly assigned GS010 in either the right or left eye. The eye assigned to GS010 received one single dose of GS010 (9E10 vg/eye) via an intravitreal (IVT) injection. The volume of the injected formula was 90 μL. The injection was performed in the vitreous humor under local anesthesia The same participants also received the sham procedure in the right or left eye, which was not assigned to receive GS010, at the same study visit Show more	All eyes that received the Sham. Each participant was randomly assigned GS010 in either the right or left eye, the eye not assigned GS010 received the sham procedure. The eye assigned to the Sham received one single sham intravitreal (IVT) injection, which was performed by applying pressure to the eye at the location of a typical IVT injection procedure, using the blunt end of a syringe without a needle The same participants also received GS010 in the right or left eye, which did not receive the sham procedure, at the same study visit Show more
Overall number of participants analyzed	37	37
Overall number of units analyzed Type of units analyzed: eyes	37	37
Week 48		
Number analyzed	37 eyes	37 eyes
[a]Least squares mean (standard error) | unit of measure: μm	−22.8 (1.0)	−24.7 (1.0)
Week 72		
Number analyzed	34 eyes[b]	34 eyes[b]

a	−25.5 (0.9)	−26.0 (0.9)
Week 96		
Number analyzed	32 eyes[c]	33 eyes[d]
a	−24.2 (0.8)	−26.1 (0.8)

[a]Least squares mean (standard error) | unit of measure: μm
[b]34 participants
[c]32 participants
[d]33 participants

7. Change from Baseline in RNFL Papillomacular Bundle Thickness
   Type: Secondary | Time Frame: Baseline; Week 48; Week 72; and Week 96

Description	Papillomacular bundle thickness was measured as a parameter of spectral domain-optical coherence tomography (SD-OCT). SD-OCT was obtained with the Spectralis® OCT (Heidelberg Engineering)
Time frame	Baseline; week 48; week 72; and week 96
Analysis population description	Intent-to-treat (ITT) population: All participants and all eyes that received study treatments, with data at both baseline and the applicable postdose visit. One participant was excluded from the ITT population due to receiving a smaller volume of study treatment than specified in the protocol. Participants received GS010 and Sham simultaneously

Arm/group title	GS010-treated eyes	Sham-treated eyes
Arm/group description	All eyes that received the study treatment, GS010. Each participant was randomly assigned GS010 in either the right or left eye. The eye assigned to GS010 received one single dose of GS010 (9E10 vg/eye) via an intravitreal (IVT) injection. The volume of the injected formula was 90 μL. The injection was performed in the vitreous humor under local anesthesia The same participants also received the sham procedure in the right or left eye, which was not assigned to receive GS010, at the same study visit Show more	All eyes that received the Sham. Each participant was randomly assigned GS010 in either the right or left eye, the eye not assigned GS010 received the sham procedure. The eye assigned to the Sham received one single sham intravitreal (IVT) injection, which was performed by applying pressure to the eye at the location of a typical IVT injection procedure, using the blunt end of a syringe without a needle The same participants also received GS010 in the right or left eye, which did not receive the sham procedure, at the same study visit Show more
Overall number of participants analyzed	37	37
Overall number of units analyzed Type of units analyzed: eyes	37	37
Week 48		

Number analyzed	37 eyes	37 eyes
[a]Least squares mean (standard error) | unit of measure: μm	−10.4 (1.0)	−12.4 (1.0)
Week 72		
Number analyzed	34 eyes[b]	34 eyes[b]
[a]	−12.8 (1.0)	−13.1 (1.0)
Week 96		
Number analyzed	32 eyes[c]	33 eyes[d]
[a]	−11.2 (1.0)	−13.3 (1.0)

[a]Least squares mean (standard error) | unit of measure: μm
[b]34 participants
[c]32 participants
[d]33 participants

8. Change from Baseline in ETDRS Total Macular Volume
   Type: Secondary | Time Frame: Baseline; Week 48; Week 72; and Week 96

Description	Early treatment diabetic retinopathy study (ETDRS) total macular volume was measured as a parameter of spectral domain-optical coherence tomography (SD-OCT). SD-OCT was obtained with the Spectralis® OCT (Heidelberg Engineering)
Time frame	Baseline; week 48; week 72; and week 96
Analysis population description	Intent-to-treat (ITT) population: All participants and all eyes that received study treatments, with data at both baseline and the applicable postdose visit. One participant was excluded from the ITT population due to receiving a smaller volume of study treatment than specified in the protocol. Participants received GS010 and Sham simultaneously

Arm/group title	GS010-treated eyes	Sham-treated eyes
Arm/group description	All eyes that received the study treatment, GS010. Each participant was randomly assigned GS010 in either the right or left eye. The eye assigned to GS010 received one single dose of GS010 (9E10 vg/eye) via an intravitreal (IVT) injection. The volume of the injected formula was 90 μL. The injection was performed in the vitreous humor under local anesthesia The same participants also received the sham procedure in the right or left eye, which was not assigned to receive GS010, at the same study visit Show more	All eyes that received the Sham. Each participant was randomly assigned GS010 in either the right or left eye, the eye not assigned GS010 received the sham procedure. The eye assigned to the Sham received one single sham intravitreal (IVT) injection, which was performed by applying pressure to the eye at the location of a typical IVT injection procedure, using the blunt end of a syringe without a needle The same participants also received GS010 in the right or left eye, which did not receive the sham procedure, at the same study visit Show more

Overall number of participants analyzed	36	37
Overall number of units analyzed Type of units analyzed: eyes	36	37
Week 48	.	
Number analyzed	36 eyes	37 eyes
[a]Least squares mean (standard error) I unit of measure: mm^3	−0.578 (0.041)	−0.708 (0.040)
Week 72		
Number analyzed	33 eyes[b]	34 eyes[c]
[a]	−0.686 (0.048)	−0.782 (0.048)
Week 96		
Number analyzed	33 eyes[b]	33 eyes[b]
[a]	−0.720 (0.050)	−0.800 (0.050)

[a]Least squares mean (standard error) I unit of measure: mm^3
[b]33 participants
[c]34 participants

9. Change from Baseline in the Foveal Threshold Sensitivities Obtained with HVF Analyzer II
   Type: Secondary I Time Frame: Baseline; Week 48; Week 72; and Week 96

Description	The assessment of standardized automated visual fields was measured using the Humphrey visual field (HVF) analyzer II. Automated visual fields included the assessment of foveal threshold sensitivities. Foveal threshold sensitivity is measured in decibels (dB), which ranges from 0 dB to 50 dB. A sensitivity threshold of 0 dB indicates not being able to see the most intense perimetric stimulus, while higher dB indicates better/normal foveal vision. A positive change from baseline indicates an improvement of symptoms
Time frame	Baseline; week 48; week 72; and week 96
Analysis population description	Intent-to-treat (ITT) population: All participants and all eyes that received study treatments, with data at both baseline and the applicable postdose visit. One participant was excluded from the ITT population due to receiving a smaller volume of study treatment than specified in the protocol. Participants received GS010 and Sham simultaneously

Arm/group title	GS010-treated eyes	Sham-treated eyes
Arm/group description	All eyes that received the study treatment, GS010. Each participant was randomly assigned GS010 in either the right or left eye. The eye assigned to GS010 received one single dose of GS010 (9E10 vg/eye) via an intravitreal (IVT) injection. The volume of the injected formula was 90 μL. The injection was performed in the vitreous humor under local anesthesia The same participants also received the sham procedure in the right or left eye, which was not assigned to receive GS010, at the same study visit Show more	All eyes that received the Sham. Each participant was randomly assigned GS010 in either the right or left eye, the eye not assigned GS010 received the sham procedure. The eye assigned to the Sham received one single sham intravitreal (IVT) injection, which was performed by applying pressure to the eye at the location of a typical IVT injection procedure, using the blunt end of a syringe without a needle The same participants also received GS010 in the right or left eye, which did not receive the sham procedure, at the same study visit Show more
Overall number of participants analyzed	11	8
Overall number of units analyzed Type of units analyzed: eyes	11	8
Week 48	.	
Number analyzed	11 eyes	7 eyes[a]
[b]Mean (standard deviation) ǀ unit of measure: decibels (dB)	3.5 (12.3)	−7.4 (12.8)
Week 72		
Number analyzed	7 eyes[a]	7 eyes[a]
[b]	6.3 (7.8)	−5.1 (11.9)
Week 96		
Number analyzed	6 eyes[c]	8 eyes
[b]	3.3 (12.7)	1.4 (19.5)

[a]7 participants
[b]Mean (standard deviation) ǀ unit of measure: decibels (dB)
[c]6 participants

10. Visual Field Mean Deviation in Decibels of Sensitivity Obtained with HVF Analyzer II
Type: Secondary | Time Frame: Baseline; Week 48; Week 72; and Week 96

Description	The assessment of standardized automated visual fields was measured using the Humphrey visual field (HVF) analyzer II. Automated visual fields included the assessment of the mean deviation (MD) in decibels (dB) of sensitivity
Time frame	Baseline; week 48; week 72; and week 96
Analysis population description	Intent-to-treat (ITT) population: All participants and all eyes that received study treatments, with data at both baseline and the applicable postdose visit. One participant was excluded from the ITT population due to receiving a smaller volume of study treatment than specified in the protocol. Participants received GS010 and Sham simultaneously

Arm/group title	GS010-treated eyes	Sham-treated eyes
Arm/group description	All eyes that received the study treatment, GS010. Each participant was randomly assigned GS010 in either the right or left eye. The eye assigned to GS010 received one single dose of GS010 (9E10 vg/eye) via an intravitreal (IVT) injection. The volume of the injected formula was 90 µL. The injection was performed in the vitreous humor under local anesthesia The same participants also received the sham procedure in the right or left eye, which was not assigned to receive GS010, at the same study visit Show more	All eyes that received the Sham. Each participant was randomly assigned GS010 in either the right or left eye, the eye not assigned GS010 received the sham procedure. The eye assigned to the Sham received one single sham intravitreal (IVT) injection, which was performed by applying pressure to the eye at the location of a typical IVT injection procedure, using the blunt end of a syringe without a needle The same participants also received GS010 in the right or left eye, which did not receive the sham procedure, at the same study visit Show more
Overall number of participants analyzed	38	38
Overall number of units analyzed Type of units analyzed: eyes	38	38
Baseline MD		
Number analyzed	38 eyes	38 eyes
[a]Mean (standard deviation) | unit of measure: decibels (dB)	−16.26 (10.59)	−16.73 (11.48)
Week 48 MD		

Number analyzed	37 eyes[b]	37 eyes[b]
[a]	−24.26 (9.37)	−23.76 (10.40)
Week 72 MD		
Number analyzed	34 eyes[c]	33 eyes[d]
[a]	−23.33 (9.41)	−22.94 (10.11)
Week 96 MD		
Number analyzed	34 eyes[c]	33 eyes[d]
[a]	−23.31 (9.41)	−22.70 (9.88)

[a]Mean (standard deviation) | unit of measure: decibels (dB)
[b]37 participants
[c]34 participants
[d]33 participants

11. Change from Baseline in Contrast Sensitivity
Type: Secondary | Time Frame: Baseline; Week 48; Week 72; and Week 96

Description	The assessment of contrast sensitivity was measured using the Pelli-Robson chart. The chart uses letters arranged in groups whose contrast varies from high to low. Participants read the letters, starting with the highest contrast, until they are unable to read two or three letters in a single group. Each eye is assigned a score based on the contrast of the last group in which two or three letters were correctly read, ranging from 0 to 2.2 "log of contrast sensitivity" (LogCS) units. A score of 2.0 LogCS represents a normal sensitivity contrast, and indicates the eye was able to detect two of the three letters with a contrast of 1 percent (contrast sensitivity = 100 percent or log 2). Scores less than 2.0 signify poorer contrast sensitivity. Pelli-Robson contrast sensitivity score of less than 1.5 is consistent with visual impairment and a score of less than 1.0 represents visual disability. A negative change from baseline indicates worsening in symptoms
Time frame	Baseline; week 48; week 72; and week 96
Analysis population description	Intent-to-treat (ITT) population: All participants and all eyes that received study treatments, with data at both baseline and the applicable postdose visit. One participant was excluded from the ITT population due to receiving a smaller volume of study treatment than specified in the protocol. Participants received GS010 and Sham simultaneously

Arm/group title	GS010-treated eyes	Sham-treated eyes
Arm/group description	All eyes that received the study treatment, GS010. Each participant was randomly assigned GS010 in either the right or left eye. The eye assigned to GS010 received one single dose of GS010 (9E10 vg/eye) via an intravitreal (IVT) injection. The volume of the injected formula was 90 µL. The injection was performed in the vitreous humor under local anesthesia. The same participants also received the sham procedure in the right or left eye, which was not assigned to receive GS010, at the same study visit. Show less	All eyes that received the Sham. Each participant was randomly assigned GS010 in either the right or left eye, the eye not assigned GS010 received the sham procedure. The eye assigned to the Sham received one single sham intravitreal (IVT) injection, which was performed by applying pressure to the eye at the location of a typical IVT injection procedure, using the blunt end of a syringe without a needle. The same participants also received GS010 in the right or left eye, which did not receive the sham procedure, at the same study visit. Show less
Overall number of participants analyzed	38	38
Overall number of units analyzed Type of units analyzed: eyes	38	38
Week 48 [a]Least squares mean (standard error) I unit of measure: LogCS	−0.35 (0.07)	−0.33 (0.07)
Week 72[a]	−0.25 (0.07)	−0.28 (0.07)
Week 96[a]	−0.27 (0.07)	−0.25 (0.07)

[a]Least squares mean (standard error) I unit of measure: LogCS

12. Change from Baseline in Color Vision
Type: Secondary I Time Frame: Baseline; Week 48; and Week 96

Description	The assessment of color vision was measured using the Farnsworth-Munsell 100-Hue Color Test. Each of the four trays consisted of 21 caps. Participants were asked to sort the randomly arranged caps following the hue order from the first to the last fixed caps. The total error score (TES) was derived by the frequency, the caps were misplaced and the severity, or distance of the misplacement Errors were made whenever caps were misplaced from the correct order. Error scores were calculated according to the distance between any two caps. The error score for each individual cap was the sum of the difference between the number of that cap and the numbers of the cap adjacent to it, minus 2. TES was the total sum of the error scores of the entire set of caps The best possible score was 0 and there is no defined upper limit to the total error score range. A lower score indicates improved color discrimination ability. A positive change from baseline indicates a worsening in symptoms
Time frame	Baseline; week 48; and week 96

Analysis population description	Intent-to-treat (ITT) population: All participants and all eyes that received study treatments, with data at both baseline and the applicable postdose visit. One participant was excluded from the ITT population due to receiving a smaller volume of study treatment than specified in the protocol. Participants received GS010 and Sham simultaneously

Arm/group title	GS010-treated eyes	Sham-treated eyes
Arm/group description	All eyes that received the study treatment, GS010. Each participant was randomly assigned GS010 in either the right or left eye. The eye assigned to GS010 received one single dose of GS010 (9E10 vg/eye) via an intravitreal (IVT) injection. The volume of the injected formula was 90 μL. The injection was performed in the vitreous humor under local anesthesia The same participants also received the sham procedure in the right or left eye, which was not assigned to receive GS010, at the same study visit Show more	All eyes that received the Sham. Each participant was randomly assigned GS010 in either the right or left eye, the eye not assigned GS010 received the sham procedure. The eye assigned to the Sham received one single sham intravitreal (IVT) injection, which was performed by applying pressure to the eye at the location of a typical IVT injection procedure, using the blunt end of a syringe without a needle The same participants also received GS010 in the right or left eye, which did not receive the sham procedure, at the same study visit Show more
Overall number of participants analyzed	21	21
Overall number of units analyzed Type of units analyzed: eyes	21	21
Week 48		
Number analyzed	18 eyes[a]	20 eyes[b]
[c]Mean (standard deviation) I unit of measure: score on a scale	133.1 (290.7)	235.6 (392.3)
Week 96		
Number analyzed	21 eyes	21 eyes
[c]	97.7 (342.2)	213.5 (393.1)

[a]18 participants
[b]20 participants
[c]Mean (standard deviation) I unit of measure: score on a scale

Adverse Events

Time Frame

From first dose to end of study (a maximum of 96 weeks)

Adverse Event Reporting Description

Safety population: All participants who were randomized and received study treatments.

Because all participants received both study treatment and the sham procedure simultaneously, adverse events (AEs) are reported overall for systemic and ocular events. Reported events include AEs associated with both GS010 and the sham procedure.

Arm/group title	All participants
Arm/group description	All participants who were enrolled and received both study treatments, GS010 and Sham. All participants in the study received both GS010 and the sham procedure simultaneously. Participants were randomly assigned to receive GS010 in either the right or left eye. The same participants also received the sham procedure in the eye not assigned to receive GS010, at the same study visit GS010: Either the right or left eye received one single dose of GS010 (9E10 vg/eye) via an intravitreal (IVT) injection. The volume of the injected formula was 90 μL. The injection was performed in the vitreous humor under local anesthesia Sham: Either the right or left eye (the eye not randomly assigned to GS010) received the sham procedure. One single sham IVT injection was performed by applying pressure to the eye at the location of a typical IVT injection procedure, using the blunt end of a syringe without a needle Show less
All-cause mortality	
Arm/group title	All participants
	Affected / at risk (%)
Total	2/39 (5.13%)
Serious adverse events	
Arm/group title	All participants
	Affected/at risk (%)
Total	3/39 (7.69%)
Hepatobiliary disorders	
Alcoholic liver disease[a,b]	1/39 (2.56%)
Injury, poisoning, and procedural complications	
Alcohol poisoning[a,b]	1/39 (2.56%)
Metabolism and nutrition disorders	
Malnutrition[a,b]	1/39 (2.56%)
Psychiatric disorders	
Alcohol withdrawal syndrome[a,b]	1/39 (2.56%)
Renal and urinary disorders	
Renal failure[a,b]	1/39 (2.56%)

a Indicates events were collected by systematic assessment b Term from vocabulary, MedDRA 20.1	
Other (not including serious) adverse events	
5% Frequency threshold for reporting other adverse events	
Arm/group title	All participants
	Affected / at risk (%)
Total	38/39 (97.44%)
Eye disorders	
Anterior chamber cell[a,b]	6/39 (15.38%)
Anterior chamber flare[a,b]	5/39 (12.82%)
Anterior chamber inflammation[a,b]	3/39 (7.69%)
Autoimmune uveitis[a,b,c]	15/39 (38.46%)
Chalazion[a,b]	2/39 (5.13%)
Conjunctival hemorrhage[a,b,d]	7/39 (17.95%)
Conjunctival hyperemia[a,b,e]	5/39 (12.82%)
Corneal disorder[a,b]	2/39 (5.13%)
Eye irritation[a,b,f]	2/39 (5.13%)
Eye pain[a,b,g]	3/39 (7.69%)
Foreign body sensation in eyes[a,b,h]	2/39 (5.13%)
Iridocyclitis[a,b,i]	18/39 (46.15%)
Iris atrophy[a,b]	3/39 (7.69%)
Iris transillumination defect[a,b]	2/39 (5.13%)
Keratic precipitates[a,b]	9/39 (23.08%)
Macular edema[a,b]	2/39 (5.13%)
Photopsia[a,b]	2/39 (5.13%)
Punctate keratitis[a,b,j]	18/39 (46.15%)
Vitreal cells[a,b]	3/39 (7.69%)
Vitreous disorder[a,b]	3/39 (7.69%)
Vitreous floaters[a,b]	3/39 (7.69%)
Vitritis[a,b]	7/39 (17.95%)
Infections and infestations	
Nasopharyngitis[a,b]	7/39 (17.95%)
Ear infection[a,b]	2/39 (5.13%)
Conjunctivitis[a,b]	2/39 (5.13%)
Investigations	

Gamma-glutamyltransferase increased[a,b]	3/39 (7.69%)
Alanine aminotransferase increased[a,b]	2/39 (5.13%)
Blood glucose increased[a,b]	2/39 (5.13%)
Neutrophil count increased[a,b]	2/39 (5.13%)
White blood cell count increased[a,b]	2/39 (5.13%)
Intraocular pressure increased[a,b,k]	13/39 (33.33%)
Nervous system disorders	
Headache[a,b]	6/39 (15.38%)
Migraine[a,b]	3/39 (7.69%)
Psychiatric disorders	
Anxiety[a,b]	3/39 (7.69%)
Depression[a,b]	2/39 (5.13%)
Social circumstances	
Alcohol use[a,b]	2/39 (5.13%)
Vascular disorders	
Hypertension[a,b]	6/39 (15.38%)

[a]Indicates events were collected by systematic assessment
[b]Term from vocabulary, MedDRA 20.1
[c]The verbatim term for all events of "autoimmune uveitis" is "intermediate uveitis."
[d]1/7 affected participants experienced this event in the sham-treated eyes
[e]4/5 affected participants experienced this event in the sham-treated eyes
[f]1/2 affected participants experienced this event in the sham-treated eyes
[g]1/3 affected participants experienced this event in the sham treated eyes.
[h]1/2 affected participants experienced this event in the sham treated eyes
[i]2/18 affected participants experienced this event in the sham-treated eyes
[j]3/18 affected participants experienced this event in the sham-treated eyes
[k]1/13 affected participants experienced this event in the sham-treated eyes

Completed

China

Safety and Efficacy Study of rAAV2-ND4 Treatment of Leber Hereditary Optic Neuropathy (LHON) (rAAV2-ND4)

ClinicalTrials.gov ID NCT01267422

Sponsor Bin Li
Information provided by Bin Li, Huazhong University of Science and Technology (Responsible Party)
Last Update Posted 2018-01-31
Study Registration Dates

First Submitted
2010-12-27

First Submitted that met QC Criteria
2010-12-27

First Posted (Estimated)
2010-12-28
Results Reporting Dates

Results First Submitted
2015-05-21

Results First Submitted that met QC Criteria
2016-03-29

Results First Posted (Estimated)
2016-05-02
Study Record Updates

Last Update Submitted that met QC Criteria
2018-01-07

Last Update Posted
2018-01-31

Last Verified
2018-01

Brief Summary
This study is meant to assess the safety and efficacy of rAAV2-ND4 treatment of Leber hereditary optic neuropathy with 11,778 LHON mutation.

Detailed Description
Leber Hereditary Optic Neuropathy (LHON) is a maternally inherited ocular disorder associated with a mutation in mtDNA. The common manifestation is visual loss which is caused by the respiratory chain enzymes complex dysfunction resulting in increased oxidative stress enzymes production.

Material and Method: Seven patients with 11,778 LHON mutation were randomly treated with a single IVT injection of recombinant adeno-associated virus-NADH dehydrogenase, subunit 4 (complex I) (rAAV2-ND4) (0.05 mL). The dose was 5×10^9 vg/0.05 mL for patients younger than 12 years old, and 1×10^{10} vg/0.05 mL for patients older than 12 years old. The visual acuity, visual evoked potential (VEP), optical coherence tomography (OCT), computerized visual field, electroretinograms (ERG), retinal nerve fiber layer (RNFL), and liver and kidney function in plasma were compared before and after treatment at 1, 3, and 6 months interval.

Official Title
Safety and Efficacy Study of a Single Intravitreal Injection of rAAV2-ND4 Treatment of Leber Hereditary Optic Neuropathy

Conditions
Leber Hereditary Optic Neuropathy

Intervention/Treatment
Drug: rAAV2-ND4

Study Start
2011-04

Primary Completion (Actual)
2015-11

Study Completion (Actual)
2015-11

Enrollment (Actual)
9

Study Type
Interventional

Phase
Not Applicable

China
Hubei Locations

Wuhan, Hubei, China, 430030
Department of Ophthalmology, Tongji Hospital, Tongji Medical College, Huazhong University of Science and Technology

Eligibility Criteria
Inclusion Criteria
- Comply with Leber hereditary optic neuropathy diagnostic criteria.
- In patients with informed consent, voluntary participation.
- Signed informed consent.
- $8 \leq$ Age ≤ 60 years old, good health, the patient can tolerate local anesthesia surgery.
- To comply with doctor's instructions, can in the time of referral.

Exclusion Criteria
- Cardiopulmonary and renal function in severe weakness, cancer, a variety of bleeding disorders, acute sensing disease, high fever, high fever disease, women during pregnancy, heart disease, such as postoperative recovery period.
- Are participating in other clinical studies of patients.
- Patients with mental disorders.

Ages Eligible for Study
8 to 60 years (Child, Adult)

Sexes Eligible for Study
All

Accepts Healthy Volunteers
No

Design Details
Primary Purpose: Treatment
Allocation: N/A
Interventional Model: Single Group Assignment
Masking: None (Open Label)

Arms and interventions

Participant group/arm	Intervention/treatment
Experimental: rAAV2-ND4 injection	Drug: rAAV2-ND4 • Iinjection • Other Names: – rAAV2-ND4 gene therapy

Primary outcome measures

Outcome measure	Measure description	Time frame
The best-corrected visual acuity (BCVA)		Up to 3 years
Results of CD3/CD4/CD8 test	The mean percentage of CD3+/CD4+/CD8+ test before and after treatment	Up to 6 months

Secondary outcome measures

Outcome measure	Measure description	Time frame
Intraocular pressure		Up to 3 years
Neutralizing antibody assay	The mean of neutralizing antibody assay of eight patients before and after treatment	Up to 3 years
Average RNFL thickness through optical coherence tomography (OCT) test	Average RNFL thickness of eight patients through optical coherence tomography(OCT) test before and after treatment	Up to 3 years
Computerized visual field (MD: mean deviation, the value close to 0 regarded normal)	MD: mean deviation, the value close to 0 regarded normal. VFI/MD:the bigger one was closer to the normal value	Up to 3 years
Computerized visual field (VFI: visual field index, the value close to 100% regarded normal)	VFI: visual field index, the value close to 100% regarded normal. VFI/MD: the bigger one was closer to the normal value	Up to 3 years

Sponsor
Bin Li

Collaborators

- Huazhong University of Science and Technology

Investigators

- Study Chair: bin Li, PhD, MD, Deputy Director of Ophthalmology

General Publications

- Carelli V, Ross-Cisneros FN, Sadun AA. Mitochondrial dysfunction as a cause of optic neuropathies. Prog Retin Eye Res. 2004 Jan;23(1):53–89. https://doi.org/10.1016/j.preteyeres.2003.10.003.
- Mackey DA, Oostra RJ, Rosenberg T, Nikoskelainen E, Bronte-Stewart J, Poulton J, Harding AE, Govan G, Bolhuis PA, Norby S. Primary pathogenic mtDNA mutations in multigeneration pedigrees with Leber hereditary optic neuropathy. Am J Hum Genet. 1996 Aug;59(2):481–5. No abstract available.
- Wallace DC, Singh G, Lott MT, Hodge JA, Schurr TG, Lezza AM, Elsas LJ second, Nikoskelainen EK. Mitochondrial DNA mutation associated with Leber's hereditary optic neuropathy. Science. 1988 Dec 9;242(4884):1427–30. https://doi.org/10.1126/science.3201231.
- Oguchi Y. [Past, present, and future in Leber's hereditary optic neuropathy]. Nippon Ganka Gakkai Zasshi. 2001 Dec;105(12):809–27. Japanese.
- Cui G, Ding H, Xu Y, Li B, Wang DW. Applications of the method of high resolution melting analysis for diagnosis of Leber's disease and the three primary mutation spectrum of LHON in the Han Chinese population. Gene. 2013 Jan 1; 512(1):108–12. https://doi.org/10.1016/j.gene.2012.09.110. Epub 2012 Oct 9.
- Mashima Y, Kigasawa K, Wakakura M, Oguchi Y. Do idebenone and vitamin therapy shorten the time to achieve visual recovery in Leber hereditary optic neuropathy? J Neuroophthalmol. 2000 Sep;20(3):166–70. https://doi.org/10.1097/00041327-200020030-00006.
- Carelli V, Barboni P, Zacchini A, Mancini R, Monari L, Cevoli S, Liguori R, Sensi M, Lugaresi E, Montagna P. Leber's Hereditary Optic Neuropathy (LHON) with 14,484/ND6 mutation in a North African patient. J Neurol Sci. 1998 Oct 8;160(2):183–8. https://doi.org/10.1016/s0022-510x(98)00239-1.
- Barnils N, Mesa E, Munoz S, Ferrer-Artola A, Arruga J. [Response to idebenone and multivitamin therapy in Leber's hereditary optic neuropathy]. Arch Soc Esp Oftalmol. 2007 Jun;82(6):377–80. https://doi.org/10.4321/s0365-66912007000600012. Spanish.
- Angebault C, Gueguen N, Desquiret-Dumas V, Chevrollier A, Guillet V, Verny C, Cassereau J, Ferre M, Milea D, Amati-Bonneau P, Bonneau D, Procaccio V, Reynier P, Loiseau D. Idebenone increases mitochondrial complex I activity in fibroblasts from LHON patients while producing contradictory effects on respiration. BMC Res Notes. 2011 Dec 22;4:557. https://doi.org/10.1186/1756-0500-4-557.

- Klopstock T, Yu-Wai-Man P, Dimitriadis K, Rouleau J, Heck S, Bailie M, Atawan A, Chattopadhyay S, Schubert M, Garip A, Kernt M, Petraki D, Rummey C, Leinonen M, Metz G, Griffiths PG, Meier T, Chinnery PF. A randomized placebo-controlled trial of idebenone in Leber's hereditary optic neuropathy. Brain. 2011 Sep;134(Pt 9):2677–86. https://doi.org/10.1093/brain/awr170. Epub 2011 Jul 25.
- Carelli V, La Morgia C, Valentino ML, Rizzo G, Carbonelli M, De Negri AM, Sadun F, Carta A, Guerriero S, Simonelli F, Sadun AA, Aggarwal D, Liguori R, Avoni P, Baruzzi A, Zeviani M, Montagna P, Barboni P. Idebenone treatment in Leber's hereditary optic neuropathy. Brain. 2011 Sep;134(Pt 9):e188. https://doi.org/10.1093/brain/awr180. Epub 2011 Aug 2. No abstract available.
- Sadun AA, Chicani CF, Ross-Cisneros FN, Barboni P, Thoolen M, Shrader WD, Kubis K, Carelli V, Miller G. Effect of EPI-743 on the clinical course of the mitochondrial disease Leber hereditary optic neuropathy. Arch Neurol. 2012 Mar;69(3):331–8. https://doi.org/10.1001/archneurol.2011.2972.
- Newman NJ. Treatment of Leber hereditary optic neuropathy. Brain. 2011 Sep;134(Pt 9):2447–50. https://doi.org/10.1093/brain/awr192. Epub 2011 Aug 22. No abstract available.
- Maguire AM, Simonelli F, Pierce EA, Pugh EN Jr., Mingozzi F, Bennicelli J, Banfi S, Marshall KA, Testa F, Surace EM, Rossi S, Lyubarsky A, Arruda VR, Konkle B, Stone E, Sun J, Jacobs J, Dell'Osso L, Hertle R, Ma JX, Redmond TM, Zhu X, Hauck B, Zelenaia O, Shindler KS, Maguire MG, Wright JF, Volpe NJ, McDonnell JW, Auricchio A, High KA, Bennett J. Safety and efficacy of gene transfer for Leber's congenital amaurosis. N Engl J Med. 2008 May 22;358(21):2240–8. https://doi.org/10.1056/NEJMoa0802315. Epub 2008 Apr 27.
- Bainbridge JW, Smith AJ, Barker SS, Robbie S, Henderson R, Balaggan K, Viswanathan A, Holder GE, Stockman A, Tyler N, Petersen-Jones S, Bhattacharya SS, Thrasher AJ, Fitzke FW, Carter BJ, Rubin GS, Moore AT, Ali RR. Effect of gene therapy on visual function in Leber's congenital amaurosis. N Engl J Med. 2008 May 22;358(21):2231–9. https://doi.org/10.1056/NEJMoa0802268. Epub 2008 Apr 27.
- Bonnet C, Kaltimbacher V, Ellouze S, Augustin S, Benit P, Forster V, Rustin P, Sahel JA, Corral-Debrinski M. Allotopic mRNA localization to the mitochondrial surface rescues respiratory chain defects in fibroblasts harboring mitochondrial DNA mutations affecting complex I or v subunits. Rejuvenation Res. 2007 Jun;10(2):127–44. https://doi.org/10.1089/rej.2006.0526.
- Ellouze S, Augustin S, Bouaita A, Bonnet C, Simonutti M, Forster V, Picaud S, Sahel JA, Corral-Debrinski M. Optimized allotopic expression of the human mitochondrial ND4 prevents blindness in a rat model of mitochondrial dysfunction. Am J Hum Genet. 2008 Sep;83(3):373–87. https://doi.org/10.1016/j.ajhg.2008.08.013. Epub 2008 Sep 4.
- Koilkonda RD, Yu H, Chou TH, Feuer WJ, Ruggeri M, Porciatti V, Tse D, Hauswirth WW, Chiodo V, Boye SL, Lewin AS, Neuringer M, Renner L, Guy J. Safety and effects of the vector for the Leber hereditary optic neuropathy gene

therapy clinical trial. JAMA Ophthalmol. 2014 Apr 1;132(4):409–20. https://doi.org/10.1001/jamaophthalmol.2013.7630.

- Koilkonda R, Yu H, Talla V, Porciatti V, Feuer WJ, Hauswirth WW, Chiodo V, Erger KE, Boye SL, Lewin AS, Conlon TJ, Renner L, Neuringer M, Detrisac C, Guy J. LHON gene therapy vector prevents visual loss and optic neuropathy induced by G11778A mutant mitochondrial DNA: biodistribution and toxicology profile. Invest Ophthalmol Vis Sci. 2014 Oct 23;55(12):7739–53. https://doi.org/10.1167/iovs.14-15388.
- Shi H, Gao J, Pei H, Liu R, Hu WK, Wan X, Li T, Li B. Adeno-associated virus-mediated gene delivery of the human ND4 complex I subunit in rabbit eyes. Clin Exp Ophthalmol. 2012 Dec;40(9):888–94. https://doi.org/10.1111/j.1442-9071.2012.02815.x. Epub 2012 Jul 2.
- Mays LE, Vandenberghe LH, Xiao R, Bell P, Nam HJ, Agbandje-McKenna M, Wilson JM. Adeno-associated virus capsid structure drives CD4-dependent CD8+ T cell response to vector encoded proteins. J Immunol. 2009 May 15;182(10):6051–60. https://doi.org/10.4049/jimmunol.0803965.
- Hsu TK, Wang AG, Yen MY, Liu JH. Leber's hereditary optic neuropathy masquerading as optic neuritis with spontaneous visual recovery. Clin Exp Optom. 2014 Jan;97(1):84–6. https://doi.org/10.1111/cxo.12100. Epub 2013 Aug 1.
- Leo-Kottler B, Christ-Adler M. [Leber optic neuropathy in women and children]. Ophthalmologe. 1999 Nov;96(11):698–701. https://doi.org/10.1007/s003470050479. German.
- Li H, Tuyishime S, Wu TL, Giles-Davis W, Zhou D, Xiao W, High KA, Ertl HC. Adeno-associated virus vectors serotype 2 induce prolonged proliferation of capsid-specific CD8+ T cells in mice. Mol Ther. 2011 Mar;19(3):536–46. https://doi.org/10.1038/mt.2010.267. Epub 2010 Dec 14.
- Giordano C, Montopoli M, Perli E, Orlandi M, Fantin M, Ross-Cisneros FN, Caparrotta L, Martinuzzi A, Ragazzi E, Ghelli A, Sadun AA, d'Amati G, Carelli V. Oestrogens ameliorate mitochondrial dysfunction in Leber's hereditary optic neuropathy. Brain. 2011 Jan;134(Pt 1):220–34. https://doi.org/10.1093/brain/awq276. Epub 2010 Oct 13.
- Testa F, Maguire AM, Rossi S, Pierce EA, Melillo P, Marshall K, Banfi S, Surace EM, Sun J, Acerra C, Wright JF, Wellman J, High KA, Auricchio A, Bennett J, Simonelli F. Three-year follow-up after unilateral subretinal delivery of adeno-associated virus in patients with Leber congenital Amaurosis type 2. Ophthalmology. 2013 Jun;120(6):1283–91. https://doi.org/10.1016/j.ophtha.2012.11.048. Epub 2013 Mar 6.
- Yang S, He H, Zhu Y, Wan X, Zhou LF, Wang J, Wang WF, Liu L, Li B. Chemical and material communication between the optic nerves in rats. Clin Exp Ophthalmol. 2015 Nov;43(8):742–8. https://doi.org/10.1111/ceo.12547. Epub 2015 Jun 25.
- Ghelli A, Porcelli AM, Zanna C, Martinuzzi A, Carelli V, Rugolo M. Protection against oxidant-induced apoptosis by exogenous glutathione in Leber hereditary optic neuropathy cybrids. Invest Ophthalmol Vis Sci. 2008 Feb;49(2):671–6. https://doi.org/10.1167/iovs.07-0880.

- Yu-Wai-Man P, Griffiths PG, Chinnery PF. Mitochondrial optic neuropathies—disease mechanisms and therapeutic strategies. Prog Retin Eye Res. 2011 Mar;30(2):81–114. https://doi.org/10.1016/j.preteyeres.2010.11.002. Epub 2010 Nov 26.
- Koilkonda RD, Guy J. Leber's Hereditary Optic Neuropathy-Gene Therapy: From Benchtop to Bedside. J Ophthalmol. 2011;2011:179412. https://doi.org/10.1155/2011/179412. Epub 2010 Dec 26.

Completed

France

Safety Evaluation of Gene Therapy in Leber Hereditary Optic Neuropathy (LHON) Patients

ClinicalTrials.gov ID NCT02064569

Sponsor GenSight Biologics
Information provided by GenSight Biologics (Responsible Party)
Last Update Posted 2020-07-01

Brief Summary
The purpose of this study is to evaluate the safety and tolerability profile of ascending doses of GS010 in Leber Hereditary Optic Neuropathy (LHON) patients.

Official Title
An Open-Label Dose Escalation Clinical Trial to Evaluate the Safety and the Tolerability of GS010 (rAAV2/2-ND4) in Patients with Leber Hereditary Optic Neuropathy Due to Mutations in the Mitochondrial NADH Dehydrogenase 4 Gene

Conditions
Leber Hereditary Optic Neuropathy

Study Type
Interventional

Enrollment (Actual)
19

Intervention/Treatment
Genetic: GS010

Phase
Phase 1 Phase 2

Other Study ID Numbers
GS-LHON/CLIN/01

Study Start (Actual)
2014-02-13

Primary Completion (Actual)
2020-06-25

Study completion (actual)
2020-06-25

France

Paris, France, 75,012
CIC du CHNO DES QUINZE-VINGTS

Eligibility Criteria
Ages Eligible for Study
18 years and older (Adult, Older Adult)

Accepts Healthy Volunteer
No

Sexes Eligible For Study
All

Inclusion Criteria
- Documented diagnosis of LHON based on a genetic test confirming the presence of the G11778A mutation in the mitochondrial ND4.
- Age 18 years old or older at the time of study entry (informed consent signature).
- Visual acuity ≤1/10 of the less functional eye.

Exclusion Criteria
- Any known allergy or hypersensibility to one of the products used during the trial.
- Contraindication to IVT surgery (anemia Hb <8 g/dl, severe cardiovascular disease, severe coagulopathy…).
- Disorder of the ocular humors and of the internal retina involving visual disability.
- Glaucoma.
- Presence of other pathology whose symptoms or associated treatments might affect the retina or the optic nerve vascular retinal occlusion.
- Narrow angle contraindicating pupillary dilation.
- Other cause of optic neuropathy (inflammatory conditions or exposure to toxins...).
- Patients presenting known mutation of other genes implicated in pathological retinal conditions.

Study Plan

Design Details
Primary Purpose: Treatment
Allocation: N/A
Interventional Model: Single Group Assignment
Masking: None (Open Label)

Arms and interventions

Participant group/arm	Intervention/treatment
Experimental: GS010	Genetic: GS010

Primary outcome measures

Outcome measure	Measure description	Time frame
Incidence of local and general adverse events and serious adverse events		Up to 48 weeks

Sponsor
GenSight Biologics

Collaborators
No information provided

Investigators
Principal Investigator: CATHERINE VIGNAL, MD, CIC CHNO DES QUINZE VINGTS

General Publications
No publications available

Not Yet Recruiting

No Location

Gene Therapy Clinical Trial for the Treatment of Leber's Hereditary Optic Neuropathy Associated with ND4 Mutations

ClinicalTrials.gov ID NCT05293626

Sponsor Neurophth Therapeutics Inc.
Information provided by Neurophth Therapeutics Inc. (Responsible Party)
Last Update Posted 2023-02-01

Brief Summary
The objective of this clinical study is to evaluate the safety and efficacy of NR082 in the treatment of LHON caused by mitochondrial ND4 gene mutation. This study will enroll subjects aged ≥18 years old and ≤75 years old to receive a single unilateral intravitreal (IVT) injection of NR082 to evaluate its safety and efficacy. The clinical manifestations of all subjects are to be reduced visual acuity caused by LHON associated with ND4 mutation, with laboratory test showing G11778A mutation (a CLIA-certified laboratory) and reduced visual acuity lasted for >6 months and <10 years.

Detailed Description

At the dose-finding stage, the principle is that the Safety Review Committee (SRC) will decide whether to make dose adjustment based on the safety data of the starting dose. The starting dose is 1.5 × 109 vg, 0.05 mL eye/dose. The safety of the starting dose will be reviewed by the SRC, and dose escalation or de-escalation is by recommendation of the SRC. The safety of the starting dose will first be performed in six evaluable subjects.

Criteria for Dose Modification

Dose Escalation

- If drug-related dose-limiting toxicity (DLT) events are observed in ≤2 of the six evaluable subjects within 6 weeks after the dosing of NR082 at the starting dose, the dose can be escalated to 4.5 × 109 vg, 0.05 mL eye/dose (high dose) after the approval by SRC.

Dose De-Escalation

If drug-related dose-limiting toxicity (DLT) events are observed in >2 of the six evaluable subjects within 6 weeks after the dosing of NR082 at the starting dose, the dose can be de-escalated to 0.5 × 109 vg, 0.05 mL eye/dose (low dose) after the approval by SRC.
If drug-related dose-limiting toxicity (DLT) events are observed in >2 of the six evaluable subjects within 6 weeks after the dosing of NR082 at the high dose, the dose can be de-escalated to 3.0 × 109 vg, 0.05 mL eye/dose (intermediate dose) after the approval by SRC.

Enrollment Sequence

- The enrollment sequence of any dose group (six subjects) is that the second subject and the third subject will be enrolled at least 7 days after the enrollment of the first subject.
- The fourth, fifth, and sixth subjects will be enrolled at least 7 days after the enrollment of the second and the third subjects.

The 7-day interval is to avoid acute safety events to the greatest possible extent.

Official Title

A Phase 1/2, Single-Arm, Open-Label, Dose-Finding Clinical Trial to Evaluate the Safety and Efficacy of Gene Therapy for Leber's Hereditary Optic Neuropathy (LHON) Associated with ND4 Mutation

Conditions

Leber Hereditary Optic Neuropathy (LHON)

Intervention/Treatment

Drug: NR082 Injection
Device: Injection needle

Study Start (Estimated)

2023-01

Primary Completion (Estimated)
2023-12

Study Completion (Estimated)
2027-08

Enrollment (Estimated)
18

Study Type
Interventional

Phase
Phase 1 Phase 2

Study Contact
Name: Bin Li
Phone Number: +8602765524119
Email: info@neurophth.com
No location data

Eligibility Criteria
Inclusion Criteria

- Age at the time of signing the informed consent form: the age of the subjects must be ≥18 years old and ≤ 75 years old.
- The clinical manifested vision loss due to LHON, and any cye BCVA ≥0.5 LogMAR.
- The genotype testing result shows the presence of G11778A mutation in the ND4 gene, and the absence of the other primary LHON-associated mutations in the mitochondrial DNA (mtDNA) (ND1 [G3460A] or ND6 [T14484C]) (confirmed by a CLIA-certified international laboratory.
- The vision loss in the eye with worse visual acuity lasted >6 months and < 10 years at screening.
- Pupils can be adequately dilated for a thorough ocular examination and visual acuity test.
- Each eye of the subject must maintain at least hand motion VA (≤ 2.3 LogMAR) as defined in the ocular/vision examination manual (operating manual for refraction and VA examinations) in this study.
- Willingness to comply with the clinical study protocol and 5 years of long-term follow-up after administration.
- Male or female.
  - A male subject must agree to take contraceptive measures at least 6 months after the treatment visit.
  - A female subject is eligible to participate if she is not pregnant, not breastfeeding, and at least one of the following conditions applies: Not a woman of childbearing potential (WOCBP); (ii) A WOCBP who agrees to follow the contraception guidance for at least 6 months after the treatment visit.

- Written informed consent form must be obtained from the subject or his/her parent/legal guardian before any study-related procedures are performed. If the subject is legally blind (> 1.0 LogMAR or the readings of decimal visual acuity chart <0.1), an impartial witness must be present throughout the informed consent process and discussion process.

Exclusion Criteria

- Any known allergy and/or hypersensitivity to the study drug or its constituents.
- Contraindication to IVT injection in any eye.
- IVT drug delivery to any eye within 30 days prior to the screening visit.
- History of vitrectomy in either eye.
- Narrow anterior chamber angle in any eye contraindicating pupillary dilation.
- Presence of disorders or diseases of the eye or adnexa, excluding LHON, which may interfere with visual or ocular assessments, including spectral-domain optical coherence tomography (SD-OCT), during the study.
- Presence of known/documented mutations, other than the LHON-related mutation, which are known to cause pathology of the optic nerve, retina or afferent visual system.
- Presence of systemic or ocular/vision diseases, disorders, or pathologies, other than LHON, known to cause or be associated with vision loss, or whose associated treatment(s) or therapy(ies) is/are known to cause or be associated with vision loss.
- Presence of optic neuropathy from any cause other than LHON.
- Presence of illness or disease that, in the opinion of the investigator, includes symptoms and/or the associated treatments that can alter visual function, for instance cancers or pathology of the central nervous system (CNS), including multiple sclerosis (diagnosis of multiple sclerosis must be based on the 2010 Revisions to the McDonald Criteria), and/or diseases or conditions that affect the safety of subjects participating in the study.
- History of recurrent uveitis (idiopathic or immune-related) or active ocular inflammation.
- Participated in another clinical study and receive an IMP within 90 days prior to the screening visit.

  (a) Exceptions: Subjects who have completed the clinical study of idebenone as IMP >90 days prior to the screening visit and have completely discontinued idebenone at least 7 days prior to dosing are still eligible to participate in the study.

- Any eye has previously received ocular gene therapy.
- Subjects who refused to stop using idebenone.
- Have undergone ocular surgery of clinical relevance (per investigator's assessment) within 90 days prior to the screening visit.
- Female subjects who are breastfeeding or plan to breastfeed within the first 6 months after the administration of NR082 injection.

- History of drug or alcohol abuse (including heavy smoking, i.e., > 20 cigarettes per day or > 20 pack-years [equivalent to one pack a day for 20 years or 2 packs a day for 10 years]).
- Human immunodeficiency virus (HIV) antibody, syphilis antibody, and HCV antibody positive are excluded; hepatitis B test that shows a clinically significant active infection requiring treatment (defined as the presence of hepatitis B core antibody [HBcAb] positive or hepatitis B surface antigen [HBsAg] positive, and hepatitis B virus deoxyribonucleic acid [HBV-DNA] > 1000 copies/mL or according to local laboratory method above lower limit of quantitative detection) is excluded.
- Unable to tolerate (e.g., immunomodulatory regimen) or unable or unwilling to comply with all the protocol requirements.
- Subjects from the study site fail to comply with or do not agree to comply with local and institutional guidelines for suspected 2019 novel coronavirus (COVID-19) infection/testing.
- Any other exclusions determined by the investigator

Ages Eligible for Study
18 Years to 75 Years (Adult, Older Adult)

Sexes Eligible for Study
All

Accepts Healthy Volunteers
No

Design Details
Primary Purpose: Treatment
Allocation: N/A
Interventional Model: Sequential Assignment
Interventional Model Description: 0.5E9 vg, 0.05 mL/eye/dose (low dose) 1.5E9 vg, 0.05 mL/eye/dose (starting dose) 3.0E9 vg, 0.05 mL/eye/dose (intermediate dose) 4.5E9 vg, 0.05 mL/eye/dose (high dose)
Masking: None (Open Label)

Arms and interventions

Participant group/arm	Intervention/treatment
Experimental: NR082 injection Potential doses at the dose-finding stage: • 0.5E9 vg, 0.05 mL/eye/dose (low dose) • 1.5E9 vg, 0.05 mL/eye/dose (starting dose) • 3.0E9 vg, 0.05 mL/eye/dose (intermediate dose) • 4.5E9 vg, 0.05 mL/eye/dose (high dose)	Drug: NR082 injection • The starting dose is 1.5E9 vg, 0.05 mL eye/dose. Dose escalation: If drug-related dose-limiting toxicity (DLT) events are observed in ≤2 of the six evaluable subjects using the starting dose within 6 weeks after the dosing of NR082, the dose can be escalated to 4.5E9 vg, 0.05 mL eye/dose (high dose) after approval by SRC. Dose de-escalation: If drug-related dose-limiting toxicity (DLT) events are observed in >2 of the six evaluable subjects using the starting dose within 6 weeks after the dosing of NR082, the dose can be de-escalated to 0.5E9 vg, 0.05 mL eye/dose (low dose) after approval by SRC. If drug-related dose-limiting toxicity (DLT) events are observed in >2 of the six evaluable subjects within 6 weeks after the dosing of NR082 at the high dose, the dose can be de-escalated to 3.0E9 vg, 0.05 mL eye/dose (intermediate dose) after the approval by SRC. Device: Injection needle • 19G 1 1/2IN TW filter needle with filter element (BD 305200), used to NR082 intraocular injection solution dose preparation; 30G 1/2IN injection needle (BD 305106), used to NR082 intraocular injection solution administration 1 mL screw top syringe (BD 309628), used to NR082 intraocular injection solution dose preparation and administration. • Other names: – Syringe

Primary outcome measures

Outcome measure	Measure description	Time frame
Incidence of adverse events (AEs)	Incidence of adverse events (AEs) within 52 weeks of NR082 intravitreal injection at different doses	52 weeks
Incidence of serious adverse events (SAEs)	Incidence of serious adverse events (SAEs) within 52 weeks of NR082 intravitreal injection at different doses	52 weeks
Incidence of dose-limiting toxicities (DLT)	Incidence of dose-limiting toxicities (DLT) (ocular and nonocular) within 52 weeks of NR082 intravitreal injection at different doses	52 weeks

Secondary outcome measures

Outcome measure	Measure description	Time frame
Proportion (percent) of subjects with an improvement of ≥0.3 logMAR from baseline in best-corrected visual acuity (BCVA) in the study eye	ETDRS visual acuity charts will used to assess proportion (percent) of subjects with an improvement of ≥0.3 logMAR from baseline in best-corrected visual acuity (BCVA)	At weeks 2, 6,12, 26, 40, 52, 78, 104, 156, 208, and 260
Mean change from baseline in BCVA (logMAR) in the study eye	ETDRS visual acuity charts will used to assess mean change from baseline in BCVA (logMAR)	At weeks 2, 6,12, 26, 40, 52, 78, 104, 156, 208, and 260
Mean change in BCVA (logMAR) compared to nadir	ETDRS visual acuity charts will be used to assess mean change in BCVA (logMAR) compared to nadir	At weeks 2, 6,12, 26, 40, 52, 78, 104, 156, 208, and 260
Change from baseline in the pattern standard deviation (PSD) in the study eye	Visual field parameters will evaluate alterations in function of different regions of the retina. The HVF analyzer is used to perform standard automated perimetry, and the kinetic visual field is measured by the Humphrey static visual field automatically detected by the computer, including the foveal and macular thresholds, as well as the central field. Change from baseline in the pattern standard deviation (PSD) in the study eye	At weeks 2, 6,12, 26, 40, 52, 78, 104, 156, 208, and 260
Change from baseline in the visual field index (VFI) in the study eye	Visual field parameters will evaluate alterations in function of different regions of the retina. The HVF analyzer is used to perform standard automated perimetry, and the kinetic visual field is measured by the Humphrey static visual field automatically detected by the computer, including the foveal and macular thresholds, as well as the central field. Change from baseline in the visual field index (VFI) in the study eye	At weeks 2, 6,12, 26, 40, 52, 78, 104, 156, 208, and 260
Change from baseline in the mean deviation (MD) in the study eye	Visual field parameters will evaluate alterations in function of different regions of the retina. The HVF analyzer is used to perform standard automated perimetry, and the kinetic visual field is measured by the Humphrey static visual field automatically detected by the computer, including the foveal and macular thresholds, as well as the central field. Change from baseline in the mean deviation (MD) in the study eye	At weeks 2, 6,12, 26, 40, 52, 78, 104, 156, 208, and 260
Change from baseline in spatial frequency parameters of contrast sensitivity in the study eye	The contrast sensitivity examination measures the subject's ability to discern targets presented at varying spatial frequencies or sizes under different contrast levels. The contrast sensitivity examination measures the full range of visual sensitivity, including brightness and contrast, and it may be used as a comprehensive assessment of visual function	At weeks 2, 6,12, 26, 40, 52, 78, 104, 156, 208, and 260

Change from baseline in visual evoked potential (VEP) parameters in the study eye	VEP is a visual electrophysiological examination used to identify possible ischemic optic neuropathy, including the P100 latency, P100 amplitude, P2 latency, P2 amplitude	At weeks 2, 6,12, 26, 40, 52, 78, 104, 156, 208, and 260
To evaluate immunogenicity	A central laboratory will be used to evaluate anti-AAV2 neutralizing antibodies in the serum samples of all subjects. These samples will be tested by the sponsor or its designee to detect anti-AAV2 neutralizing antibodies in the samples and report the titer of confirmed positive samples. Samples confirmed positive for anti-AAV2 neutralizing antibodies will also be evaluated for the presence of neutralizing antibodies	At weeks 1, 2, and 6
To evaluate immunogenicity	The interferon gamma enzyme-linked immunospot (ELISpot) assay will be performed to measure the proliferative response of lymphocytes to AAV2 antigen and ND4 peptide. The number of activated cells in the sample were calculated	At weeks 1, 2, 6, 12, 26, 40, and 52
To evaluate vector shedding	Assessment of vector DNA shedding in tears (both eyes). Samples were analyzed to determine the presence of viral DNA in tears	At weeks 1, 2, 6, 12, 26, 40, and 52
To evaluate biodistribution	Assessment of biodistribution in whole blood. Samples were analyzed to determine the presence of viral DNA in whole blood	At weeks 1, 2, 6, 12, 26, 40, and 52
To evaluate the improvement in BCVA of the study eye (< 0.3 logMAR)	ETDRS visual acuity charts will used to assess proportion (percent) of subjects with an improvement of ≥0.2 logMAR and ≥ 0.1 logMAR from baseline in BCVA Proportion (percent) of subjects with visual acuity of >1.0 logMAR before and after treatment	At weeks 52, 78, 104, 156, 208, and 260
To evaluate the change from baseline in VFQ-25	VFQ-25 is a 25-item short form version of the 51-item National Eye Institute Visual Function Questionnaire (NEI VFQ), which can effectively measure patient-reported outcomes (including quality of life, QoL). It consists of 25 items from 12 dimensions. The total score and the score of each dimension are the mean values of nonmissing items of corresponding dimensions or items, with the score range from 0 to 100, higher scores mean a worse outcome	At weeks 2, 26, 52, 104, 156, 208, and 260

To evaluate the change from baseline in quality of SF-36	The SF-36 questionnaire is a universal tool for evaluating patient-reported QoL outcome. SF-36 comprises 36 questions which cover eight domains of health: (1) limitations in physical activities because of health problems; (2) limitations in social activities because of physical or emotional problems; (3) limitations in usual role activities because of physical health problems; (4) bodily pain; (5) general mental health (psychological distress and well-being); (6) limitations in usual role activities because of emotional problems; (7) vitality (energy and fatigue); and (8) general health perceptions. The scale score of each domain will be calculated based on the total score of the items included in the said domain and readjusted to 0–100, higher scores mean a worse outcome	At weeks 2, 26, 52, 104, 156, 208, and 260
Change from baseline in retinal nerve fiber layer (RNFL) thickness of the study eye	OCT is an imaging technology to investigate the ocular fundus by using the basic principle of low-coherence light interferometry. It detects the reflection or diffusion signals of biological tissue layers of different depths by inputting low-coherence light and obtains the images and quantitative results of the microscopic structure of the retina	At weeks 2, 6,12, 26, 52, 104, 156, 208, and 260
Change from baseline in retinal ganglion cell complex thickness of the study eye	OCT is an imaging technology to investigate the ocular fundus by using of the basic principle of low-coherence light interferometry. It detects the reflection or diffusion signals of biological tissue layers of different depths by inputting low-coherence light and obtains the images and quantitative results of the microscopic structure of the retina	At weeks 2, 6,12, 26, 52, 104, 156, 208, and 260
To evaluate the visual function improvement after NR082 treatment	Early treatment diabetic retinopathy study (ETDRS) visual acuity charts will be used to assess proportion (percent) of subjects with an improvement of ≥0.3 logMAR from baseline in best-corrected visual acuity (BCVA) of the nonstudy eye	At weeks 2, 6,12, 26, 52, 104, 156, 208, and 260

Sponsor
Neurophth Therapeutics Inc.

Collaborators
No information provided

Investigators
No information provided

General Publications
No publications available

Active, Not Recruiting

United States/Europe

Safety Study of an Adeno-Associated Virus Vector for Gene Therapy of Leber's Hereditary Optic Neuropathy (LHON)

ClinicalTrials.gov ID NCT02161380

Sponsor Byron Lam
Information provided by Byron Lam, University of Miami (Responsible Party)
Last Update Posted 2023-04-25

Brief Summary

Hypotheses
The primary hypothesis being tested is that there will be no toxicity resulting in loss of vision to no light perception in injected eyes.

Official Title
An Open-Label Dose Escalation Study of an Adeno-Associated Virus Vector (scAAV2-P1ND4v2) for Gene Therapy of Leber Hereditary Optic Neuropathy (LHON) Caused by the G11778A Mutation in Mitochondrial DNA

Conditions
Leber Hereditary Optic Neuropathy

Intervention/Treatment
Drug: injection of scAAV2-P1ND4v2 $1.18 \times 10e^{9}$ vg (Low)
Drug: injection of scAAV2-P1ND4v2 $5.81 \times 10e^{9}$ vg (Med)
Drug: injection of scAAV2-P1ND4v2 $2.4 \times 10e^{10}$ vg (High)
Drug: injection of scAAV2-P1ND4v2 $1.0 \times 10e^{11}$ vg (Higher)

Study Start (Actual)
2014-07-14

Primary Completion (Actual)
2023-03-31

Study Completion (Estimated)
2024-03-31

Enrollment (Actual)
28

Study Type
Interventional

Phase
Phase 1

United States
Florida Locations

Miami, Florida, United States, 33136
Bascom Palmer Eye Institute, University of Miami

Eligibility Criteria
Inclusion Criteria

- Age 15 or older.
- Patients with LHON and the G11778A mitochondrial DNA mutation. A previous CLIA-certified genetic lab result showing the LHON G11778A mutation will be accepted for inclusion.
- Ability to perform tests of visual and retinal function.
- Ability to comply with research procedures.
- Able and willing to provide informed consent before undergoing any study related procedures.
- Good general health as based on the investigator's assessment of the history, physical examination, and laboratory testing performed at the baseline examination.

Exclusion Criteria

- Unwilling or unable to give consent.
- Unable or unlikely to return for scheduled protocol visits.
- Pregnant or nursing women or unwillingness for subject with childbearing potential to use contraception during the first year of the study.
- Optic disc drusen on exam or in previous history.
- Ocular diseases or visual dysfunction conditions other than refractive error (e.g., amblyopia, glaucoma, etc.) in the eye selected for the injection.
- Previous eye surgery in the eye selected for injection.
- Aspartate transaminase (AST)/alanine transaminase (ALT) >5.0 × upper limit of normal (ULN); total bilirubin >3 x ULN; hemoglobin <8 g/dL; neutrophil count <1.0 × 109/L; or platelet count <50 × 109/L.

  (a) Any laboratory screening test that meets the abnormality criteria stated above can be repeated once between Baseline 1 to Baseline 2.

- Type I diabetes or the presence of diabetic retinopathy.
- History of neurodegenerative conditions (e.g., multiple sclerosis, neuromyelitis optica, Parkinson disease).
- History of autoimmune conditions (e.g., systemic lupus erythematosus).
- History of systemic diseases having ocular manifestations likely to confound assessment of study results.
- History of cancer within 5 years other than localized basal or squamous cell carcinoma not near the orbital area. Patients with a prior history of cancer will need documentation from their cancer specialist that the cancer was cured at least 5 years before study entry.
- Allergy to pupil dilating drops or narrow angles precluding safe dilation.
- No Light Perception (NLP) vision in either eye.

Ages Eligible for Study
15 Years and older (Child, Adult, Older Adult)

Sexes Eligible for Study
All

Accepts Healthy Volunteers
No

Design Details
Primary Purpose: Treatment
Allocation: Nonrandomized
Interventional Model: Single Group Assignment
Masking: None (Open Label)

Arms and interventions

Participant group/arm	Intervention/treatment
Experimental: 1 Chronic bilateral severe vision loss injection of scAAV2-P1ND4v2	Drug: injection of scAAV2-P1ND4v2 1.18x10e9 vg (low) • Injection of total volume of each intravitreal injection is 200 μL Drug: injection of scAAV2-P1ND4v2 5.81 X10e9 vg (med) • Injection of total volume of each intravitreal injection is 200 μL Drug: injection of scAAV2-P1ND4v2 2.4 X10e10vg (high) • Injection of total volume of each intravitreal injection is 100 μL Drug: injection of scAAV2-P1ND4v2 1.0 X10e11vg (higher) • Injection of total volume of each intravitreal injection is 100 μL
Experimental: 2 Acute bilateral severe vision loss injection of scAAV2-P1ND4v2	Drug: injection of scAAV2-P1ND4v2 1.18x10e9 vg (low) • Injection of total volume of each intravitreal injection is 200 μL Drug: injection of scAAV2-P1ND4v2 5.81 X10e9 vg (med) • Injection of total volume of each intravitreal injection is 200 μL Drug: injection of scAAV2-P1ND4v2 1.0 X10e11vg (higher) • Injection of total volume of each intravitreal injection is 100 μL
Experimental: 3 Acute unilateral severe vision loss injection of scAAV2-P1ND4v2	Drug: injection of scAAV2-P1ND4v2 1.18x10e9 vg (low) • Injection of total volume of each intravitreal injection is 200 μL Drug: injection of scAAV2-P1ND4v2 5.81 X10e9 vg (med) • Injection of total volume of each intravitreal injection is 200 μL Drug: injection of scAAV2-P1ND4v2 1.0 X10e11vg (higher) • Injection of total volume of each intravitreal injection is 100 μL

Primary outcome measures

Outcome measure	Measure description	Time frame
Assessment of primary endpoint—toxicity	Incidence of local and general adverse events and serious adverse events	3 year

Secondary outcome measures

Outcome measure	Measure description	Time frame
Assessment of secondary endpoint—safety & efficacy	Visual acuity change from baseline 2	3 year

Sponsor
Byron Lam

Collaborators
- National Eye Institute (NEI)

Investigators
- Principal Investigator: Byron Lam, MD, Bascom Palmer Eye Institute, Miller School of Medicine, University of Miami, Miami, FL 33136

General Publications
No publications available

Active, Not Recruiting

Efficacy & Safety Study of Bilateral IVT Injection of GS010 in LHON Subjects Due to the ND4 Mutation for up to 1 Year (REFLECT)

ClinicalTrials.gov ID NCT03293524

Sponsor GenSight Biologics
Information provided by GenSight Biologics (Responsible Party)
Last Update Posted 2022-08-03

Brief Summary
The goal of this clinical trial is to assess the safety and efficacy of GS010, a gene therapy, in improving the retina functional & structural outcomes in subjects with LHON due to the G11778A ND4 mitochondrial mutation when vision loss duration is present up to 1 year.

Detailed Description
GS-LHON-CLIN-05 is a Phase III, global, multicenter randomized, double-masked for the primary analysis, placebo-controlled, clinical study. As LHON is a neurodegenerative disease, the goal is to administer GS010 as soon as possible upon confirmation of the LHON diagnosis and the causative mutation.

Official Title

Efficacy and Safety of Bilateral Intravitreal Injection of GS010: A Randomized, Double-Masked, Placebo-Controlled Trial in Subjects Affected with G11778A ND4 Leber Hereditary Optic Neuropathy for up to 1 Year

Conditions

Leber Hereditary Optic Neuropathy

Intervention/Treatment

Genetic: GS010
Drug: Placebo

Study Start (Actual)

2018-03-12

Primary Completion (Estimated)

2024-06-30

Study Completion (Estimated)

2024-06-30

Enrollment (Estimated)

90

Study Type

Interventional

Phase

Phase 3

United States
California Locations

Pasadena, California, United States, 91105
Doheny Eye Center UCLA Pasadena

Colorado Locations

Aurora, Colorado, United States, 80045
University of Colorado Health Eye Center

Georgia Locations

Atlanta, Georgia, United States, 30322
Emory Healthcare—The Emory Clinic

Massachusetts Locations

Boston, Massachusetts, United States, 02114
Massachusetts Eye and Ear Infirmary

New York Locations

New York, New York, United States, 10029

Icahn School of Medicine at Mount Sinai

Pennsylvania Locations

Philadelphia, Pennsylvania, United States, 19107
Wills Eye Institute—Ocular Oncology Service

Tennessee Locations

Nashville, Tennessee, United States, 37232
Vanderbilt Eye Institute

Belgium

Gent, Belgium, 9000
Universitair Ziekenhuis Gent

France

Paris, France, 75,012
CHNO Les Quinze Vingts

Italy

Bologna, Italy, 40139
IRCCS Istituto delle Scienze Neurologiche di Bologna UOC Clinica Neurologica

Spain

Madrid, Spain, 28034
Hospital Universitario Ramon y Cajal

Taiwan

Taipei, Taiwan, 11217
Taipei Veterans General Hospital

United Kingdom
Greater London Locations

London, Greater London, United Kingdom, EC1V 2PD
Moorfields Eye Hospital

Eligibility Criteria
Main Selection Criteria

- Age 15 years or older on the date of signed informed consent.
- Clinically manifested vision loss due to ND4 LHON, to any extent, in at least one eye.
- Vision loss duration of ≤365 days (i.e., ≤ 1 year) in each affected eye at Inclusion Visit (Visit 2).

Main Nonselection Criteria

- Contraindication to intravitreal injection in any eye.
- Subjects refusing to discontinue idebenone.
- Previous vitrectomy in either eye.
- Narrow angle in any eye contraindicating pupillary dilation.
- Presence of known/documented mutations, other than the G11778A ND4 LHON-causing mutation, which are known to cause pathology of the optic nerve, retina or afferent visual system.
- History of recurrent uveitis (idiopathic or immune-related) or active ocular inflammation.

Main Inclusion Criteria

- Vision loss duration of ≤365 days (i.e., ≤1 year) in each affected eye at Inclusion Visit (Visit 2).
- Each eye of the subject must maintain at least Hand Motion (HM) visual acuity, as defined by the study's SOP for visual acuity testing.
- Documented results of genotyping showing the presence of the G11778A mutation in the ND4 gene and the absence of the other primary LHON-associated mutations (ND1 or ND6) in the subject's mitochondrial DNA.

Main Exclusion Criteria

- Light Perception (LP) or No Light Perception (NLP) visual acuity in any eye, as defined by the study's standard operating procedure (SOP) for visual acuity testing.
- Presence of active infectious conjunctivitis, keratitis, scleritis or endophthalmitis in either eye.
- Presence of alcoholism, alcohol dependence, or alcohol or drug abuse (excluding nicotine).

Ages Eligible for Study
15 Years and older (Child, Adult, Older Adult)

Sexes Eligible for Study
All

Accepts Healthy Volunteers
No

Design Details
Primary Purpose: Treatment
Allocation: Randomized
Interventional Model: Parallel Assignment
Masking: Double (Participant Investigator)

Arms and interventions

Participant group/arm	Intervention/treatment
Experimental: treatment arm 1 Subjects will be randomized to treatment arm 1 or treatment arm 2 in a 1:1 allocation. Subjects in treatment arm 1 will receive intravitreal GS010 in both eyes.	Genetic: GS010 • GS010 is a recombinant adeno-associated viral vector serotype 2 (rAAV2/2) containing the wild-type ND4 gene (rAAV2/2-ND4). GS010 will be administrated via intravitreal injection containing 9E10 viral genomes in 90 μL balanced salt solution (BSS) as a single baseline intravitreal injection • Other names: – Lenadogene nolparvovec
Placebo comparator: treatment arm 2 Subjects will be randomized to treatment arm 1 or treatment arm 2 in a 1:1 allocation. Subjects in treatment arm 2 will receive GS010 in one eye and placebo intravitreal injection in the other eye	Genetic: GS010 • GS010 is a recombinant adeno-associated viral vector serotype 2 (rAAV2/2) containing the wild-type ND4 gene (rAAV2/2-ND4). GS010 will be administrated via intravitreal injection containing 9E10 viral genomes in 90 μL balanced salt solution (BSS) as a single baseline intravitreal injection • Other names: – Lenadogene nolparvovec Drug: placebo • The placebo is a BSS, sterile, apyrogenic solution and used for ocular surgery. The placebo will be administered via intravitreal injection in a volume of 90 μL

Primary outcome measures

Outcome measure	Measure description	Time frame
Best-corrected visual acuity (BCVA) reported using Log of the minimal angle of resolution (logMAR)—1 year	The primary efficacy endpoint will be the change from baseline (visit 2) BCVA reported with logMAR at 1.5 years posttreatment in second affected/not yet affected eyes of ND4 LHON subjects with vision loss up to 1 year. The change from baseline (visit 2) in second affected/not yet affected eyes receiving GS010 and placebo will be the primary response of interest. LogMAR BCVA will be used to represent BCVA	At 1.5 year postbaseline treatment

Secondary outcome measures

Outcome measure	Measure description	Time frame
Best-corrected visual acuity (BCVA) reported with logMAR—2 years	Change from baseline in logMAR BCVA at each timepoint of the follow-up period and at 2 years posttreatment.	At 1.5- and 2-years postbaseline treatment

Responder Analysis	Response status at each timepoint of the follow-up period and at 2 years posttreatment. Definitions of responder eyes include: 1. Eyes whose logMAR BCVA improves (i.e., decreases) by ≥0.3 logMAR (equivalent to a gain of ≥15 ETDRS letters) compared to baseline 2. Eyes whose logMAR BCVA does not increase (i.e., worsen) by ≥0.3 logMAR (equivalent to eyes that lose ≤15 ETDRS letters) compared to baseline 3. Eyes whose logMAR visual acuity is <1.0 (i.e., better than logMAR 1.0, equivalent to better than Snellen acuity of 20/200)	At 1.5- and 2-years postbaseline treatment
Spectral domain-optical coherence tomography (SD-OCT) parameter	Parameters measured with SD-OCT over time and at 1.5 and 2-years postbaseline treatment. The change from baseline will be the response. Analysis will be performed mainly for second affected/not yet affected eyes treated with GS010 versus placebo and also for first affected eyes receiving GS010 as well	At 1.5- and 2-years postbaseline treatment
Humphrey visual field (HVF) parameter	Parameters measured with HVF 30–2 over time and at 1.5 and 2-years postbaseline treatment. The change from baseline will be the response. Analysis will be performed mainly for second affected/not yet affected eyes treated with GS010 versus placebo and also for first affected eyes receiving GS010 as well	At 1.5- and 2-years postbaseline treatment
Pelli Robson low vision contrast sensitivity parameter	Parameters measured with Pelli Robson low vision contrast sensitivity over time and at 1.5- and 2-years postbaseline treatment. The change from baseline will be the response. Analysis will be performed mainly for second affected/not yet affected eyes treated with GS010 versus placebo and also for first affected eyes receiving GS010 as well	At 1.5- and 2-years postbaseline treatment
Quality of life: visual functioning questionnaire-25	Visual functioning questionnaire-25 at 1.5- and 2-years posttreatment	At 1.5- and 2-years postbaseline treatment
Quality of life: 36-item short form health survey, version 2 questionnaire	36-item short form health survey, version 2 questionnaire at 1- and 2-years posttreatment	At 1.5- and 2-years postbaseline treatment

Other outcome measures

Outcome measure	Measure description	Time frame
Adverse events (AEs) and serious adverse events (SAEs)	Adverse events (AEs) and serious adverse events (SAEs), including those that are treatment-emergent and nontreatment-emergent, throughout the study period and at each study visit. Incidence and severity of systemic and local (ocular) AEs and SAEs will be determined at each clinical site and for the entire study cohort	Up to 2-years postbaseline treatment
Physical examinations	Results of physical examinations	At 2-years postbaseline treatment
Electrocardiograms	Results of electrocardiograms (ECGs)	At 2-years postbaseline treatment
Laboratory results	Results of laboratory tests from blood collection	At 2-years postbaseline treatment
Immune response evaluations	Results of immune response evaluations 1. Time course of the humoral immune response measured with neutralizing antibodies (Nab) against adeno-associated virus vector 2 (AAV2) 2. Time course of the cellular immune response against AAV2	Up to 2-years postbaseline treatment
Blood bio-dissemination of AAV2 vector DNA	Results of bio-dissemination testing up to 4-weeks posttreatment	Up to 4 weeks posttreatment

Sponsor
GenSight Biologics

Collaborators
No information provided

Investigators

- Principal Investigator: Nancy Newman, MD, Emory University Hospital Atlanta, Georgia, United States, 30,322

General Publications
No publications available

Active, Not Recruiting

China

A Single Intravitreal Injection of rAAV2-ND4 for the Treatment of Leber's Hereditary Optic Neuropathy

ClinicalTrials.gov ID NCT03153293

Sponsor Huazhong University of Science and Technology
Information provided by Bin Li, Huazhong University of Science and Technology (Responsible Party)
Last Update Posted 2020-09-17

Brief Summary
This study is meant to evaluate the safety and efficacy of rAAV2-ND4 treatment for Leber hereditary optic neuropathy with the G11778A mutation in mitochondrial DNA.

Detailed Description
Leber Hereditary Optic Neuropathy (LHON) is a maternally inherited ocular disorder primarily associated with mutations in mitochondrial DNA. The disease is a common cause of blindness in both eyes of affected teenagers and young adults. There is currently no approved effective treatment for LHON.

In 2011, the first LHON gene therapy investigator-initiated study was conducted (registered in December 2010 with ClinicalTrials.gov Identifier NCT01267422) to explore the safety and efficacy of gene therapy for LHON. The gene therapy was a recombinant adeno-associated virus serotype 2 containing human mitochondrial ND4 (MT-ND4) gene (rAAV2-ND4). By 36 months of follow-up, six out of nine patients who received the rAAV2-ND4 intravitreal injection experienced clinically significant vision improvement and no adverse events were observed.

This is an open-label, single-arm, multicenter study to further evaluate the safety and efficacy of rAAV-ND4 in the treatment of LHON patients with G11778A mutation. All patients will be treated with a single intravitreal injection rAAV-ND4, with dose 1 × 10^10 vg/0.05 mL in one of the eyes.

Official Title
A Single Intravitreal Injection of rAAV2-ND4 for the Treatment of Leber Hereditary Optic Neuropathy

Conditions
Leber Hereditary Optic Neuropathy

Intervention/Treatment
Drug: rAAV2-ND4

Study Start (Actual)
2017-12-27

Primary Completion (Actual)
2020-01-15

Study Completion (Estimated)
2025-01-15

Enrollment (Actual)
159

Study Type
Interventional

Phase
Phase 2 Phase 3

China
Hubei Locations

Wuhan, Hubei, China, 430,030
Department of Ophthalmology, Tongji Hospital, Tongji Medical College, Huazhong University of Science and Technology

Eligibility Criteria
Inclusion Criteria

- Patients carry the mitochondrial point mutation at 11778, which is consistent with the diagnostic criteria for LHON.
- No apparent eye sight improvement in LHON patients or any other treatment within the past year.
- Eyesight of both eyes is below 0.3.
- Patients signed written informed consent.
- Patients are between the ages of 10 and 65 years old and able to tolerate the gene therapy procedure which includes local anesthesia.
- Patients are willing to follow the doctor's instructions and to consult the doctor at prescribed times.
- Patient's physical examination results are all normal, including liver function, kidney function, routine blood test, routine urine test, complete immunological test, and humoral immune response.

Exclusion Criteria

- Patients who are wearing a cardiac pacemaker, suffering from severe heart, lung or kidney function failure, various hemorrhagic diseases, acute infectious diseases, high fever, or convalescing after heart surgery or who are pregnant are excluded.
- Patients who are participating in other clinical studies are excluded.
- Patients who suffer from a diagnosed mental problem are excluded.
- Patients who suffer from chronic diseases such as diabetes and hypertension are excluded.

- Patients who show abnormal test results such as positive AAV2 humoral immune response (positive means that the AAV2 neutralizing antibody assay of patient was significant different when comparing free serum with 1:20 serum concentrations) and abnormal human T lymphocyte subsets CD3+, CD3+/CD4+, and CD3+/CD8+ prior to gene therapy surgery are excluded.

Ages Eligible for Study
10 to 65 years (Child, Adult, Older Adult)

Sexes Eligible for Study
All

Accepts Healthy Volunteers
No

Design Details
Primary Purpose: Treatment.
Allocation: N/A
Interventional Model: Single Group Assignment
Masking: None (Open Label)

Arms and interventions

Participant group/arm	Intervention/treatment
Experimental: rAAV2-ND4 A single IVT injection of recombinant adeno-associated virus-NADH dehydrogenase, subunit 4 (complex I) (rAAV2-ND4) (0.05 mL). The dose is 1×10^{10} vg/0.05 mL for test groups.	Drug: rAAV2-ND4 • A single IVT injection

Primary outcome measures

Outcome measure	Measure description	Time frame
BCVA	The best-corrected visual acuity	Change from baseline at 12 months
Computerized visual field		Change from baseline at 12 months

Secondary outcome measures

Outcome measure	Measure description	Time frame
VEP	Visual evoked potential	Change from baseline at 12 months
RNFL	Retinal nerve fiber layer	Change from baseline at 12 months
Liver function in plasma		Change from baseline at 12 months
Kidney function in plasma		Change from baseline at 12 months

Sponsor
Huazhong University of Science and Technology

Collaborators
- Taihe Hospital

Investigators
- Study Chair: Bin Li, PhD, MD, Deputy Director of Ophthalmology, Tongji Hospital
- Principal Investigator: Yong Zhang, PhD, MD, Director of Ophthalmology, Shiyan Taihe Hospital

General Publications
No publications available

Unknown Status

China

Efficacy Study of Gene Therapy for the Treatment of Acute LHON Onset Within Three Months (LHON)

ClinicalTrials.gov ID NCT03428178

Sponsor Bin Li
Information provided by Bin Li, Huazhong University of Science and Technology (Responsible Party)
Last Update Posted 2020-07-29

Brief Summary
Efficacy Study of Gene Therapy for The Treatment of Acute Leber's Hereditary Optic Neuropathy (LHON) onset within three months.

Detailed Description
Leber Hereditary Optic Neuropathy (LHON) is a maternally inherited ocular disorder associated with a mutation in mtDNA. The disease is a common cause of teenaged blindness in both eyes for which there is currently no effective treatment.

In 2008, the investigators recognized that gene therapy for LHON could be performed not only theoretically but technically. The investigators have been carrying out a series of basic and clinical studies from constructing the vectors to identifying and mitigating safety issues. After performing several animal experiments, the investigators had moved into clinical trials. In 2011, the investigators performed the first LHON gene therapy trial in the world, which was registered in December 2010 at ClinicalTrials.gov (Registration number: CT01267422) and was a preliminary study to verify the safety and efficacy of gene therapy for LHON. In the 36-month follow-up, the investigators found that six out of nine patients have vision improvement obviously and no adverse events were observed.

This is a multicenter, prospective study of 120 patients with the G11778A mutation in Mt-DNA. This clinical trial recruited 20 patients with the 11,778 mutation of MT-DNA onset within 3 months, 20 between 3 and 6 months, 20 between 6 and 12 months, 20 between 12 and 24 months, 20 between 24 and 60 months, and 20 over 60 months. All patients will be treated with a single vitreous cavity injection of recombinant adeno-associated virus-NADH dehydrogenase, subunit 4 (complex I) (rAAV2-ND4) (0.05 mL), with dose 1 × 10^10 vg/0.05 mL. The eye of treatment is up to the time of onset.

The visual acuity, visual field, visual evoked potential (VEP), optical coherence tomography (OCT), electroretinograms (ERG), retinal nerve fiber layer (RNFL), and liver and kidney functions in plasma were compared after treatment at 1, 2, 3, 6, and 12 months interval.

Official Title
Efficacy Study of Gene Therapy for the Treatment of Acute LHON Onset Within 3 Months

Conditions
Acute LHON
Onset Within 3 Months
Onset Between 3 –6and Months
Onset Between 6 and 12 Months
Onset Between 12 and 24 Months
Onset Between 24 and 60 Months
Onset Over 60 Months

Intervention/Treatment
Drug: rAAV2-ND4

Study Start (Actual)
2018-01-08

Primary Completion (Actual)
2018-12-06

Study Completion (Estimated)
2020-12-30

Enrollment (Actual)
120

Study Type
Interventional

Phase
Not Applicable

China
Hubei Locations

Wuhan, Hubei, China, 430030
Department of Ophthalmology, Tongji Hospital, Tongji Medical College, Huazhong University of Science and Technology

Eligibility Criteria
Inclusion Criteria

- Patients carry the mitochondrial point mutation at 11778, which is consistent with the diagnostic criteria for LHON.
- The vision falls within 3 months, onset between 3 and 6 months, onset between 6 and 12 months, onset between 12 and 24 months, onset between 24 and 60 months, and onset over 60 months.
- Patients signed written informed consent.
- Patients are between the ages of 8 and 60 years old and able to tolerate the gene therapy procedure which includes local anesthesia.
- Patients are willing to follow the doctor's instructions and to consult the doctor at prescribed times.
- Patient's physical examination results are all normal, including liver function, kidney function, routine blood test, routine urine test, complete immunological test, and humoral immune response.

Exclusion Criteria

- Patients who are wearing a cardiac pacemaker, suffering from severe heart, lung or kidney function failure, various hemorrhagic diseases, acute infectious diseases, high fever, or convalescing after heart surgery or who are pregnant are excluded.
- Patients who are participating in other clinical studies are excluded.
- Patients who suffer from a diagnosed mental problem are excluded.
- Patients who suffer from chronic diseases such as diabetes and hypertension are excluded.
- Patients who show abnormal test results such as positive AAV2 humoral immune response (positive means that the AAV2 neutralizing antibody assay of patient was significant different when comparing free serum with 1:20 serum concentrations) and abnormal human T lymphocyte subsets CD3+, CD3+/CD4+, and CD3+/CD8+ prior to gene therapy surgery are excluded.

Ages Eligible for Study
8 to 60 years (Child, Adult)

Sexes Eligible for Study
All

Accepts Healthy Volunteers
Yes

Design Details
Primary Purpose: Treatment
Allocation: N/A
Interventional Model: Single Group Assignment
Interventional Model Description: 20 patients of Leber Hereditary Optic Neuropathy (LHON) onset within 3 months, 20 between 3 and 6 months, 20 between 6 and 12 months, 20 between 12 and 24 months, 20 between 24 and 60 months, and 20 over 24 months.
Masking: None (Open Label)

Arms and interventions

Participant group/arm	Intervention/treatment
Experimental: rAAV2-ND4 A single IVT of recombinant adeno-associated virus-NADH dehydrogenase, subunit 4 (complex I) (rAAV2-ND4) (0.05 mL). The dose is 1×10^{10} vg/0.05 mL for test groups.	Drug: rAAV2-ND4 • rAAV2-ND4 of vitreous cavity injection • Other names: – rAAV2-ND4 gene therapy

Primary outcome measures

Outcome measure	Measure description	Time frame
BCVA	The best-corrected visual acuity	Change from baseline at 12 months

Secondary outcome measures

Outcome measure	Measure description	Time frame
Computerized visual field	Visual field index	Change from baseline at 12 months
Computerized visual field	Mean defect	Change from baseline at 12 months
VEP	Visual evoked potential	Change from baseline at 12 months
RNFL	Retinal nerve fiber layer	Change from baseline at 12 months
Liver function in plasma	Before and after the treatment. Liver function in plasma will be checked	Before treatment and in the first, third, sixth, and twelfth month after the treatment
Kidney function in plasma	Before and after the treatment, kidney function in plasma will be checked	Before treatment and in the first, third, sixth, and twelfth month after the treatment

Sponsor

Bin Li

Collaborators

No information provided

Investigators

No information provided

General Publications

- Yang S, Ma SQ, Wan X, He H, Pei H, Zhao MJ, Chen C, Wang DW, Dong XY, Yuan JJ, Li B. Long-term outcomes of gene therapy for the treatment of Leber's hereditary optic neuropathy. EBioMedicine. 2016 Aug;10:258–68. https://doi.org/10.1016/j.ebiom.2016.07.002. Epub 2016 Jul 6.
- Yang S, Yang H, Ma SQ, Wang SS, He H, Zhao MJ, Li B. Evaluation of Leber's hereditary optic neuropathy patients prior to a gene therapy clinical trial. Medicine (Baltimore). 2016 Oct;95(40):e5110. doi: https://doi.org/10.1097/MD.0000000000005110.

- Ran R, Yang S, He H, Ma S, Chen Z, Li B. A retrospective analysis of characteristics of visual field damage in patients with Leber's hereditary optic neuropathy. Springerplus. 2016 Jun 23;5(1):843. https://doi.org/10.1186/s40064-016-2540-7. eCollection 2016.
- Wan X, Pei H, Zhao MJ, Yang S, Hu WK, He H, Ma SQ, Zhang G, Dong XY, Chen C, Wang DW, Li B. Efficacy and Safety of rAAV2-ND4 Treatment for Leber's Hereditary Optic Neuropathy. Sci Rep. 2016 Feb 19;6:21587. https://doi.org/10.1038/srep21587.
- Yang S, He H, Zhu Y, Wan X, Zhou LF, Wang J, Wang WF, Liu L, Li B. Chemical and material communication between the optic nerves in rats. Clin Exp Ophthalmol. 2015 Nov;43(8):742–8. https://doi.org/10.1111/ceo.12547. Epub 2015 Jun 25.
- Pei H, Wan X, Hu W, Dong X, Li B. Construction and detection of a novel type of recombinant human rAAV2/2-ND4. Eye Sci. 2013 Jun;28(2):55–9.
- Cui G, Ding H, Xu Y, Li B, Wang DW. Applications of the method of high resolution melting analysis for diagnosis of Leber's disease and the three primary mutation spectrum of LHON in the Han Chinese population. Gene. 2013 Jan 1;512(1):108–12. https://doi.org/10.1016/j.gene.2012.09.110. Epub 2012 Oct 9.
- Shi H, Gao J, Pei H, Liu R, Hu WK, Wan X, Li T, Li B. Adeno-associated virus-mediated gene delivery of the human ND4 complex I subunit in rabbit eyes. Clin Exp Ophthalmol. 2012 Dec;40(9):888–94. https://doi.org/10.1111/j.1442-9071.2012.02815.x. Epub 2012 Jul 2.
- Feuer WJ, Schiffman JC, Davis JL, Porciatti V, Gonzalez P, Koilkonda RD, Yuan H, Lalwani A, Lam BL, Guy J. Gene Therapy for Leber Hereditary Optic Neuropathy: Initial Results. Ophthalmology. 2016 Mar;123(3):558–70. https://doi.org/10.1016/j.ophtha.2015.10.025. Epub 2015 Nov 19.
- Erickson RP. Leber's optic atrophy, a possible example of maternal inheritance. Am J Hum Genet. 1972 May;24(3):348–9. No abstract available.
- Wallace DC, Singh G, Lott MT, Hodge JA, Schurr TG, Lezza AM, Elsas LJ second, Nikoskelainen EK. Mitochondrial DNA mutation associated with Leber's hereditary optic neuropathy. Science. 1988 Dec 9;242(4884):1427–30. https://doi.org/10.1126/science.3201231.
- Huoponen K, Vilkki J, Aula P, Nikoskelainen EK, Savontaus ML. A new mtDNA mutation associated with Leber hereditary optic neuroretinopathy. Am J Hum Genet. 1991 Jun;48(6):1147–53.
- Mackey D, Howell N. A variant of Leber hereditary optic neuropathy characterized by recovery of vision and by an unusual mitochondrial genetic etiology. Am J Hum Genet. 1992 Dec;51(6):1218–28.
- Maguire AM, Simonelli F, Pierce EA, Pugh EN Jr., Mingozzi F, Bennicelli J, Banfi S, Marshall KA, Testa F, Surace EM, Rossi S, Lyubarsky A, Arruda VR, Konkle B, Stone E, Sun J, Jacobs J, Dell'Osso L, Hertle R, Ma JX, Redmond TM, Zhu X, Hauck B, Zelenaia O, Shindler KS, Maguire MG, Wright JF, Volpe NJ, McDonnell JW, Auricchio A, High KA, Bennett J. Safety and efficacy of gene transfer for Leber's congenital amaurosis. N Engl J Med. 2008 May 22;358(21):2240–8. https://doi.org/10.1056/NEJMoa0802315. Epub 2008 Apr 27.

- Bainbridge JW, Smith AJ, Barker SS, Robbie S, Henderson R, Balaggan K, Viswanathan A, Holder GE, Stockman A, Tyler N, Petersen-Jones S, Bhattacharya SS, Thrasher AJ, Fitzke FW, Carter BJ, Rubin GS, Moore AT, Ali RR. Effect of gene therapy on visual function in Leber's congenital amaurosis. N Engl J Med. 2008 May 22;358(21):2231–9. https://doi.org/10.1056/NEJMoa0802268. Epub 2008 Apr 27.
- Hauswirth WW, Aleman TS, Kaushal S, Cideciyan AV, Schwartz SB, Wang L, Conlon TJ, Boye SL, Flotte TR, Byrne BJ, Jacobson SG. Treatment of leber congenital amaurosis due to RPE65 mutations by ocular subretinal injection of adeno-associated virus gene vector: short-term results of a phase I trial. Hum Gene Ther. 2008 Oct;19(10):979–90. https://doi.org/10.1089/hum.2008.107.
- Hufnagel RB, Ahmed ZM, Correa ZM, Sisk RA. Gene therapy for Leber congenital amaurosis: advances and future directions. Graefes Arch Clin Exp Ophthalmol. 2012 Aug;250(8):1117–28. https://doi.org/10.1007/s00417-012-2028-2. Epub 2012 May 29.
- Howell N, Bindoff LA, McCullough DA, Kubacka I, Poulton J, Mackey D, Taylor L, Turnbull DM. Leber hereditary optic neuropathy: identification of the same mitochondrial ND1 mutation in six pedigrees. Am J Hum Genet. 1991 Nov;49(5):939–50.
- Zhang Y, Tian Z, Yuan J, Liu C, Liu HL, Ma SQ, Li B. The Progress of Gene Therapy for Leber's Optic Hereditary Neuropathy. Curr Gene Ther. 2017;17(4):320–326. https://doi.org/10.2174/1566523218666171129204926.

Chapter 4
Other Treatment Studies for Optic Nerve Disease

Recruiting

United States

Electrical Stimulation for the Treatment of Optic Neuropathies (rtACS)

ClinicalTrials.gov ID NCT05626426

Sponsor Stanford University
Information provided by Jeffrey L Goldberg, Stanford University (Responsible Party)
Last Update Posted 2023-03-08

Brief Summary
The overall aim of this study is to see whether long-term electrical stimulation with a home-stimulation device works well and is safe for the treatment of open-angle glaucoma. Open-Angle Glaucoma is a disease where the nerves in the back of your eye die off faster than expected regardless of your eye pressure.

Detailed Description
This is a concurrent open-label study for patients who are deemed safe to participate in the electrical stimulation trial but do not fit the exact criteria for the randomized clinical trial.

Official Title
An Open-Label Study to Evaluate the Safety and Efficacy of Repetitive, Transorbital Alternating Current Stimulation (rtACS) for the Treatment of Optic Neuropathies

J. N. Weiss, *Clinical Trials in Optic Nerve Disease Treatment*,
https://doi.org/10.1007/978-3-031-58815-0_4

Conditions
Glaucoma
Glaucoma, Open-Angle
Optic Nerve Diseases

Intervention/Treatment
- Device: Repetitive, Transorbital Alternating Current Stimulation (rtACS)

Other Study ID Numbers
- 68207

Study Start (Actual)
2023-02-27

Primary Completion (Estimated)
2024-12

Study Completion (Estimated)
2024-12

Enrollment (Estimated)
20

Study Type
Interventional

Phase
Not Applicable

United States
California Locations

Palo Alto, California, United States, 94303
Recruiting
Byers Eye Institute

Contact
Zac Wennberg-Smith
650-497-5942 zacwenn@stanford.edu

Eligibility Criteria
Description

Inclusion Criteria
- Participant must be at least 18.
- Participant must have the ability to comply with the requirements of the study and complete the schedule of events (SOEs).
- Participant's clinical diagnosis must be consistent with glaucoma characterized by the following features: Mean deviation (MD) worse than −3 on Humphrey Visual Field 24-2 testing. Reliable visual field measures, fixation losses do not exceed 20%, and false positives do not exceed 20%.

- In the opinion of the investigator, the participant's eye pressure must be clinically stable.
- If a participant has two eyes meeting study criteria, the worse eye as determined by mean deviation. If both eyes qualify and have the same MD, the patient may choose which eye they are willing to enter, or else a randomization procedure will assign one eye to the study.
- Participant must understand and sign the informed consent. If the participant's vision is impaired to the point where he/she cannot read the informed consent document, the document will be read to the participant in its entirety.

Exclusion Criteria

- Participant is unable to comply with study procedures or follow-up visits.
- Participant has a history of ocular herpes zoster.
- Participant has pathological nystagmus
- Participant has evidence of visually significant retinopathy including but not limited to Diabetic retinopathy or retinitis pigmentosa.
- Participant has evidence of corneal opacification or lack of optical clarity.
- Participant has uveitis or other ocular inflammatory disease.
- Participant has any electric or electronic implants such as a pacemaker.
- Participant has acute conjunctivitis.
- Participant has an acute autoimmune disease.
- Participant is pregnant or lactating.
- Participant has, in the opinion of the investigator, any physical or mental condition that would increase the risk of participation in the study or may interfere with the study procedures, evaluations, and outcome assessments, including but not limited to all forms of dementia.
- Unresected brain tumors.
- Implanted intracranial magnetic metals (metallic implants in the head/skull such as clamps, coils, ventriculo-peritoneal shunts, endoprostheses, etc.), which are not MRI-compatible. Note: metallic dental implants and titanium screws or plates are acceptable
- Patients with any skin damage.
- Children and comatose patients.
- Patients with a history of epileptic seizure within the last 10 years.
- Patients with uncontrolled systemic hypertension or uncontrolled diabetes.
- Participant is not able to travel, to comply with the requirements of the study or not willing to complete the schedule of events (SOEs) and/or unable to confirm follow-up participation.
- Prior participation in a vision training/stimulation study in the last 12 months

Ages Eligible for Study

18 Years and older (Adult, Older Adult)

Sexes Eligible for Study

All

Accepts Healthy Volunteers
No

Design Details
Primary Purpose: Treatment
Allocation: N/A
Interventional Model: Single Group Assignment
Masking: None (Open Label)

Arms and interventions

Participant group/arm	Intervention/treatment
Experimental: active SASm Patients will receive active treatment with the device every other day over 8 weeks	Device: Repetitive, Transorbital Alternating Current Stimulation (rtACS) • Patients receive treatment every other day via a headband that delivers electrical stimulation to the retina • Other names: – Electrical stimulation

Primary outcome measures

Outcome measure	Measure description	Time frame
Change from baseline in visual field assessed by Humphrey Visual Field Index (VFI)		Baseline through 6 months
Change from baseline in visual field assessed by Humphrey Mean Deviation (MD)		Baseline through 6 months

Secondary outcome measures

Outcome measure	Measure description	Time frame
Change from baseline in ganglion cell layer as measured by optical coherence tomography (OCT, visible light, and/or infrared)		Baseline through 6 months
Change from baseline in nerve fiber layer thickness as measured by optical coherence tomography (OCT, visible light, and/or infrared)		Baseline through 6 months
Change from baseline in visual acuity as assessed by the Snellen visual acuity test	The Snellen test is a standard eye chart test used to test eyesight	Baseline through month 6
Change from baseline in visual evoked potential		Baseline through month 6

Outcome measure	Measure description	Time frame
Change from baseline in retinal metabolic analysis (RMA)/ OcuMet imaging	There are two index measures of retinal metabolism and a normative database; change from baseline with a statistically significant difference from test-retest variability will be the exploratory endpoint measured here	Baseline through month 6
Change from baseline in adaptive optics retinal imaging	There are no index measures for adaptive optics retinal imaging in this disease; change from baseline will be the exploratory endpoint measured here	Baseline through month 6
Change from baseline in laser speckle flowgraphy	There is one index measure of retinal blood flow response to light stimulation; change from baseline with a statistically significant difference from test-retest variability will be the exploratory endpoint measured here	Baseline through month 6
Change from baseline in OCT angiography	There are 3 index measures of retinal blood flow in OCT-A; change from baseline with a statistically significant difference from test-retest variability will be the exploratory endpoint measured here	Baseline through month 6

Sponsor
Stanford University

Collaborators
- NYU Langone Health
- Otto-von-Guericke University Magdeburg

Investigators
- Principal Investigator: Jeffrey L Goldberg, MD PhD, Stanford University

General Publications
No publications available

Recruiting

China

Targeted Shortwave Diathermy Combined with Perceptual Training for Patients with Severe Traumatic Optic Neuropathy

ClinicalTrials.gov ID NCT05140486

Sponsor Hunan Provincial People's Hospital
Information provided by Qingping Tang, Hunan Provincial People's Hospital (Responsible Party)
Last Update Posted 2021-12-01

Brief Summary

Purpose: Patients with severe traumatic optic neuropathy (TON) have limited improvement in visual function despite therapy. The hypothesis of the study is that the targeted shortwave diathermy combined with perceptual training may enhance visual function in patients with severe TON after endoscopic optic nerve decompression (EOND) surgery.

Design: Clinical trial Subjects: Twenty-two subjects with severe TON after EOND surgery were randomly assigned to either a rehabilitation (Reh) group or nonrehabilitation (Nreh) group.

Methods: High-resolution computed tomography and MRI were used to locate the impaired nerve. The subjects in the Reh group received targeted shortwave diathermy therapy 5 days per week for 4 weeks and perceptual training 5 days per week for 10 weeks.

Main Outcome Measures: A thorough evaluation of visual function, visual evoked potential, and diffusion tensor imaging was executed.

Detailed Description

Study sample description Indirect traumatic optic neuropathy (TON) was diagnosed by a history of blunt head or facial trauma combined with decreased visual acuity, color vision, and a relative afferent pupillary defect with a normal fundus during the early period of post-trauma. The investigators excluded cases with direct trauma to optic nerve identified by high-resolution CT scan of the orbital and optic canal. The patients with indirect TON were intravenously administered methylprednisolone (30 mg/kg per day) every day for 3 consecutive days. All consecutive subjects with indirect TON who were admitted to Xiangya Hospital and managed with endoscopic optic nerve decompression surgery were recruited. The subjects were randomly assigned to either a rehabilitation group or a nonrehabilitation group. Since there were no grading criteria in evaluating the severity of indirect TON, TON with Best-corrected visual acuity equal to or more than 1.85 LogMAR after endoscopic optic nerve decompression surgery was considered severe TON and those patients were recruited in this study. The subjects in the rehabilitation group will receive shortwave diathermy therapy and perceptual training after endoscopic optic nerve decompression surgery. The subjects in the nonrehabilitation group will not receive any rehabilitation treatment after endoscopic optic nerve decompression surgery.

Endoscopic ON decompression surgery: All operations were performed under general anesthesia by a surgeon (Hua Zhang). Briefly, a routine endoscopic endonasal sphenoethmoidectomy was performed to expose and resect the posterior ethmoidal lamina papyracea. After the optic canal was exposed, the upper, medial, and partial lower surfaces of the whole range of the optic canal wall were removed. Finally, the ON sheath from the annulus of the Zinn to the cranial cavity, along with the annulus of the Zinn, was incised, and the surface of the ON was covered with a piece of gelatin sponge filled with methylprednisolone solution (40 mg/mL).

Shortwave diathermy therapy The Shortwave diathermy (SWD) device applied in this study was DL-CII (Dajia®, Shantou, China). This therapeutic apparatus is delivered at a frequency of approximately 27.12 ± 0.6% MHz in continuous modes with a power of 50 W ± 20%. In our study, 2 sets of circular capacitive electrodes were used with a diameter of 80 mm for adults and 50 mm for children. The fracture areas were located using a high-resolution CT scan. One electrode was applied in the temporal area of the ipsilateral side of the injured nerve identified by a three-dimensional alignment procedure through a high-resolution CT scan. This area was not only a shorter distance from the skin to the injured nerve but was also as far away from the crystalline lens as possible. To decrease the negative effects of SWD on the nerve systems, another circular electrode of SWD was applied in the frontal area of the ipsilateral side of the injured nerve. In the acute stage of the TON (within 10 days after injury), the athermal mode of the SWD was applied to the marked areas for a 10-min daily session. Ten days after injury, the microthermal mode was used for a 15-min daily session. All subjects in the rehabilitation group received SWD therapy 5 days per week for 4 weeks.

Perceptual training Perceptive learning sessions were composed of a series of training procedures. First, sensory stimulations including touch, stroking, tapping, and pressing on the local area of the ipsilateral eye as well as surface location of the injured ON were offered.

Second, light stimulation was applied at different intensities of bright based on evaluation of the pupillary light reflex of the subject, 1–5 s each time, 10–15 times a day, and avoiding glare and longtime light stimulation on eye when training. Additionally, the subjects were instructed to enter the bright room from the dark room when the participants were wearing an eye patch in the intact eye. Third, differentiation of the shapes and objects in dynamic or static states with different colors, different sizes, and different shapes was performed. Either real objects or pictures could be selected in the training session. Fourth, different written words with different sizes and different distances were discriminated in the different directions of the eye.

Based on evaluation of the visual acuity, the training sequence was from large words to small, from simple words to complex, and from proximal to distal distance of the eye. Fifth, color vision was trained using real objects or pictures. The subjects were instructed to select the color from the single and bright to multiple and dark color. The color contrast was initiated from maximum to minimal contrast. Finally, the visual field training was scattered in the above training methods. Each training media including the light, objects, words, and color was input from the anterior, superior, inferior, nasal, and temporal sides of the eye. These trainings started from the center of the normal visual field to the terminal of the visual field. When the training media reached the terminal of the visual field in every direction, ocular fixation with 2–5 s was performed to increase the scope of the visual field. Each stimulation was given 5–10 times for each direction. In the early periods of the training, when the visual acuity was a complete loss, the training sections were relatively independent. When the visual acuity of subjects was partially recovered, the training sections were mixed. In addition, many training techniques were used in this study. First, visual imagery training was used when the patients had complete or severe visual loss. Visual imagery training can be defined as "a dynamic state during which the representation of a specific object is internally reactivated within visual memory without any overt visual input and that is governed by the principles of central visual control". The intervention of the VI training was as follows: the subjects used the intact eye to observe the object for 5 s, then the participants closed their eyes and imagined viewing the object using the injured eye for 10 s for 10 repetitions. Additionally, proprioceptive training, including going over the barriers, going up and downstairs, walking the slope, and training the balance, was executed. Finally, constraint-induced perceptive therapy was performed when the visual lesion partially recovered. The subjects wore an eye patch on the intact eye for 30 min in one section, 2–4 h a day, 7 days per week. In constraint-induced perceptive training, activities of daily living (ADL), natural environmental training, and fun games with colorful objects were executed, and the subjects were instructed to complete the ADL, play gobang, watch the green leaves, and colorful flowers from proximal to distal distance. All the subjects in the Reh group received perceptive learning therapy 5 days per week for 10 weeks except constraint-induced perceptive therapy.

Official Title

Targeted Shortwave Diathermy Combined With Perceptual Training for Patients With Severe Traumatic Optic Neuropathy After Endoscopic Optic Nerve Decompression: a Preliminary Clinical Trial

Conditions

Traumatic Optic Neuropathy

Intervention/Treatment

- Procedure: Rehabilitation: shortwave diathermy and perceptual training

Other Study ID Numbers

- HunanPPH

Study Start (Actual)

2017-01-20

Primary Completion (Estimated)
2022-12-31

Study Completion (Estimated)
2022-12-31

Enrollment (Estimated)
60

Study Type
Interventional

Phase
Not Applicable

Study Contact
Name: Qingping Tang
Phone Number: +86-073185232387
Email: tqingping111@126.com

China

Changsha, China, 410008
Recruiting
Tang

Contact
Qingping Tang
+86-073185232387

Eligibility Criteria
Description

Inclusion Criteria

- The indications for endoscopic optic nerve decompression surgery included no improvement after intravenous treatment for 24 h, no evidence of injury in the intracranial portion of the optic nerve, and the presence of bony fragments or hematoma compressing the optic nerve.
- TON with best-corrected visual acuity equal to or more than 1.85 logMAR after surgery was considered as severe TON, and those patients managed with endoscopic optic nerve decompression surgery were recruited in this study.
- Eligible criteria for the participants were as follows: (1) not receiving other physical therapy regimens aside from this intervention; (2) age 3–60 years old; (3) ability to execute simple verbal instructions; (4) not being delirious; (5) having stable vital signs and medical conditions.

Exclusion Criteria

- The exclusion criteria included severe diffuse brain damage, and/or severe cardiac and pulmonary disease, which were contraindicated in rehabilitation procedure.

Ages Eligible for Study
3 Years to 60 Years (Child, Adult)

Sexes Eligible for Study
All

Accepts Healthy Volunteers
No

Design Details
Primary Purpose: Treatment
Allocation: Randomized
Interventional Model: Parallel Assignment
Masking: Single (Outcomes Assessor)

Arms and interventions

Participant group/arm	Intervention/treatment
Experimental: shortwave diathermy and perceptual training The subjects in this group will receive shortwave diathermy 5 days per week for 4 weeks and perceptual training 5 days per week for 10 weeks after endoscopic optic nerve decompression surgery	Procedure: rehabilitation: shortwave diathermy and perceptual training • All subjects in the rehabilitation group received shortwave diathermy therapy 5 days per week for 4 weeks and perceptual training 5 days per week for 10 weeks
No intervention: nonrehabilitation The subjects in the nonrehabilitation group will not only receive any rehabilitation therapy after endoscopic optic nerve decompression surgery	

Primary outcome measures

Outcome measure	Measure description	Time frame
MRI	A 32-channel head coil on a 3.0 T MRI system (Philips, Ltd., Best, the Netherlands) was used for the acquisition of imaging data. T1- and T2-weighted, fat-suppressed images were obtained axially through the orbit and some parts of the brain, including the intracranial portion of the optic nerve, postoperatively and 10 weeks after rehabilitation	15 min
Diffusion tensor imaging	Optic nerve diffusion tensor imaging images were obtained using single-shot echoplanar imaging sequences. The images were acquired from the optic papilla to the orbital apex of the optic nerve with 40 contiguous slices. The region of interest was manually placed over the optic nerve at the anterior, middle, and posterior segments on the non-diffusion-weighted image. The fraction anisotropy, mean diffusivity, axial diffusivity, and radial diffusivity of optic nerves were measured	15 min

Secondary outcome measures

Outcome measure	Measure description	Time frame
Visual evoked potential	Pattern visual evoked potential testing was recorded using an MEB-9404C (Nihon Kohden Corp, Tokyo, Japan). The latency and amplitude of the P100 wave in the VEP testing were collected for analysis	30 min
Best-corrected visual acuity	Best-corrected visual acuity was measured by a standardized Snellen visual chart. Visual results were converted into logMAR units for the convenience of statistical analysis. Hand motion, light perception, and no light perception were converted to 2.3, 2.5, and 3 logMAR units, respectively	5 min
Color vision	Color vision was evaluated using the Ishihara color vision test 24 plate. The exclusion criterion of the color vision test was congenital color vision deficiency. The number of correct answers in a set of 24 plates was recorded as the color vision score	5 min

Sponsor
Hunan Provincial People's Hospital

Collaborators
No information provided

Investigators
- Study Chair: Xiao Ye Wang, Brain Hospital of Hunan Province, Hunan University of Chinese Medicine

General Publications
No publications available

Completed

United States

Vision Restoration Therapy (VRT) to Treat Non-arteritic Anterior Ischemic OpticNeuropathy

ClinicalTrials.gov ID NCT00140491

Sponsor Emory University
Information provided by Valerie Biousse, Emory University (Responsible Party)
Last Update Posted 2013-10-23

Brief Summary

The goal of this pilot study is to evaluate the effect of Vision Restoration Therapy, VRT, on the visual function of patients with unilateral or bilateral AION, who have good central vision (at least 20/60) and altitudinal visual field defects.

Detailed Description

Anterior ischemic optic neuropathy (AION) is one of the most common causes of optic neuropathy after the age of 50. There is currently no available treatment and although up to 40% of patients have some spontaneous improvement within the first few months, most patients remain visually devastated. About 50% of patients retain relatively spared central visual acuity with an inferior altitudinal visual field defect. These patients usually complain of difficulty reading and loss of depth perception.

Recently, training-induced enlargement of visual field defects has been demonstrated in some patients with VF defects secondary to lesions of the retrochiasmal visual pathways. This computer-based Vision Restoration Therapy (VRT) was developed in Germany and has been FDA-cleared in the United States for the past 1 year.

VRT is currently available at Emory for patients with homonymous hemianopia. Patients work on personally designed software (on a laptop at home) twice daily (30 min each) for 6 months. Zones of partially damaged neurons, which are usually located between the intact and damaged area of the visual field (transition zone), are deliberately stimulated by VRT. There is only anecdotal evidence that this visual restoration therapy may be helpful in enlarging the visual field of patients with optic neuropathies.

The goal of this pilot study is to evaluate the effect of VRT on the visual function of patients with unilateral or bilateral AION, who have good central vision (at least 20/60) and altitudinal visual field defects. The effect of VRT will be evaluated by visual acuity, color vision, stereo vision, Humphrey VF (24-2 SITA standard) testing, and scales evaluating reading speed and vision-based quality of life. These measures will be repeated before VRT, at 3 months, at 6 months, and at 1 year after VRT. Twenty patients will be included in the study. Patients will be randomized at inclusion between VRT and sham (placebo)-training (ten in each group). The 10 patients receiving sham training will then receive VRT for the following 6 months if they so choose. All data will be analyzed in a blinded fashion. The company developing VRT in the United States (NOVAVISION) has agreed to provide VRT and sham-training.

Official Title

Visual Field Defects in Non-Arteritic Anterior Ischemic Optic Neuropathy: Effect of Vision Restoration Therapy (VRT)

Conditions

Non-Arteritic Anterior Ischemic Optic Neuropathy

InterventionsTreatment

- Device: Vision Restoration Therapy (NOVAVISION)

Other Study ID Numbers
- 0435-2005
- Valerie Biousse 404-778-5158

Study Start
2005-08

Primary Completion (Actual)
2007-04

Study Completion (Actual)
2007-04

Enrollment
20

Study Type
Interventional

Phase
Not Applicable

United States
Georgia Locations

Atlanta, Georgia, United States, 30322
Emory Eye Center

Eligibility Criteria
Description

Inclusion Criteria
- Patients seen by Dr. Biousse or Dr. Newman in the Neuro-Ophthalmology Unit at Emory University.
- Age ≥30 years.
- Diagnosis of non-arteritic ischemic optic neuropathy at least 6 months prior to inclusion.
- Uni- or bilateral AION (in case of bilateral AION, only one eye will be included in the study).
- Best corrected visual acuity of at least 20/60 in the study eye
- Altitudinal or arcuate visual field defect, splitting fixation by >10-decibel difference above and below the horizontal meridian.
- Stable visual function was demonstrated by more than two stable visual acuity measurements and two automated visual field testings prior to inclusion in the study.
- Patient willing, and able, to spend 60 minutes-a-day for 6 months working on a computer.

Exclusion Criteria

- Patient cognitively or physically unable to perform reliable automated perimetry testing (on the 24-2 SITA Standard program) (which is grossly equivalent to the effort and attention needed to perform VRT daily at home).
- Other causes of optic neuropathy.
- Associated ocular disease requiring treatments or responsible for visual loss (such as untreated significant cataract, glaucoma, age-related macular degeneration, etc.…).
- Visual acuity worse than 20/60 in the study eye.
- Non-stable visual field defect on previous evaluations.
- Epilepsy.

Ages Eligible for Study
30 Years and older (Adult, Older Adult)

Sexes Eligible for Study
All

Accepts Healthy Volunteers
No

Design Details
Primary Purpose: Treatment
Allocation: Randomized
Interventional Model: Parallel Assignment
Masking: Double

Arms and interventions

Intervention/treatment
Device: Vision Restoration Therapy (NOVAVISION)

Primary outcome measures

Outcome measure	Measure description	Time frame
Visual function		

Sponsor
Emory University

Collaborators
No information provided

Investigators

- Principal Investigator: Valerie Biousse, MD, Emory Eye Center

General Publications
No publications available

No Results Posted

Completed

A New Medicine to Treat Nonarteritic Anterior Ischemic Optic Neuropathy (NAION) (Ampyra)

ClinicalTrials.gov ID NCT01975324

Sponsor Neuro-Ophthalmologic Associates, PC
Information provided by Mark L. Moster, M.D., Neuro-Ophthalmologic Associates, PC (Responsible Party)
Last Update Posted 2016-01-25

Brief Summary
Determine whether dalfampridine (Ampyra) can improve visual function in patients who have had nonarteritic ischemic optic neuropathy (NAION) with stable visual impairment.

Detailed Description
The aim of this study is to determine whether dalfampridine can improve visual function in patients who have had nonarteritic ischemic optic neuropathy (NAION) with stable visual impairment.

The objective of this double-masked crossover study is to determine whether visual function can be improved in numerous parameters. This includes high contrast visual acuity, low contrast visual acuity, visual field, visual quality of life (VFQ-39), electrophysiology, multifocal electro retinography (mERG), visual evoked potential (VEP), and structure, spectral domain optical coherence tomography (OCT).

Based on the promising results of the use of dalfampridine in Multiple Sclerosis (MS) and in stroke, we hypothesize that the patients with chronic stable deficits after nonarteritic ischemic optic neuropathy (NAION) will have improved visual function with the administration of dalfampridine.

Official Title
Dalfampridine Treatment for Nonarteritic Anterior Ischemic Optic Neuropathy (NAION)

Conditions
Non-Arteritic Ischemic Optic Neuropathy

Intervention/Treatment
- Drug: dalfampridine
- Drug: Placebo

Other Study ID Numbers
- Dalfampridine 13-265

Study Start
2013-07

Primary Completion (Actual)
2015-12

Study Completion (Actual)
2015-12

Enrollment (Actual)
20

Study Type
Interventional

Phase
Phase 4

United States
Pennsylvania Locations

Philadelphia, Pennsylvania, United States, 19107
Neuro-Ophthalmologic Associates, PC

Eligibility Criteria
Description

Inclusion Criteria
- NAION 6 months prior to enrollment
- visual acuity of 20/40 or worse

Exclusion Criteria
Current use of Dalfampridine (Ampyra)
  - Pregnancy
  - History of seizures
  - Renal Failure
  - Not able to perform testing

Ages Eligible for Study
40 Years and older (Adult, Older Adult)

Sexes Eligible for Study
All

Accepts Healthy Volunteers
No

Sponsor
Neuro-Ophthalmologic Associates, PC

Collaborators
- Acorda Therapeutics

Investigators
- Principal Investigator: Mark L Moster, MD, Neuro-Ophthalmologic Associates, PC

General Publications

- Newman NJ, Scherer R, Langenberg P, Kelman S, Feldon S, Kaufman D, Dickersin K; Ischemic Optic Neuropathy Decompression Trial Research Group. The fellow eye in NAION: report from the ischemic optic neuropathy decompression trial follow-up study. Am J Ophthalmol. 2002 Sep;134(3):317–28. https://doi.org/10.1016/s0002-9394(02)01639-2.
- The ischemic optic neuropathy decompression trial (IONDT): design and methods. Control Clin Trials. 1998 Jun;19(3):276–96. https://doi.org/10.1016/s0197-2456(98)00003-8.
- Bever CT Jr. 10 questions about 4-aminopyridine and the treatment of multiple sclerosis. Neurologist. 2009 May;15(3):161–2. https://doi.org/10.1097/NRL.0b013e3181679be5. No abstract available.
- Davis FA, Stefoski D, Rush J. Orally administered 4-aminopyridine improves clinical signs in multiple sclerosis. Ann Neurol. 1990 Feb;27(2):186–92. https://doi.org/10.1002/ana.410270215.
- Jones RE, Heron JR, Foster DH, Snelgar RS, Mason RJ. Effects of 4-aminopyridine in patients with multiple sclerosis. J Neurol Sci. 1983 Aug-Sep;60(3):353–62. https://doi.org/10.1016/0022-510x(83)90145-4.
- Stefoski D, Davis FA, Faut M, Schauf CL. 4-Aminopyridine improves clinical signs in multiple sclerosis. Ann Neurol. 1987 Jan;21(1):71–7. https://doi.org/10.1002/ana.410210113.
- van Diemen HA, van Dongen MM, Dammers JW, Polman CH. Increased visual impairment after exercise (Uhthoff's phenomenon) in multiple sclerosis: therapeutic possibilities. Eur Neurol. 1992;32(4):231–4. https://doi.org/10.1159/000116830.
- Bever CT Jr., Young D, Anderson PA, Krumholz A, Conway K, Leslie J, Eddington N, Plaisance KI, Panitch HS, Dhib-Jalbut S, et al. The effects of 4-aminopyridine in multiple sclerosis patients: results of a randomized, placebo-controlled, double-blind, concentration-controlled, crossover trial. Neurology. 1994 Jun;44(6):1054–9. https://doi.org/10.1212/wnl.44.6.1054.
- Stefoski D, Davis FA, Fitzsimmons WE, Luskin SS, Rush J, Parkhurst GW. 4-Aminopyridine in multiple sclerosis: prolonged administration. Neurology. 1991 Sep;41(9):1344–8. https://doi.org/10.1212/wnl.41.9.1344.
- Polman CH, Bertelsmann FW, de Waal R, van Diemen HA, Uitdehaag BM, van Loenen AC, Koetsier JC. 4-Aminopyridine is superior to 3,4-diaminopyridine in the treatment of patients with multiple sclerosis. Arch Neurol. 1994 Nov;51(11):1136–9. https://doi.org/10.1001/archneur.1994.00540230074016.
- Strupp M, Brandt T. Pharmacological advances in the treatment of neuro-otological and eye movement disorders. Curr Opin Neurol. 2006 Feb;19(1):33–40. https://doi.org/10.1097/01.wco.0000196156.00481.e1.
- Goodman AD, Brown TR, Krupp LB, Schapiro RT, Schwid SR, Cohen R, Marinucci LN, Blight AR; Fampridine MS-F203 Investigators. Sustained-release oral fampridine in multiple sclerosis: a randomised, double-blind, controlled trial. Lancet. 2009 Feb 28;373(9665):732–8. https://doi.org/10.1016/S0140-6736(09)60442-6.

- Goodman AD, Brown TR, Edwards KR, Krupp LB, Schapiro RT, Cohen R, Marinucci LN, Blight AR; MSF204 Investigators. A phase 3 trial of extended release oral dalfampridine in multiple sclerosis. Ann Neurol. 2010 Oct;68(4):494–502. https://doi.org/10.1002/ana.22240.
- Ho PW, Reutens DC, Phan TG, Wright PM, Markus R, Indra I, Young D, Donnan GA. Is white matter involved in patients entered into typical trials of neuroprotection? Stroke. 2005 Dec;36(12):2742–4. https://doi.org/10.1161/01.STR.0000189748.52500.a7. Epub 2005 Nov 3.

No Results Posted

Completed

Ranibizumab Therapy for Non-arteritic Ischemic Optic Neuropathy (NAION)

ClinicalTrials.gov ID NCT00561834

Sponsor University of Colorado, Denver
Information provided by University of Colorado, Denver (Responsible Party)
Last Update Posted 2016-09-30

Brief Summary
The purpose of this study was to explore the safety and efficacy of ranibizumab to treat non-arteritic ischemic optic neuropathy based on clinical and anatomical findings.

Detailed Description
Nonarteritic anterior ischemic optic neuropathy (NAION) is the most common acute optic neuropathy in people older than 50 years. It is characterized by sudden partial loss of vision in one eye and has an increased risk of vision loss in the fellow eye. Although the cause has not been determined, NAION is thought to occur following an idiopathic ischemic event involving the short posterior ciliary arteries that supply blood to the most anterior part of the optic nerve. A complete loss of vision is rare, but partial loss of visual field or acuity can result from NAION in the affected eye(s).

Patients who have a 'disc at risk' or 'crowded disc' (small cup: disc ratio) are at increased risk for developing NAION. Other risk factors for NAION include age >50 years and white race (estimated 95% of cases). Hypertension and diabetes also predispose to NAION development. Other factors that have been associated with NAION include high cholesterol, arteriosclerosis, stroke, cardiac and intraocular surgery, tobacco use, nocturnal hypotension, blood loss, glaucoma, elevated homocysteine, and sleep apnea. The association between NAION and hypertension, high cholesterol, and diabetes is stronger in individuals younger than 50 years than in older persons.

Patients with NAION caused by ischemia leading to swelling of the optic nerve and rapidly progressing visual loss have had limited results with therapy such as corticosteroids, brimonidine, levodopa, or surgery, such as optic nerve sheath decompression, in the past. Currently, there is no standard of care for these patients.

Although the role of vascular endothelial growth factor (VEGF) in NAION has not been established, ischemic conditions may lead to VEGF production which could be the cause of edema and swelling. This possibility suggests that VEGF may be a target for therapeutic intervention by ranibizumab. Ranibizumab has demonstrated an effect on edema and vascular permeability. In animal studies, it has shown a concentration-dependent effect of blunting the vascular permeability induced by VEGF. Of the more than 5000 subjects with age-related macular degeneration in current and completed clinical trials, vascular permeability, and edema have decreased with the use of ranibizumab.

Official Title
Ranibizumab Therapy for Non-Arteritic Ischemic Optic Neuropathy (NAION)

Conditions
Nonarteritic Anterior Ischemic Optic Neuropathy

Intervention/Treatment
- Drug: ranibizumab

Other Study ID Numbers
- 07-0446
- genentech FVF4256s (Other Identifier) (OTHER: genentech)

Study Start
2007-11

Primary Completion (Actual)
2009-04

Study Completion (Actual)
2009-04

Enrollment (Actual)
2

Study Type
Interventional

Phase
Phase 1

United States
Colorado Locations

Aurora, Colorado, United States, 80045-0510
Rocky Mountain Lions Eye Institute

Eligibility Criteria
Description

Inclusion Criteria

- Provide written informed consent
- 21 years of age or older
- New onset, within 14 days, of ischemia and vision loss
- Best Corrected Visual Acuity (BCVA) 20/40 or worse

Exclusion Criteria

- Pregnancy or lactation
- Proliferative diabetic retinopathy,
- Diabetic macular edema,
- Uveitis,
- History of ocular trauma,
- Severe glaucoma,
- Age-related macular degeneration.
- Prior or concomitant treatment of oral steroids within 30 days,
- Participation in any studies of investigational drugs within 30 days,
- Participation in a ranibizumab clinical trial or,
- Prior treatment intravitreally or intravenously of Avastin or steroids.

Ages Eligible for Study
21 Years and older (Adult, Older Adult)

Sexes Eligible for Study
All

Accepts Healthy Volunteers
No

Design Details
Primary Purpose: Treatment
Allocation: N/A
Interventional Model: Single Group Assignment
Masking: None (Open Label)

Arms and interventions

Participant group/arm	Intervention/treatment
Experimental: ranibizumab To determine the mean change in best-corrected visual acuity (BCVA) using the Early Treatment Diabetic Retinopathy Study testing system at 6 months in NAION patients treated as needed (PRN) with ranibizumab	Drug: ranibizumab • All patients ($n = 15$) will be treated with open-label 0.5 mg ranibizumab given intravitreally monthly as needed for 6 months

Primary outcome measures

Outcome measure	Measure description	Time frame
Change in visual acuity	The mean change in best-corrected Snellen visual acuity at 6 months in NAION patients treated as needed with ranibizumab	Baseline and 6 months

Sponsor
University of Colorado, Denver

Collaborators
- Genentech, Inc.

Investigators
- Principal Investigator: Naresh Mandava, MD, Rocky Mountain Lions Eye Institute, University of Colorado Health Sciences Center

General Publications
No publications available

Results
Outcome Measures

1. Change in Visual Acuity
   Type: Primary | Time Frame: Baseline and 6 months

Description	The mean change in best-corrected Snellen visual acuity at 6 months in NAION patients treated as needed with ranibizumab
Time frame	Baseline and 6 months
Analysis population description	[Not Specified]

Arm/group title	Ranibizumab
Arm/group description	Ranibizumab: 0.5 mg ranibizumab given intravitreally as needed after initial treatment
Overall number of participants analyzed	2
Lines change in visual acuity subject 1 [a]Measure type: number | unit of measure: lines change in Snellen chart	4
Lines change in visual acuity-subject 2[a]	3

[a] Measure type: number | unit of measure: lines change in Snellen chart

Adverse Events
Time Frame
1 year 5 months
Adverse Event Reporting Description
[Not Specified]

Arm/group title	Ranibizumab
Arm/group description	Ranibizumab: 0.5 mg ranibizumab given intravitreally as needed after initial treatment
All-cause mortality	
Arm/group title	Ranibizumab
	Affected/at risk (%)
Total	--/--
Serious adverse events	
Arm/group title	Ranibizumab
	Affected/at risk (%)
Total	0/2 (0.00%)
Other (not including serious) adverse events	
0% Frequency threshold for reporting other adverse events	
Arm/group title	Ranibizumab
	Affected/at risk (%)
Total	0/2 (0.00%)

Completed

A Study Investigating the Safety, Tolerability, and Efficacy of Elamipretide Topical Ophthalmic Solution for Treatment of Leber's Hereditary Optic Neuropathy

ClinicalTrials.gov ID NCT02693119

Sponsor Stealth BioTherapeutics Inc.
Information provided by Stealth BioTherapeutics Inc. (Responsible Party)
Last Update Posted 2021-11-30

Brief Summary
This is a Phase 2, prospective, randomized, double-masked, vehicle-controlled, single-center study in approximately 12 subjects with LHON to evaluate safety, tolerability, and efficacy of elamipretide (MTP-131) topical ophthalmic solution in this patient population. At the conclusion of 52 weeks of treatment, subjects will be

offered the opportunity to enter an Open-Label Extension for up to 48 additional weeks of treatment.

Detailed Description
This was a prospective, randomized, double-masked (DM), vehicle-controlled, single-center study plus open-label extension period (OLE) in which approximately 12 subjects with LHON having the genetic mtDNA mutation m.11778G > A were randomized in a masked manner into 1 of 3 groups in a 1:1:1 ratio: one drop of elamipretide 1.0% topical ophthalmic solution twice daily (BID) in the: left eye, right eye, or both eyes.

After completion of the 52-week treatment period or the Week 56 follow-up period, subjects were invited to participate in the OLE period for up to 108 weeks. During the OLE, participants received 1% topical ophthalmic elamipretide in both eyes (OU) daily. If a subject did not consent to the OLE, he/she completed the study at the Week 56 (±7 days) visit. There were 4 periods in this study: (1) screening period (up to 6 weeks); (2) double-masked treatment period (52 weeks); (3) OLE period (up to 108 weeks), and (4) follow-up period (4 weeks) after completion of End-of-Treatment (EOT) visit.

Official Title

A Prospective, Randomized, Double-Masked, Vehicle Controlled, Phase 2 Clinical Study to Evaluate the Safety, Tolerability, and Efficacy of Elamipretide Topical Ophthalmic Solution in Subjects With Leber's Hereditary Optic Neuropathy (LHON)

Conditions

Leber's Hereditary Optic Neuropathy

Intervention/Treatment
- Drug: elamipretide (MTP-131) 1% topical ophthalmic solution
- Drug: Vehicle topical ophthalmic solution

Other Study ID Numbers
- SPILH-201

Study Start
2016-03

Primary Completion (Actual)
2019-09

Study Completion (Actual)
2019-12

Enrollment (Actual)
12

Study Type
Interventional

Phase
Phase 2

United States
California Locations

Pasadena, California, United States, 91105
Doheny Eye Center

Eligibility Criteria
Description

Inclusion Criteria
- Adults ≥18 and ≤50 years old at the time of loss of vision in the second eye.
- Able to provide informed consent and willing to comply with all study visits and examinations.
- Diagnosis of LHON based on clinical and ophthalmic functional/anatomic test findings, and satisfactory documentation of the mitochondrial DNA mutation m.11778G > A.
- Loss of vision in both eyes of ≥1 year and ≤10 years at the time of the Screening Visit and current clinically stable visual function (as assessed by the Investigator).
- Able to self-administer eye drops as demonstrated at screening or having a care provider who can do so.
- Documentation of having satisfactorily completed at least two previous Humphrey automated visual field tests prior to screening.
- Women of childbearing potential must agree to use birth control as specified in the protocol from the date they sign the informed consent form.

Exclusion Criteria
- Any other ocular pathology requiring treatment with prescription topical ophthalmic drops (e.g., glaucoma, dry eye)
- Cup to disc ratio of >0.8 in either eye
- Media opacity, suboptimal pupillary dilatation, or refractive error that interferes with adequate retinal imaging
- Known to be immunocompromised or receiving systemic immunosuppression
- Any disease or medical condition that in the opinion of the Investigator would prevent the subject from participating in the study or might confound study results
- Participation in other investigational drug or device clinical trials within 30 days prior to enrollment, or planning to participate in any other investigational drug or device clinical trials within 30 days of study completion
- Women who are pregnant or lactating

Other protocol-defined inclusion/exclusion criteria may apply.

Ages Eligible for Study
18 Years to 50 Years (Adult)

Sexes Eligible for Study
All

Accepts Healthy Volunteers
No

Design Details
Primary Purpose: Treatment
Allocation: Randomized
Interventional Model: Parallel Assignment
Masking: Quadruple (Participant Care Provider Investigator Outcomes Assessor)

Arms and interventions

Participant group/arm	Intervention/treatment
Experimental: group 1 One drop elamipretide (MTP-131) 1% topical ophthalmic solution BID applied to the left eye (OS) and one drop of vehicle topical ophthalmic solution BID in the fellow eye	Drug: elamipretide (MTP-131) 1% topical ophthalmic solution • Other names: – MTP-131 – Bendavia Drug: vehicle topical ophthalmic solution
Experimental: group 2 One drop elamipretide (MTP-131) 1% topical ophthalmic solution BID applied to the right eye (OD) and one drop of vehicle topical ophthalmic solution BID in the fellow eye	Drug: elamipretide (MTP-131) 1% topical ophthalmic solution • Other names: – MTP-131 – Bendavia Drug: vehicle topical ophthalmic solution
Experimental: group 3 One drop elamipretide (MTP-131) 1% topical ophthalmic solution BID applied to both eyes (OU)	Drug: elamipretide (MTP-131) 1% topical ophthalmic solution • Other names: – MTP-131 – Bendavia
Experimental: OLE One drop elamipretide (MTP-131) 1% topical ophthalmic solution BID applied to both eyes (OU)	Drug: elamipretide (MTP-131) 1% topical ophthalmic solution • Other names: – MTP-131 – Bendavia

Primary outcome measures

Outcome measure	Measure description	Time frame
Double-masked period: incidence of ocular TEAEs	The incidence of ocular treatment-emergent adverse events (TEAEs)	Assessed at each visit: baseline, Day 5 Visit, Weeks 4, 8, 12, 16, 20, 24, 28, 32, 36, 40, 44, 48, 52 (end of treatment visit), and Week 56 (follow-up visit)
Open-label extension: incidence of ocular TEAEs	Open-label extension: the incidence of ocular treatment-emergent adverse events (TEAEs)	Assessed at Week 68, 84, 100, 116, 132, 148, 152, Week 160/ (end of treatment visit)
Double-masked period: severity of ocular TEAEs	The severity of ocular treatment-emergent adverse events (TEAEs)	Assessed at each visit: baseline, Day 5 Visit, Weeks 4, 8, 12, 16, 20, 24, 28, 32, 36, 40, 44, 48, 52 (end of treatment visit) and Week 56 (follow-up visit)

Outcome measure	Measure description	Time frame
OLE: severity of ocular TEAEs	The severity of ocular treatment-emergent adverse events (TEAEs)	Assessed at Weeks 68, 84, 100, 116, 132, 148, 152, and Week 160 (end of treatment visit)
Double-masked period: best corrected visual Acuity (BCVA)	Double-masked period: best corrected visual acuity (BCVA) using the early treatment diabetic retinopathy study (ETDRS) scale by visit. ETDRS charts present a series of five letters of equal difficulty on each row, with standardized spacing between letters and rows; there is a total of 14 lines (70 letters), with letter size increasing further geometrically and equivalently in every line by a factor of 1.2589 (or 0.1 log unit), moving up the chart. Minimum score of zero, maximum score of 100. Change from baseline: a more negative score is a worse outcome, and a more positive score is better outcome. A lower score means less letters were read correctly (worse outcome), and a higher score means more letters were read correctly (better outcome)	Assessed at each visit: baseline, Day 5 Visit, Weeks 4, 8, 12, 16, 20, 24, 28, 32, 36, 40, 44, 48, 52 (end of treatment visit), and Week 56 (follow-up visit)
Open-label extension period: best corrected visual acuity (BCVA) using the using the early treatment diabetic retinopathy study (ETDRS) scale	Open-label extension period: best corrected visual acuity (BCVA) using the using the early treatment diabetic retinopathy study (ETDRS) scale by visit. ETDRS charts present a series of five letters of equal difficulty on each row, with standardized spacing between letters and rows; there is a total of 14 lines (70 letters), with letter size increasing further geometrically and equivalently in every line by a factor of 1.2589 (or 0.1 log unit), moving up the chart. Minimum score of 0, maximum score of 100. Change from baseline: a more negative score is a worse outcome, and a more positive score is better outcome. A lower score means less letters were read correctly (worse outcome), and a higher score means more letters were read correctly (better outcome)	Assessed at each visit from baseline from Week 68 to Week 160 (follow-up visit)

Secondary outcome measures

Outcome measure	Measure description	Time frame
Double-masked period: photopic negative response electroreti-nography (PhNR-ERG) A-wave amplitude	Change from baseline in photopic negative response electroretinography (PhNR-ERG) a-wave amplitude by visit. Photopic negative response electroretinography (PhNR-ERG) assesses retinal cell function. A decrease in the amplitude of the a-wave is associated with worse outcomes. Change from baseline in a-wave amplitude: a more positive number equals a decrease in amplitude, and therefore, a worse outcome, a more negative number means a better outcome	Assessed at each visit from baseline to Week 56 (follow-up visit), except for Day 5 visit
Open-label extension period: photopic negative response electroreti-nography (PhNR-ERG) A-wave amplitude	Change from baseline in photopic negative response electroretinography (PhNR-ERG) a-wave amplitude by visit. Photopic negative response electroretinography (PhNR-ERG) assesses retinal cell function. A decrease in the amplitude of the a-wave is associated with worse outcomes. Change from baseline in a-wave amplitude: a more positive number equals a decrease in amplitude, and therefore, a worse outcome, a more negative number means a better outcome	Assessed at each visit from baseline from Week 68 to Week 160
Double-masked period: photopic negative response electroreti-nography (PhNR-ERG) B-wave amplitude	Change from baseline in photopic negative response electroretinography (PhNR-ERG) b-wave amplitude by visit. Photopic negative response electroretinography (PhNR-ERG) assesses retinal cell function. A decrease in the amplitude of the b-wave is associated with worse outcomes. Change from baseline in b-wave amplitude: a more negative number equals a decrease in amplitude, and therefore, a worse outcome, a more positive number means a better outcome	Assessed at each visit from baseline to Week 56 (follow-up visit), except for Day 5 visit
Open-label extension period: PhNR-ERG B-wave amplitude	Change from baseline in photopic negative response electroretinography (PhNR-ERG) b-wave amplitude by visit. Photopic negative response electroretinography (PhNR-ERG) assesses retinal cell function. A decrease in the amplitude of the b-wave is associated with worse outcomes. Change from baseline in b-wave amplitude: a more negative number equals a decrease in amplitude, and therefore, a worse outcome, a more positive number means a better outcome	Assessed at each visit from baseline from Week 68 to Week 160
Double-masked period: PhNR amplitude	Double-masked period: change from baseline in PhNR amplitude by visit. Photopic negative response electroretinography (PhNR-ERG) assesses retinal cell function. A decrease in PhNR amplitude means worse outcome. Change from baseline: a more negative number means a better outcome, and a more positive number means a worse outcome	Assessed at each visit from baseline to Week 56 (follow-up visit), except for Day 5 visit

Outcome measure	Measure description	Time frame
Open-label extension period: PhNR amplitude	Open-label extension period: change from baseline in PhNR amplitude by Visit. Photopic negative response electroretinography (PhNR-ERG) assesses retinal cell function. A decrease in PhNR amplitude means worse outcome. Change from baseline: a more negative number means a better outcome, and a more positive number means a worse outcome	Assessed at each visit from baseline from Week 68 to Week 160
Double-masked period: PhNR/B-wave amplitude ratio	Double-masked period: change from baseline in PhNR/b-wave amplitude ratio by visit. Photopic negative response electroretinography (PhNR) assesses retinal cell function. A decrease in PhNR amplitude means worse outcome	Assessed at each visit from baseline to Week 56 (follow-up visit), except for Day 5 visit
Open-label extension period: change from baseline by visit PhNR/b wave amplitude ratio	Open-label extension period: change from baseline by visit PhNR/b wave amplitude ratio by visit. A reduced amplitude ratio equals a worse outcome	Assessed at each visit from baseline from Week 68 to Week 160
Double-masked period: change from baseline by visit PhNR peak to trough adjusted for A-wave amplitude	Double-masked period: change from baseline by visit in PhNR peak to trough adjusted for a-wave amplitude by visit. Calculated as (b-wave amplitude - PhNR amplitude)/a-wave amplitude. A reduced amplitude ratio equals aworse outcome	Assessed at each visit from baseline to Week 56 (follow-up visit), except for Day 5 visit
Open-label extension period: change from baseline by visit PhNR peak to trough adjusted for A-wave amplitude	Open-label extension period: change from baseline by visit in PhNR peak to trough adjusted for a-wave amplitude by visit. [Calculated by b-wave amplitude – PhNR amplitude)/a-wave amplitude.] Photopic negative response electroretinography (PhNR-ERG) assesses retinal cell function. A decrease in the amplitude of the a-wave is associated with worse outcomes. A reduced amplitude ratio equals a worse outcome	Assessed at each visit from baseline from Week 68 to Week 160
Double-masked period: PhNR peak to trough amplitude (unadjusted) from baseline	Double-masked period: change from baseline in PhNR Peak to trough amplitude (unadjusted) by visit. Calculated as b-wave amplitude – PhNR amplitude. Photopic negative response electroretinography (PhNR-ERG) assesses retinal cell function. A decrease in amplitude is associated with worse outcomes	Assessed at each visit from baseline to Week 56 (follow-up visit), except for Day 5 visit
Open-label extension period: PhNR peak to trough amplitude (unadjusted)	Open-label extension period: change from baseline in PhNR peak to trough amplitude (unadjusted) by visit. b-wave amplitude – PhNR amplitude. Photopic negative response electroretinography (PhNR-ERG) assesses retinal cell function. A decrease in the amplitude of the a-wave is associated with worse outcomes	Assessed at each visit from baseline from Week 68 to Week 160

Outcome measure	Measure description	Time frame
Double-masked: VFQ-39 composite	Double-masked: change from baseline in visual function questionnaire (VFQ-39) composite score by visit. National Eye Institute VFQ-39 measures health-related quality of life in 12 domains: general vision, ocular pain, near activities, distance activities, vision-specific social functioning, vision-specific mental health, vision-specific role difficulties, vision-specific dependency, driving, color vision, peripheral vision, and composite score. For each domain, the lowest and highest possible scores are 0 and 100 points, respectively. Higher score means higher functioning. Scores represent the achieved percentage of the total possible score, e.g. a score of 50 represents 50% of the highest possible score. For the composite score, the vision-targeted sub-scale scores are averaged, excluding the general health questions. Domain scores from each cohort are averaged, and the change from baseline per domain is calculated	Assessed at baseline, Week 52 (end-of-treatment visit) and Week 56 (follow-up visit)
Open-label extension period: VFQ-39 composite score	Change from baseline in visual function questionnaire (VFQ-39) composite score. National Eye Institute VFQ-39 measures health-related quality of life in 12 domains: general vision, ocular pain, near activities, distance activities, vision-specific social functioning, vision-specific mental health, vision-specific role difficulties, vision-specific dependency, driving, color vision, peripheral vision, and composite score. For each domain: the lowest and highest possible scores are 0 and 100 points, respectively. Higher score means higher functioning. Scores represent the achieved percentage of the total possible score, e.g. a score of 50 represents 50% of the highest possible score. For the composite score, the vision-targeted sub-scale scores are averaged, excluding the general health questions. Domain scores from each cohort are averaged, and the change from baseline per domain is calculated	Assessed at baseline, Week 160 (end of OLE period)
Open-label extension period: VFQ-39 general health score	Change from baseline in visual function questionnaire (VFQ-39) general health score. National Eye Institute VFQ-39 score measures the health-related quality of life of subjects with visual impairment, in 12 domains: general vision, ocular pain, near activities, distance activities, vision-specific social functioning, vision-specific mental health, vision-specific role difficulties, vision-specific dependency, driving, color vision, and peripheral vision and 1 composite score. Each domain is converted to a 0–100 scale; the lowest and highest possible scores are set at 0 and 100 points, respectively. Higher score means higher functioning. Scores represent the achieved percentage of the total possible score, e.g. a score of 50 represents 50% of the highest possible score. For the composite score, the vision-targeted sub-scale scores are averaged, excluding the general health questions. Domain scores from each cohort are averaged, and the change from baseline per domain is calculated	Assessed at baseline, Week 160 (end of OLE period)

Outcome measure	Measure description	Time frame
Double-masked: VFQ-39 general vision score	Change from baseline in VFQ-39 general vision score. National Eye Institute VFQ-39 score measures the health-related quality of life of subjects with visual impairment, in 12 domains: general vision, ocular pain, near activities, distance activities, vision-specific social functioning, vision-specific mental health, vision-specific role difficulties, vision-specific dependency, driving, color vision, and peripheral vision and 1 composite score. Each domain is converted to a 0–100 scale; the lowest and highest possible scores are set at 0 and 100 points, respectively. Higher score means higher functioning. Scores represent the achieved percentage of the total possible score, e.g. a score of 50 represents 50% of the highest possible score. For the composite score, the vision-targeted sub-scale scores are averaged, excluding the general health questions. Domain scores from each cohort are averaged, and the change from baseline per domain is calculated	Assessed at baseline, Week 52 (end-of-treatment visit) and Week 56 (follow-up visit)
Open-label extension period: VFQ-39 general vision score	Change from baseline in VFQ-39 general vision score. National Eye Institute VFQ-39 score measures the health-related quality of life of subjects with visual impairment, in 12 domains: general vision, ocular pain, near activities, distance activities, vision-specific social functioning, vision-specific mental health, vision-specific role difficulties, vision-specific dependency, driving, color vision, and peripheral vision and 1 composite score. Each domain is converted to a 0–100 scale; the lowest and highest possible scores are set at 0 and 100 points, respectively. Higher score means higher functioning. Scores represent the achieved percentage of the total possible score, e.g. a score of 50 represents 50% of the highest possible score. For the composite score, the vision-targeted sub-scale scores are averaged, excluding the general health questions. Domain scores from each cohort are averaged, and the change from baseline per domain is calculated	Assessed at baseline, Week 160 (end of OLE period)
Double-masked: VFQ-39 ocular pain score	Change from baseline in VFQ-39 ocular pain score. National Eye Institute VFQ-39 measures health-related quality of life in 12 domains: general vision, ocular pain, near activities, distance activities, vision-specific social functioning, vision-specific mental health, vision-specific role difficulties, vision-specific dependency, driving, color vision, peripheral vision, and composite score. For each domain: the lowest and highest possible scores are 0 and 100 points, respectively. Higher score means higher functioning. Scores represent the achieved percentage of the total possible score, e.g. a score of 50 represents 50% of the highest possible score. For the composite score, the vision-targeted sub-scale scores are averaged, excluding the general health questions. Domain scores from each cohort are averaged, and the change from baseline per domain is calculated	Assessed at baseline, Week 52 (end-of-treatment visit) and Week 56 (follow-up visit)

Outcome measure	Measure description	Time frame
Open-label extension period: VFQ-39 ocular pain score	Change from baseline in VFQ-39 ocular pain score by visit. National Eye Institute VFQ-39 measures health-related quality of life in 12 domains: general vision, ocular pain, near activities, distance activities, vision-specific social functioning, vision-specific mental health, vision-specific role difficulties, vision-specific dependency, driving, color vision, peripheral vision, and composite score. For each domain, the lowest and highest possible scores are 0 and 100 points, respectively. Higher score means higher functioning. Scores represent the achieved percentage of the total possible score, e.g. a score of 50 represents 50% of the highest possible score. For the composite score, the vision-targeted sub-scale scores are averaged, excluding the general health questions. Domain scores from each cohort are averaged, and the change from baseline per domain is calculated	Assessed at baseline, Week 160 (end of OLE period)
Double-masked: VFQ-39 near activities score	Change from baseline in VFQ-39 near activities score from baseline. National Eye Institute VFQ-39 measures health-related quality of life in 12 domains: general vision, ocular pain, near activities, distance activities, vision-specific social functioning, vision-specific mental health, vision-specific role difficulties, vision-specific dependency, driving, color vision, peripheral vision, and composite score. For each domain, the lowest and highest possible scores are 0 and 100 points, respectively. Higher score means higher functioning. Scores represent the achieved percentage of the total possible score, e.g. a score of 50 represents 50% of the highest possible score. For the composite score, the vision-targeted sub-scale scores are averaged, excluding the general health questions. Domain scores from each cohort are averaged, and the change from baseline per domain is calculated	Assessed at baseline, Week 52 (end-of-treatment visit) and Week 56 (follow-up visit)
Open-label extension period: VFQ-39 near activities	Change from baseline in visual function questionnaire (VFQ-39) near activities score. National Eye Institute VFQ-39 score measures the health-related quality of life of subjects with visual impairment, in 12 domains: general vision, ocular pain, near activities, distance activities, vision-specific social functioning, vision-specific mental health, vision-specific role difficulties, vision-specific dependency, driving, color vision, and peripheral vision and 1 composite score. Each domain is converted to a 0–100 scale; score ranges from 0 and 100 points, respectively. Higher score means higher functioning. Scores represent the achieved percentage of the total possible score, e.g. a score of 50 represents 50% of the highest possible score. For the composite score, the vision-targeted sub-scale scores are averaged, excluding the general health questions. Domain scores from each cohort are averaged, and the change from baseline per domain is calculated	Assessed at baseline, Week 160 (end of OLE period)

Outcome measure	Measure description	Time frame
Double-masked period: mean retinal nerve fiber (RNFL) layer thickness	Change from baseline in retinal nerve fiber layer thickness by spectral domain optical coherence tomography (SD-OCT). RNFL measures the loss of retinal ganglion cell axons. RNFL thickness decreases as disease progresses. A positive number, or, absence of change from baseline reflects a good clinical outcome, a negative number reflects loss of thickness, or a bad outcome	Assessed at baseline and Week 52 (end-of-treatment visit)
Open-label extension period: retinal nerve fiber layer thickness	Open-label extension period: change from baseline in retinal nerve fiber layer thickness by SD-OCT by visit. Change from baseline in retinal nerve fiber layer thickness by spectral domain optical coherence tomography (SD-OCT). RNFL measures the loss of retinal ganglion cell axons. RNFL thickness decreases as the disease progresses. A positive number, or, absence of change from baseline reflects a good clinical outcome, a negative number reflects loss of thickness or a bad outcome	Assessed at baseline, Week 148
Double-masked period: visual field mean deviation as measured by Humphrey automated visual field testing stimulus III	Change from baseline in visual field mean deviation (MD) as measured by Humphrey automated visual field testing stimulus III by visit. The Humphrey visual field test measures the entire area of peripheral vision that can be seen while the eye is focused on a central point. Mean deviation (MD) is the mean deviation in the patient's results compared to those expected from the age-matched normative database. Lower/more negative scores mean worse outcome, higher/more positive score means better outcome	Assessed at each visit from baseline to Week 56 (follow-up visit), except for Day 5 visit
Open-label extension period: visual field mean deviation (dB) measured by Humphrey from baseline	Change from baseline in visual field mean deviation (MD) as measured by Humphrey automated visual field testing stimulus III by visit. The Humphrey visual field test measures the entire area of peripheral vision that can be seen while the eye is focused on a central point. Mean deviation (MD) is the mean deviation in the patient's results compared to those expected from the age-matched normative database. Lower/More negative scores mean worse outcome, and higher/more positive score means better outcome	Assessed at each visit from baseline from Week 68 to Week 160
Double-masked period: color discrimination—number of plates	Double-masked period: change from baseline in color discrimination—number of plates from baseline by a visit by Ishihara test. Score range: 0–38. Higher number equals better color discrimination equals better outcome. Lower number equals worse color discrimination equals worse outcome	Assessed at each visit from baseline to Week 56 (follow-up visit)
Open-label extension period: change from baseline in color discrimination—number of plates by visit	Open-label extension period: change from baseline in color discrimination—number of plates from baseline by a visit by Ishihara test. Score range: 0–38. Higher number equals better color discrimination equals better outcome. Lower number equals worse color discrimination equals worse outcome	Assessed at each visit from baseline from Week 68 to Week 160

Outcome measure	Measure description	Time frame
Double-masked period: change from baseline in contrast sensitivity by Pelli-Robson contrast sensitivity chart by visit	Letters are arranged on a 60 × 85 cm chart in sets of triplets which contain the same contrast, decreasing in log 10 contrast from top to bottom and left to right as the participant progresses from one triplet to the other. Each group of three letters is decreased in contrast by a factor of 0.71 ($1/\sqrt{2}$) (log contrast 0.15) of the proceeding set. Participant reads letters, starting with the highest contrast, until unable to read letters in a single group. Score is based on the contrast of the last group read correctly. The size of the letters on the chart subtend 0.5° at 3 m, The test is scored in LogCS units, where each set of triplets advances in steps of 0.15 log units ranging from LogCS of 0.00 (approx. 100% contrast) to LogCS 2.25 (approx. 0.56% contrast). Change from baseline: the more negative the number means poor outcome, the more positive the number means better outcome	Assessed at each visit from baseline to Week 56 (follow-up visit)
Open-label extension period: change from baseline in contrast sensitivity by visit	Letters are arranged on a 60 × 85 cm chart in sets of triplets which contain the same contrast, decreasing in log10 contrast from top to bottom and left to right as the participant progresses from one triplet to the other. Each group of three letters is decreased in contrast by a factor of 0.71 ($1/\sqrt{2}$) (log contrast 0.15) of the proceeding set. Participant reads letters, starting with highest contrast, until unable to read letters in a single group. Score is based on the contrast of the last group read correctly. The size of the letters on the chart subtend 0.5° at 3 m, The test is scored in LogCS units, where each set of triplets advances in steps of 0.15 log units ranging from LogCS of 0.00 (approx. 100% contrast) to LogCS 2.25 (approx. 0.56% contrast). Change from baseline: the more negative the number means poor outcome, the more positive the number means better outcome	Assessed at each visit from baseline from Week 68 to Week 160
Double-masked change from baseline in retinal ganglion cell layer thickness	Change from baseline in retinal ganglion cell layer thickness by SD-OCT from baseline by visit	Assessed at baseline and Week 52 (end-of-treatment visit)
Open-label extension period: change from baseline in retinal ganglion cell layer thickness	Open-label extension period: change from baseline in retinal ganglion cell layer thickness by SD-OCT by SD-OCT by visit	Assessed at baseline, Week 148

Outcome measure	Measure description	Time frame
Double-masked: VFQ-39 distance activities score	Change from baseline in visual function questionnaire (VFQ-39) distance activities score. National Eye Institute VFQ-39 score measures the health-related quality of life of subjects with visual impairment, in 12 domains: general vision, ocular pain, near activities, distance activities, vision-specific social functioning, vision-specific mental health, vision-specific role difficulties, vision-specific dependency, driving, color vision, and peripheral vision and 1 composite score. Each domain is converted to a 0–100 scale; the lowest and highest possible scores are set at 0 and 100 points, respectively. Higher score means higher functioning. Scores represent the achieved percentage of the total possible score, e.g. a score of 50 represents 50% of the highest possible score. For the composite score, the vision-targeted sub-scale scores are averaged, excluding the general health questions. Domain scores from each cohort are averaged, and the change from baseline per domain is calculated	Assessed at baseline, Week 52 (end-of-treatment visit), and Week 56 (follow-up visit)
Open-label extension period: VFQ-39 distance activities score	Change in visual function questionnaire (VFQ-39) distance activities score. National Eye Institute VFQ-39 score measures the health-related quality of life of subjects with visual impairment, in 12 domains: general vision, ocular pain, near activities, distance activities, vision-specific social functioning, vision-specific mental health, vision-specific role difficulties, vision-specific dependency, driving, color vision, and peripheral vision and 1 composite score. Each domain is converted to a 0–100 scale; the lowest and highest possible scores are set at 0 and 100 points, respectively. Higher score means higher functioning. Scores represent the achieved percentage of the total possible score, e.g. a score of 50 represents 50% of the highest possible score. For the composite score, the vision-targeted sub-scale scores are averaged, excluding the general health questions. Domain scores from each cohort are averaged, and the change from baseline per domain is calculated	Assessed at baseline, Week 160 (end of OLE period)

Outcome measure	Measure description	Time frame
Open-label extension period: VFQ-39 social functioning score	Change from baseline in visual function questionnaire (VFQ-39) social functioning score. National Eye Institute VFQ-39 score measures the health-related quality of life of subjects with visual impairment, in 12 domains: general vision, ocular pain, near activities, distance activities, vision-specific social functioning, vision-specific mental health, vision-specific role difficulties, vision-specific dependency, driving, color vision, and peripheral vision and 1 composite score. Each domain is converted to a 0–100 scale; the lowest and highest possible scores are set at 0 and 100 points, respectively. Higher score means higher functioning. Scores represent the achieved percentage of the total possible score, e.g. a score of 50 represents 50% of the highest possible score. For the composite score, the vision-targeted sub-scale scores are averaged, excluding the general health questions. Domain scores from each cohort are averaged and, the change from baseline per domain is calculated	Assessed at baseline, Week 160 (end of OLE period)
Double-masked: VFQ-39 social functioning score	Change from baseline in visual function questionnaire (VFQ-39) social functioning score. National Eye Institute VFQ-39 score measures the health-related quality of life of subjects with visual impairment, in 12 domains: general vision, ocular pain, near activities, distance activities, vision-specific social functioning, vision-specific mental health, vision-specific role difficulties, vision-specific dependency, driving, color vision, and peripheral vision and 1 composite score. Each domain is converted to a 0–100 scale; the lowest and highest possible scores are set at 0 and 100 points, respectively. Higher score means higher functioning. Scores represent the achieved percentage of the total possible score, e.g. a score of 50 represents 50% of the highest possible score. For the composite score, the vision-targeted sub-scale scores are averaged, excluding the general health questions. Domain scores from each cohort are averaged, and the change from baseline per domain is calculated	Assessed at baseline, Week 52 (end-of-treatment visit), and Week 56 (follow-up visit)

Outcome measure	Measure description	Time frame
Double-masked: VFQ-39 mental health score	Change from baseline in visual function questionnaire (VFQ-39) mental health score. National Eye Institute VFQ-39 score measures the health-related quality of life of subjects with visual impairment, in 12 domains: general vision, ocular pain, near activities, distance activities, vision-specific social functioning, vision-specific mental health, vision-specific role difficulties, vision-specific dependency, driving, color vision, and peripheral vision and 1 composite score. Each domain is converted to a 0–100 scale; the lowest and highest possible scores are set at 0 and 100 points, respectively. Higher score means higher functioning. Scores represent the achieved percentage of the total possible score, e.g. a score of 50 represents 50% of the highest possible score. For the composite score, the vision-targeted sub-scale scores are averaged, excluding the general health questions. Domain scores from each cohort are averaged, and the change from baseline per domain is calculated	Assessed at baseline, Week 52 (end-of-treatment visit), and Week 56 (follow-up visit)
Open-label extension period: VFQ-39 mental health score	Change from baseline in visual function questionnaire (VFQ-39) mental health score. National Eye Institute VFQ-39 score measures the health-related quality of life of subjects with visual impairment, in 12 domains: general vision, ocular pain, near activities, distance activities, vision-specific social functioning, vision-specific mental health, vision-specific role difficulties, vision-specific dependency, driving, color vision, and peripheral vision and 1 composite score. Each domain is converted to a 0–100 scale; the lowest and highest possible scores are set at 0 and 100 points, respectively. Higher score means higher functioning. Scores represent the achieved percentage of the total possible score, e.g. a score of 50 represents 50% of the highest possible score. For the composite score, the vision-targeted sub-scale scores are averaged, excluding the general health questions. Domain scores from each cohort are averaged, and the change from baseline per domain is calculated	Assessed at baseline, Week 160 (end of OLE Period)

Outcome measure	Measure description	Time frame
Double-masked: VFQ-39 role difficulties score	Change from baseline in visual function questionnaire (VFQ-39) role difficulties score National Eye Institute VFQ-39 score measures health-related quality of life of subjects with visual impairment, in 12 domains: general vision, ocular pain, near activities, distance activities, vision-specific social functioning, vision-specific mental health, vision-specific role difficulties, vision-specific dependency, driving, color vision, and peripheral vision and 1 composite score. Each domain is converted to a 0–100 scale; the lowest and highest possible scores are set at 0 and 100 points, respectively. Higher score means higher functioning. Scores represent the achieved percentage of the total possible score, e.g. a score of 50 represents 50% of the highest possible score. For the composite score, the vision-targeted sub-scale scores are averaged, excluding the general health questions. Domain scores from each cohort are averaged, and the change from baseline per domain is calculated	Assessed at baseline, Week 52 (end-of-treatment visit), and Week 56 (follow-up visit)
Open-label extension period: VFQ-39 role difficulties score	Change from baseline in visual function questionnaire (VFQ-39) role difficulties score. National Eye Institute VFQ-39 score measures the health-related quality of life of subjects with visual impairment, in 12 domains: general vision, ocular pain, near activities, distance activities, vision-specific social functioning, vision-specific mental health, vision-specific role difficulties, vision-specific dependency, driving, color vision, and peripheral vision and 1 composite score. Each domain is converted to a 0–100 scale; the lowest and highest possible scores are set at 0 and 100 points, respectively. Higher score means higher functioning. Scores represent the achieved percentage of the total possible score, e.g. a score of 50 represents 50% of the highest possible score. For the composite score, the vision-targeted sub-scale scores are averaged, excluding the general health questions. Domain scores from each cohort are averaged, and the change from baseline per domain is calculated	Assessed at baseline, Week 160 (end of OLE period)

Outcome measure	Measure description	Time frame
Open-label extension period: VFQ-39 dependency score	Change from baseline in visual function questionnaire (VFQ-39) dependency score. National Eye Institute VFQ-39 score measures the health-related quality of life of subjects with visual impairment, in 12 domains: general vision, ocular pain, near activities, distance activities, vision-specific social functioning, vision-specific mental health, vision-specific role difficulties, vision-specific dependency, driving, color vision, and peripheral vision and 1 composite score. Each domain is converted to a 0–100 scale; the lowest and highest possible scores are set at 0 and 100 points, respectively. Higher score means higher functioning. Scores represent the achieved percentage of the total possible score, e.g. a score of 50 represents 50% of the highest possible score. For the composite score, the vision-targeted sub-scale scores are averaged, excluding the general health questions. Domain scores from each cohort are averaged, and the change from baseline per domain is calculated	Assessed at baseline, Week 160 (end of OLE Period)
Double-masked: VFQ-39 dependency score	Change from baseline in visual function questionnaire (VFQ-39) dependency score. National Eye Institute VFQ-39 score measures the health-related quality of life of subjects with visual impairment, in 12 domains: general vision, ocular pain, near activities, distance activities, vision-specific social functioning, vision-specific mental health, vision-specific role difficulties, vision-specific dependency, driving, color vision, and peripheral vision and 1 composite score. Each domain is converted to a 0–100 scale; the lowest and highest possible scores are set at 0 and 100 points, respectively. Higher score means higher functioning. Scores represent the achieved percentage of the total possible score, e.g. a score of 50 represents 50% of the highest possible score. For the composite score, the vision-targeted sub-scale scores are averaged, excluding the general health questions. Domain scores from each cohort are averaged, and the change from baseline per domain is calculated	Assessed at baseline, Week 52 (end-of-treatment visit), and Week 56 (follow-up visit)

Outcome measure	Measure description	Time frame
Double-masked: VFQ-39 color vision score	Change from baseline in visual function questionnaire (VFQ-39) color vision score. National Eye Institute VFQ-39 score measures the health-related quality of life of subjects with visual impairment, in 12 domains: general vision, ocular pain, near activities, distance activities, vision-specific social functioning, vision-specific mental health, vision-specific role difficulties, vision-specific dependency, driving, color vision, and peripheral vision and 1 composite score. Each domain is converted to a 0–100 scale; the lowest and highest possible scores are set at 0 and 100 points, respectively. Higher score means higher functioning. Scores represent the achieved percentage of the total possible score, e.g. a score of 50 represents 50% of the highest possible score. For the composite score, the vision-targeted sub-scale scores are averaged, excluding the general health questions. Domain scores from each cohort are averaged, and the change from baseline per domain is calculated	Assessed at baseline, Week 52 (end-of-treatment visit), and Week 56 (follow-up visit)
Open-label extension period: VFQ-39 color vision score	Change from baseline in visual function questionnaire (VFQ-39) color vision score. National Eye Institute VFQ-39 score measures the health-related quality of life of subjects with visual impairment, in 12 domains: general vision, ocular pain, near activities, distance activities, vision-specific social functioning, vision-specific mental health, vision-specific role difficulties, vision-specific dependency, driving, color vision, and peripheral vision and 1 composite score. Each domain is converted to a 0–100 scale; the lowest and highest possible scores are set at 0 and 100 points, respectively. Higher score means higher functioning. Scores represent the achieved percentage of the total possible score, e.g. a score of 50 represents 50% of the highest possible score. For the composite score, the vision-targeted sub-scale scores are averaged, excluding the general health questions. Domain scores from each cohort are averaged, and the change from baseline per domain is calculated	Assessed at baseline, Week 160 (end of OLE Period)

Outcome measure	Measure description	Time frame
Double-Masked: VFQ-39 peripheral score	Change from baseline in visual function questionnaire (VFQ-39) peripheral score. National Eye Institute VFQ-39 score measures the health-related quality of life of subjects with visual impairment, in 12 domains: general vision, ocular pain, near activities, distance activities, vision-specific social functioning, vision-specific mental health, vision-specific role difficulties, vision-specific dependency, driving, color vision, and peripheral vision and 1 composite score. Each domain is converted to a 0–100 scale; the lowest and highest possible scores are set at 0 and 100 points, respectively. Higher score means higher functioning. Scores represent the achieved percentage of the total possible score, e.g. a score of 50 represents 50% of the highest possible score. For the composite score, the vision-targeted sub-scale scores are averaged, excluding the general health questions. Domain scores from each cohort are averaged, and the change from baseline per domain is calculated	Assessed at baseline, Week 52 (end-of-treatment visit), and Week 56 (follow-up visit)
Open--label extension period: visual function questionnaire (VFQ-39) peripheral score	Change from baseline in visual function questionnaire (VFQ-39) peripheral score. National Eye Institute VFQ-39 score measures the health-related quality of life of subjects with visual impairment, in 12 domains: general vision, ocular pain, near activities, distance activities, vision-specific social functioning, vision-specific mental health, vision-specific role difficulties, vision-specific dependency, driving, color vision, and peripheral vision and 1 composite score. Each domain is converted to a 0–100 scale; the lowest and highest possible scores are set at 0 and 100 points, respectively. Higher score means higher functioning. Scores represent the achieved percentage of the total possible score, e.g. a score of 50 represents 50% of the highest possible score. For the composite score, the vision-targeted sub-scale scores are averaged, excluding the general health questions. Domain scores from each cohort are averaged, and the change from baseline per domain is calculated	Assessed at baseline, Week 160 (end of OLE period)
Double-masked period: change in intraocular pressure (IOP)	Double-masked period: change in intraocular pressure (IOP) in mmHg from baseline by visit	Assessed at each visit: baseline, Day 5 visit, Weeks 4, 8, 12, 16, 20, 24, 28, 32, 36, 40, 44, 48, 52 (end of treatment visit), and Week 56 (follow-up visit)
Open-label extension period: intraocular pressure (IOP)	Change from baseline in intraocular pressure (IOP) in mmHg by visit	Assessed at baseline, Week 68, 84, 100, 116, 132, 148, 152, Week 160/ (end of treatment visit)

Outcome measure	Measure description	Time frame
OLE: slit lamp examination (SLE)-vehicle eye	Open-label extension: shift in slit lamp examination from baseline by visit: number of eyes that changed from normal or abnormal not clinically significant, to abnormal clinically significant for vehicle eyes	Assessed at baseline, Week 68, 84, 100, 116, 132, 148, 152, Week 160/ (end of treatment visit)
OLE: slit lamp examination (SLE)-elamipretide eye	Open-label extension: shift in slit lamp examination from baseline by visit: number of eyes that changed from normal or abnormal not clinically significant, to abnormal clinically significant for elamipretide eyes	Assessed at baseline, Week 68, 84, 100, 116, 132, 148, 152, Week 160/ (end of treatment visit)
Double-masked: slit lamp changes from baseline: vehicle eye and elamipretide eye	Incidence of change from normal or abnormal, clinically insignificant to normal clinically significant	Assessed at each visit: baseline, Day 5 visit, Weeks 4, 8, 12, 16, 20, 24, 28, 32, 36, 40, 44, 48, 52 (end of treatment visit), and Week 56 (follow-up visit)
Double-masked: dilated fundus changes from baseline: vehicle eye and elamipretide eyes	Double-masked: dilated fundus changes from baseline: vehicle eye and elamipretide eyes incidence of change from normal or abnormal-clinically insignificant, to normal clinically significant	Assessed at each visit: baseline, Day 5 Visit, Weeks 4, 8, 12, 16, 20, 24, 28, 32, 36, 40, 44, 48, 52 (end of treatment visit) and Week 56 (follow-up visit)
Open-label extension period: dilated fundus changes from baseline: vehicle eye and elamipretide eyes	Incidence of change from normal or abnormal-clinically insignificant, to normal clinically significant	Assessed at baseline, Week 68, 84, 100, 116, 132, 148, 152, Week 160/ (end of treatment visit)
Double-masked: VFQ-39 general health score	Change from baseline in visual function questionnaire (VFQ-39) general health score. National Eye Institute VFQ-39 score measures the health-related quality of life of subjects with visual impairment, in 12 domains: general vision, ocular pain, near activities, distance activities, vision-specific social functioning, vision-specific mental health, vision-specific role difficulties, vision-specific dependency, driving, color vision, and peripheral vision and 1 composite score. Each domain is converted to a 0–100 scale; the lowest and highest possible scores are set at 0 and 100 points, respectively. Higher score means higher functioning. Scores represent the achieved percentage of the total possible score, e.g. a score of 50 represents 50% of the highest possible score. For the composite score, the vision-targeted sub-scale scores are averaged, excluding the general health questions. Domain scores from each cohort are averaged, and the change from baseline per domain is calculated	Assessed at baseline, Week 52 (end-of-treatment visit), and Week 56 (follow-up visit)

Collaborators and Investigators
This is where you will find people and organizations involved with this study.

Sponsor
Stealth BioTherapeutics Inc.

Collaborators
No information provided

Investigators
- Principal Investigator: Alfredo Sadun, MD, PhD, University of California, Los Angeles

General Publications
No publications available

Teas Reported

Completed

Study to Assess the Efficacy and Safety of Raxone in LHON Patients (LEROS)

ClinicalTrials.gov ID NCT02774005

Sponsor Santhera Pharmaceuticals
Information provided by Santhera Pharmaceuticals (Responsible Party)
Last Update Posted 2023-04-21

Brief Summary
LEROS is an open-label interventional Phase IV study, designed to further assess the efficacy and safety of Raxone® in the long-term treatment of LHON patients.

Official Title
External Natural History Controlled, Open-Label Intervention Study to Assess the Efficacy and Safety of Long-Term Treatment With Raxone® in Leber's Hereditary Optic Neuropathy (LHON)

Conditions
Leber's Hereditary Optic Neuropathy (LHON)

Intervention/Treatment
- Drug: Idebenone

Other Study ID Numbers
- SNT-IV-005

Study Start
2016-05

Primary Completion (Actual)
2021-03-29

Study Completion (Actual)
2021-03-29

Enrollment (Actual)
199

Study Type
Interventional

Phase
Phase 4

United States
Arizona Locations

Phoenix, Arizona, United States
Retinal Consultants of Arizona

California Locations

Palo Alto, California, United States, 94040-2833
Palo Alto Medical Foundation

Stanford, California, United States, 94303
Stanford Byers Eye Institute

Colorado Locations

Aurora, Colorado, United States
University of Colorado Health Eye Center

Georgia Locations

Atlanta, Georgia, United States, 30322
Emory University Hospital

Maryland Locations

Bethesda, Maryland, United States
Bethesda Neurology, LLC

Missouri Locations

Saint Louis, Missouri, United States, 63110
Washington University

New York Locations

New York, New York, United States, 10003
New York Eye and Ear Infirmary

Virginia Locations

Charlottesville, Virginia, United States, 22903
University of Virginia

Austria

Wien, Austria
AKH - Medizinische Universitaet Wien

Belgium

Brussels, Belgium
CHU Saint-Pierre

Brussels, Belgium
Cliniques Universitaire Saint-Luc

Leuven, Belgium
UZ Leuven - Campus Sint-Rafaël

Liège, Belgium
C. H. U. Sart Tilman

Bulgaria

Sofia, Bulgaria
UMHAT "Alexandrovska" EAD

Germany

Muenchen, Germany
Friedrich-Baur-Institut

Italy

Bologna, Italy
Università di Bologna-Clinica Neurologica-Dipartimento di Scienze Neurologiche

Poland

Krakow, Poland, 31-501
SPZOZ Spital Uniwersytecki w Krakowie, Oddzial Kliniczny Okulistyki i Onkologii Okulistycznej

Poznań, Poland
Szpital Kliniczny Przemienienia Panskiego Uniwersytetu Medycznego im. Karola Marcinkowskiego

Szczecin, Poland
Samodzielny Publiczny Szpital Kliniczny Nr 2 PUM w Szczecinie

Warszawa, Poland
Samodzielny Publiczny Kliniczny Szpital Okulistyczny

Wrocław, Poland

Uniwersytecki Szpital Kliniczny

Portugal

Porto, Portugal
Centro Hospitalar de São João, EPE

Spain

Barcelona, Spain
Institut Catala de Retina

Madrid, Spain
Hospital Universitario Ramon y Cajal

United Kingdom

Cardiff, United Kingdom
University Hospital of Wales

London, United Kingdom
Moorfields Eye Hospital

Manchester, United Kingdom
Manchester Royal Eye Hospital

Romford, United Kingdom
Queen's Hospital

Eligibility Criteria
Description

Inclusion Criteria
- Impaired visual acuity in affected eyes due to LHON
- No explanation for visual loss besides LHON
- Age more or equal 12 years
- Onset of symptoms ≤5 years of Baseline
- Confirmation of either G11778A, G3460A or T14484C LHON mtDNA (for the Intent-to Treat (ITT) population, not required for enrolment)
- Written informed consent obtained from the patient
- Ability and willingness to comply with study procedures and visits
- Women of Childbearing Potential (WCBP) who have a negative urine or serum pregnancy test at Baseline visit and who are willing to use a highly effective contraceptive measure and maintain it until treatment discontinuation.

Exclusion Criteria
- Patient has provided natural history data to the Case Record Survey (SNT-CRS-002)
- Any previous use of idebenone
- Any other cause of visual impairment (e.g. glaucoma, diabetic retinopathy, AIDS-related visual impairment, cataract, macular degeneration, etc.) or any

active ocular disorder (uveitis, infections, inflammatory retinal disease, thyroid eye disease, etc.)
- Known history of clinically significant elevations (greater than three times the upper limit of normal) of aspartate aminotransferase (AST), alanine transaminase (ALT), or creatinine
- Patient has a condition or is in a situation which, in an investigator's opinion may put the patient at significant risk, may confound study results, or may interfere significantly with the patient's participation in the study
- Participation in another clinical trial of any investigational drug within 3 months prior to Baseline
- Hypersensitivity to the active substance or to any of the following excipients: Lactose monohydrate, Microcrystalline cellulose, Croscarmellose sodium, Povidone K25, Magnesium stearate, Colloidal silica, Macrogol 3350, Poly(vinyl alcohol), Talc, Titanium dioxide, Sunset yellow FCF (E110).
- Women who are pregnant or have a positive pregnancy test at Baseline visit
- Women who are breastfeeding

Ages Eligible for Study
12 Years and older (Child, Adult, Older Adult)

Sexes Eligible for Study
All

Accepts Healthy Volunteers
No

Design Details
Primary Purpose: Treatment
Allocation: N/A
Interventional Model: Single Group Assignment
Masking: None (Open Label)

Arms and interventions

Participant group/arm	Intervention/treatment
Experimental: raxone	Drug: idebenone • Other names: – Raxone

Primary outcome measures

Outcome measure	Measure description	Time frame
Proportion (number) of eyes with clinically relevant recovery of visual acuity from baseline	Proportion (number) of eyes with clinically relevant recovery of visual acuity (VA) from baseline or in which baseline VA better than 1.0 logMAR was maintained at month 12 in patients treated with Raxone® ≤1 year after the onset of symptoms, compared to matching external natural history control group	12 months

Secondary outcome measures

Outcome measure	Measure description	Time frame
Components of the primary endpoint: proportion of eyes with clinically relevant recovery (CRR) of VA from baseline at month 12 compared to matching external national history (NH) control group	CRR is defined as: • Improvement from "off-chart" (the equivalent of counting fingers, hand motion, light perception, or no light perception) visual acuity to at least 1.6 logMAR value, OR • Improvement of at least 0.2 logMAR value within "on-chart" visual acuity A patient had a CRR if at least one eye had CRR logMAR = logarithm of the minimum angle of resolution	12 months
Components of the primary endpoint: proportion of eyes in which baseline visual acuity (VA) better than 1.0 logMAR was maintained at month 12 (clinically relevant stabilization) compared to matching external NH control group	For the proportion of eyes in which baseline VA better than 1.0 logMAR was maintained at month 12 (CRS) compared to matching external NH control group only patients having VA <1.0 at baseline are taking into account Clinically relevant stabilization (CRS) was defined as maintenance of VA <1.0 logMAR in eyes with VA <1.0 logMAR at baseline A patient had a CRS if at least one eye had CRS logMAR = logarithm of the minimum angle of resolution	12 months

Sponsor
Santhera Pharmaceuticals

Collaborators
No information provided

Investigators
No information provided

General Publications
No publications available

Drug Efficacy Not Reported

Completed

Lipoic Acid as a Treatment for Acute Optic Neuritis

ClinicalTrials.gov ID NCT01294176

Sponsor Oregon Health and Science University
Information provided by Vijayshree Yadav, Oregon Health and Science University (Responsible Party)
Last Update Posted 2019-04-26

Brief Summary
The purpose of this study is to determine if oral lipoic acid can safely help relieve permanent optic nerve injury in patients diagnosed with acute optic neuritis. It will also explore how the body absorbs and breaks down the study drug, and what effects it has on the immune system.

Detailed Description
Oral lipoic acid is an antioxidant that helps proteins work in the body. It is available in oral and intravenous formulations and has been used in the past to treat nerve damage like that seen in diabetes and some other metabolic disorders. It is available as a dietary supplement in the United States.

Patients with a diagnosis of acute optic neuritis who are enrolled in the study will undergo medical and nervous system examinations, and blood draws. The study doctor will take a medical history and perform physical examinations. Research assistants at the MS Center, who are trained in blood draws, will perform the blood draws. Patients will also undergo Optical coherence tomography (OCT) examination at Casey Eye Institute and receive two MRIs at Oregon Health and Science University (OHSU). Because it is a placebo-controlled trial, subjects will have a 50:50 chance of receiving either placebo (inactive) or study drug. If enrolled in the study, patients will take two gel capsules of the study drug or placebo at the same time every day for 6 weeks.

Official Title
Lipoic Acid as a Treatment for Acute Optic Neuritis: A Pilot Study

Conditions
Optic Neuritis

Intervention/Treatment
- Drug: Lipoic Acid

Other Study ID Numbers
- OHSU IRB00005634

Study Start
2011-01

Primary Completion (Actual)
2016-11

Study Completion (Actual)
2016-11

Enrollment (Actual)
31

Study Type
Interventional

Phase
Phase 1

United States
Oregon Locations

Portland, Oregon, United States, 97239
Oregon Health & Science University

Eligibility Criteria
Description

Inclusion Criteria
- Diagnosis of acute, unilateral AON with visual symptoms (vision loss) of 14 days or less
- 18–65 years of age, inclusive
- AON as a first event (possibly idiopathic) or in relationship to clinically isolated syndrome or to MS according to McDonald criteria
- No previous history of optic neuritis or ophthalmoscopic signs of optic atrophy in the affected eye
- Subject is available for treatment initiation within 14 days of onset of AON symptoms

Exclusion Criteria
- Other causes of visual loss in the affected eye (e.g. amblyopia or glaucoma)
- OCT is non-evaluable at screening visit due to edema.
- AON symptoms improve before administration of study medication.
- Subject has fever or active infection at time of enrollment.
- Subject is pregnant or breastfeeding.
- Subject has diabetes mellitus.
- Subject has another significant health problem (e.g. active coronary heart disease, liver disease, significant pulmonary disease).

Ages Eligible for Study
18 Years to 65 Years (Adult, Older Adult)

Sexes Eligible for Study
All

Accepts Healthy Volunteers

No

Study Plan

Design Details

Primary Purpose: Treatment
Allocation: Randomized
Interventional Model: Parallel Assignment
Masking: Quadruple (Participant Care Provider Investigator Outcomes Assessor)

Arms and interventions

Participant group/arm	Intervention/treatment
Active comparator: oral lipoic acid Lipoic acid is a natural antioxidant available as an oral dietary supplement. A higher than average dose of 1200 mg will be administered in this trial	Drug: lipoic acid • Lipoic acid will be administered orally, in two 600 mg capsules, for a total 1200 mg dose. The dose will be administered daily for a 6-week treatment period
Placebo comparator: Avicel™ The placebo is Avicel™ (microcellulose crystal) and 4.3 mg quercetin (a bioflavanoid)	Drug: lipoic acid • Lipoic acid will be administered orally, in two 600 mg capsules, for a total 1200 mg dose. The dose will be administered daily for a 6-week treatment period

Primary outcome measures

Outcome measure	Measure description	Time frame
The primary outcome measure will be the difference from baseline in retinal nerve fiber layer (RNFL) thickness of the affected optic nerve, as determined by OCT, at 12 and 24 weeks post-LA treatment	Individual data will be assessed at the last study visit (6 months postbaseline). Group data cannot be assessed until all participants have exited the study. The time frame for final assessment of the primary outcome measure is dependent on how quickly the recruitment goal is met	Baseline, Week 24

Secondary outcome measures

Outcome measure	Measure description	Time frame
Secondary outcome measures to assess optic nerve injury will be changed from baseline in the RNFL thickness at Week 24, and changes from baseline in low- and high-contrast visual acuity, contrast sensitivity, and visual field changes at Weeks 12 and 24	Individual data will be assessed at the last study visit (6 months postbaseline). Group data cannot be assessed until all participants have exited the study. The time frame for final assessment of the primary outcome measure is dependent on how quickly the recruitment goal is met	Baseline, Week 24

Sponsor
Oregon Health and Science University

Collaborators
No information provided

Investigators
No information provided

General Publications
No publications available

No Results Posted

Completed

Single Oral Doses Study of Nerispirdine on Visual Function in Patients with Multiple Sclerosis

ClinicalTrials.gov ID NCT00772525

Sponsor Sanofi
Information provided by Sanofi (Responsible Party)
Last Update Posted 2016-02-26

Brief Summary
The primary objective of the study was to evaluate the effect of Nerispirdine (50 or 400 mg) and placebo given orally as a single dose once a week in a crossover design on the latency of Visual Evoked Potentials (VEP) P100 in optic nerves.

Secondary objectives included evaluation of the effect of Nerispirdine on VEP amplitude and other visual parameters including visual acuity and contrast, as well as evaluation of the safety and tolerability of Nerispirdine in patients with Multiple Sclerosis (MS).

Contrast sensitivity and visual acuity examinations (in addition to Optical Coherence Tomography [OCT] and VEPs) were needed during the screening period for defining etiologic relationships (if non-MS-related impairment) and for assessing the effect of treatment of age-related eye disease versus the MS-related vision impairment.

Detailed Description
The crossover design included 3 treatment periods 1 week apart and 6 treatment sequences. Study participation was to be 5 weeks.

Official Title

A Double-blind, Placebo-controlled, Randomized Crossover, Activity Study of Single Oral Doses of 50 and 400 mg Nerispirdine on Visual Function in Patients With Multiple Sclerosis

Conditions

Multiple Sclerosis
Optic Nerve
Neuritis

Intervention/Treatment

- Drug: Nerispirdine
- Drug: Placebo

Other Study ID Numbers

- ACT10573

Study Start

2008-09

Primary Completion (Actual)

2009-06

Study Completion (Actual)

2009-06

Enrollment (Actual)

31

Study Type

Interventional

Phase

Phase 2

United States
New Jersey Locations

Bridgewater, New Jersey, United States, 08807
Sanofi-Aventis Administrative Office

Eligibility Criteria
Description

Inclusion Criteria

- Clinically definite MS (McDonald criteria), which includes patients with remitting-relapsing, secondary progressive, progressive-relapsing, or primary progressive MS who have had a past history of Optic Neuritis.

Exclusion Criteria

- Multiple sclerosis exacerbation within 60 days of the Screening Visit and the relapse involved the visual fields or visual acuity
- No eye with appropriate degree of lesions for this study as defined by criteria based on degree of visual acuity deficit, refractive error, VEP P100 latency, and average retinal nerve fiber layer thickness as measured by Optical Coherence Tomography (OCT)
- Any MS-unrelated prior ophthalmological impairment (e.g., compressive, ischemic, toxic, or nutritional optic neuropathies, Leber's hereditary optic atrophy)
- Previously exposed to 3,4-diaminopyridine or 4-aminopyridine

The above information is not intended to contain all considerations relevant to a patient's potential participation in a clinical trial.

Ages Eligible for Study
18 Years and older (Adult, Older Adult)

Sexes Eligible for Study
All

Accepts Healthy Volunteers
No

Design Details
Primary Purpose: Treatment
Allocation: Randomized
Interventional Model: Crossover Assignment
Masking: Triple (Participant Care Provider Investigator)

Arms and interventions

Participant group/arm	Intervention/treatment
Experimental: sequence 1 Placebo, 1 day treatment period 1 50 mg nerispirdine, 1 day treatment period 2 400 mg nerispirdine, 1 day treatment period 3	Drug: nerispirdine • Form: tablet Route: oral • Other names: – HP184 Drug: placebo • Form: tablet Route: oral
Experimental: sequence 2 Placebo, 1 day treatment period 1 400 mg nerispirdine, 1 day treatment period 2 50 mg nerispirdine, 1 day treatment period 3	Drug: nerispirdine • Form: tablet Route: oral • Other names: – HP184 Drug: placebo • Form: tablet Route: oral

Participant group/arm	Intervention/treatment
Experimental: sequence 3 50 mg nerispirdine, 1 day treatment period 1 Placebo, 1 day treatment period 2 400 mg nerispirdine, 1 day treatment period 3	Drug: nerispirdine • Form: tablet Route: oral • Other names: – HP184 Drug: placebo • Form: tablet Route: oral
Experimental: sequence 4 50 mg nerispirdine, 1 day treatment period 1 400 mg nerispirdine, 1 day treatment period 2 Placebo, 1 day treatment period 3	Drug: nerispirdine • Form: tablet Route: oral • Other names: – HP184 Drug: placebo • Form: tablet Route: oral
Experimental: sequence 5 400 mg nerispirdine, 1 day treatment period 1 Placebo, 1 day treatment period 2 50 mg nerispirdine, 1 day treatment period 3	Drug: nerispirdine • Form: tablet Route: oral • Other names: – HP184 Drug: placebo • Form: tablet Route: oral
Experimental: sequence 6 400 mg nerispirdine, 1 day treatment period 1 50 mg nerispirdine, 1 day treatment period 2 Placebo, 1 day treatment period 3	Drug: nerispirdine • Form: tablet Route: oral • Other names: – HP184 Drug: placebo • Form: tablet Route: oral

Primary outcome measures

Outcome measure	Measure description	Time frame
Visual evoked potential (P100) latency		Pre-dose and post-dose of each treatment intake (3)

Secondary outcome measures

Outcome measure	Measure description	Time frame
Pelli-Robson contrast sensitivity score		Pre-dose and post-dose of each treatment intake (3)
Early treatment diabetic retinopathy study (EDTRS) visual acuity score		Pre-dose and post-dose of each treatment intake (3)
Visual evoked potential (VEP) amplitude		Pre-dose and post-dose of each treatment intake (3)

Sponsor
Sanofi

Collaborators
No information provided

Investigators
- Principal Investigator: Robert SERGOTT, MD, Wills Eye Institute, Thomas Jefferson University, Philadelphia Pennsylvania, USA

General Publications
No publications available

No Results Posted

Completed

Intravenous Immunoglobulin Therapy in Optic Neuritis

ClinicalTrials.gov ID NCT00000117

Sponsor National Eye Institute (NEI)
Information provided by National Eye Institute (NEI)
Last Update Posted 2009-09-17

Brief Summary
To determine whether high-dose intravenous immunoglobulin (IVIg) is more effective than placebo in restoring lost visual function (visual acuity) in optic neuritis (ON).

To determine the time course of recovery following IVIg administration. If the reports of IVIg-associated clinical improvement occurring within 3–6 months following treatment can be confirmed, this would provide indirect evidence that IVIg may promote central nervous system (CNS) remyelination in optic neuritis and multiple sclerosis (MS).

Detailed Description
Optic neuritis is the leading cause of transient, spontaneous, reversible visual loss in young adults. Characteristically, patients present with central visual loss that peaks within a few days and is often associated with eye pain. Visual loss may be complete. Spontaneous recovery usually begins within 4 weeks, and marked recovery occurs within 1–3 months in most patients. Although clinical improvement is the rule, not all patients recover fully, and many are left with residual symptoms. Although there are limited pathological studies in inflammatory ON, the pathological changes are thought to be virtually identical with those seen in MS, with disruption of the blood-nerve (brain) barrier; primary demyelination with axonal sparing; variable degrees of lymphocytic infiltration; an abundance of macrophages around

the inflammatory demyelination lesion; various degrees of remyelination; and, later, oligodendrocyte loss, axonal loss, and gliosis.

Remyelination by oligodendrocytes occurs early in the MS lesion, as documented by myelin sheaths that are abnormally thin relative to axon diameter. These thin myelin sheaths are often seen prominently at the edge of demyelinated plaques. A recent series of studies has shown that within weeks of the initial event, there is extensive oligodendrocyte regeneration and remyelination. These immature oligodendrocytes express a series of developmentally restricted antigens. This finding has been interpreted to suggest that the cells that repopulate the acute plaque and that affect remyelination are newly generated and not residual, mature oligodendrocytes. These observations support the possibility that factors that promote remyelination could be used to improve clinical recovery in ON and MS.

Work at the Mayo Clinic has shown that both immunoglobulin G (IgG) directed against spinal cord antigens and purified polyclonal mouse IgG administered systemically promote extensive remyelination in SJL mice chronically infected with Theiler's virus. In addition, tissue culture studies suggest that IgG directed against CNS components may promote oligodendroglial proliferation and differentiation. Thus, experimental evidence exists for the concept that immunoglobulins may stimulate the proliferation and differentiation of oligodendrocytes. It is possible that myelin components on the surface of oligodendrocytes could function as receptors or components of receptors. Antibodies could mimic endogenous ligands, thereby inducing the proliferation or differentiation of these cells.

In a preliminary, open-label pilot study of patients with chronic, steroid-unresponsive ON, Drs. van Engelen, Hommes, and colleagues suggested that improvement in visual recovery could be seen following IgG treatment in patients with chronic, stable ON. These encouraging but preliminary basic and clinical studies have prompted us to design a double-blind and placebo-controlled clinical trial of IVIg in patients with recently acquired but apparently permanent muscle paralysis from MS (NS31506) and to develop this NEI-funded ON study (U10EY1096301).

In this randomized, placebo-controlled, double-blind clinical trial, 60 patients were assigned to receive either IVIg or a placebo over a period of 3 months. In order to be eligible, patients who meet the inclusion criteria needed to have a stable loss of visual function (unchanged between the pre-enrollment screening visit and the enrollment visit). All patients were re-examined at 3, 6, 9, and 12 months, with the primary outcome being the impact of treatment on visual acuity at 6 months as determined by measurements on a retroilluminated Early Treatment Diabetic Retinopathy Study chart at 4 m.

One group of patients received 0.4 g/kg Gammimmune N intravenously daily for 5 days, and thereafter once a month for 3 months (total: 8 infusions). The other group of patients received infusions of 0.1% human serum albumin in 10% maltose (placebo) according to the identical protocol used for Gammimmune N.

The primary outcome measure was an improvement in Logmar visual acuity by an average of 0.2 at 6 months. The secondary outcome measures included change in visual acuity at 3, 9, and 12 months, as determined on a retroilluminated ETDRS chart at 4 m; change in visual fields at 6 and 12 months; change in visual evoked responses at 3, 6, and 12 months; and change in neurological examination (EDSS, FS, AI) at 3, 6, 9, and 12 months.

Conditions
Optic Neuritis

Intervention/Treatment
- Drug: Immunoglobulin

Other Study ID Numbers
- NEI-13

Study Start
1995-08

Primary Completion

Study Completion (Actual)
1997-12

Enrollment

Study Type
Interventional

Phase
Phase 3

United States
Minnesota Locations

Rochester, Minnesota, United States
Mayo Clinic, Department of Neurology

Rochester, Minnesota, United States
Mayo Clinic

Eligibility Criteria
Description

To be eligible, patients must have a history of one or more episodes of previous demyelinating optic neuritis occurring in the setting of classic, adult-onset definite MS (clinically definite or laboratory-supported definite MS, or cranial MRI changes consistent with MS). In most cases, the onset of MS will have occurred between the ages of 18 and 45. Patients must be younger than 50 years and must have apparently irreversible loss of visual acuity that meets the following criteria:

Visual acuity must be worse than 20/40 for at least 6 months. Patients must be able to read at least one letter on the 1-m eye chart. Patients with no light perception or hand movement vision only are not eligible.

The above level of visual dysfunction must be observed on at least two serial examinations (separated by at least 1 month) in the Department of Ophthalmology at the Mayo Clinic.

Optic disc pallor must be present.

Patients must have impairment in the affected eye(s) on perimetry consistent with optic nerve dysfunction and must have a visual field mean deviation of less than −4.00.

Patients must not have received ACTH or corticosteroids within the preceding 2 months.

Ages Eligible for Study
Up to 50 Years (Child, Adult)

Sexes Eligible for Study
All

Design Details
Primary Purpose: Treatment
Allocation: Randomized
Masking: Double

Arms and interventions

Intervention/treatment
Drug: immunoglobulin

Sponsor
National Eye Institute (NEI)

Collaborators
No information provided

Investigators
No information provided

General Publications
No publications available

No Results Posted

Completed

A Pilot Study of Mitoxantrone for the Treatment of Recurrent Neuromyelitis Optica (Devic's Disease)

ClinicalTrials.gov ID NCT00304291

Sponsor State University of New York at Buffalo
Information provided by Bianca Weinstock-Guttman, State University of New York at Buffalo (Responsible Party)
Last Update Posted 2020-12-28

Brief Summary

Neuromyelitis optica (NMO) is a severe demyelinating disease that selectively involves the optic nerves and the spinal cord but usually spares the brain. NMO is considered to have a B cell-induced pathogenesis. Mitoxantrone (MITO, Novantrone®), a synthetic anthracenedione approved for worsening relapsing-remitting multiple sclerosis (MS) and secondary progressive MS, has been shown to primarily suppress the humoral response. We conducted a prospective 2-year study to evaluate the benefit of MITO in five relapsing NMO patients.

Detailed Description

The treatment protocol consisted of monthly 12 mg/m^2 MITO intravenous infusions for 6 months followed by 3 additional treatments every 3 months. Neurological assessment including the determination of the Expanded Disability Status Scale (EDSS) score was performed every 3 months and during relapses. Orbital, brain, and spinal cord MRI was performed at baseline, 3, 6, 12, 18, and 24 months. Visual evoked potentials and ophthalmologic evaluations were performed at baseline and annually.

Official Title

A Pilot Study of Mitoxantrone for the Treatment of Recurrent Neuromyelitis Optica (Devic's Disease)

Conditions

Neuromyelitis Optica
Myelitis, Transverse
Demyelinating Autoimmune Diseases, CNS
Autoimmune Diseases of the Nervous System

Intervention/Treatment

- Drug: Mitoxantrone

Other Study ID Numbers

- JNI-NMO-101

Study Start

2001-08

Primary Completion

Study Completion

2004-05

Enrollment

5

Study Type

Interventional

Phase
Phase 4

United States
New York Locations

Buffalo, New York, United States, 14203
Baird Multiple Sclerosis Center

Eligibility Criteria
Description

Inclusion Criteria

- Recurrent longitudinal myelitis (>3 segments of spinal cord involvement by MRI) with or without recurrent ON (unilateral or bilateral) but with normal brain MRI.
- Patients with recurrent longitudinally extensive myelitis without optic neuritis have an underlying pathology and serology similar to NMO, and it is appropriate to consider this a form of NMO10.
- Cerebrospinal fluid required no intrathecal IgG synthesis or oligoclonal bands.
- Age was required to be 18–55 years.
- Extended Disability Status Score ≤7.

Exclusion Criteria

- Cardiac risk factors (e.g. history of congestive heart failure and left ventricular ejection fraction (LVEF) <50%
- Systemic diseases such as lupus, Sjogren's syndrome, anti-phospholipid antibody syndrome, sarcoidosis, rheumatoid arthritis, or vitamin B12 deficiency
- Previous treatment with mitoxantrone or anthracyclines

Ages Eligible for Study
18 Years to 55 Years (Adult)

Sexes Eligible for Study
All

Accepts Healthy Volunteers
No

Study Plan

Design Details
Primary Purpose: Treatment
Allocation: Non-Randomized
Interventional Model: Single Group Assignment
Masking: None (Open Label)

Arms and interventions

Intervention/treatment
Drug: mitoxantrone

Primary outcome measures

Outcome measure	Measure description	Time frame
Relapse rate		

Secondary outcome measures

Outcome measure	Measure description	Time frame
Safety		

Sponsor
State University of New York at Buffalo

Collaborators
- EMD Serono

Investigators
- Study Director: Bianca Weinstock-Guttman, M.D., Baird Multiple Sclerosis Center

General Publications
No publications available

No Results Posted

Completed

Efficacy and Safety Study of Satralizumab (SA237) as Add-On Therapy to Treat Participants with Neuromyelitis Optica (NMO) and NMO Spectrum Disorder (NMOSD)

ClinicalTrials.gov ID NCT02028884

Sponsor Hoffmann-La Roche
Information provided by Hoffmann-La Roche (Responsible Party)
Last Update Posted 2023-04-18

Brief Summary
The objective of this study was to evaluate the efficacy, safety, pharmacodynamic, pharmacokinetic, and immunogenic profiles of satralizumab, compared with placebo, in addition to baseline immunosuppressive treatment in participants with NMO and NMOSD.

Official Title

A Multicenter, Randomized, Addition to Baseline Treatment, Double-Blind, Placebo-Controlled, Phase 3 Study to Evaluate the Efficacy and Safety of Satralizumab (SA237) in Patients With Neuromyelitis Optica (NMO) and NMO Spectrum Disorder (NMOSD)

Conditions

Neuromyelitis Optica (NMO)
NMO Spectrum Disorder (NMOSD)

Intervention/Treatment

- Drug: Satralizumab
- Drug: Placebo
- Drug: Baseline Treatment

Other Study ID Numbers

- BN40898
- 2013-003752-21 (EudraCT Number)
- SA-307JG (Other Identifier) (Other: Chugai Pharmaceutical)

Study Start (Actual)

2014-02-20

Primary Completion (Actual)

2018-06-06

Study Completion (Actual)

2021-12-23

Enrollment (Actual)

85

Study Type

Interventional

Phase

Phase 3

United States
Alabama Locations

Birmingham, Alabama, United States, 35233
Children's Hospital of Alabama

France

Strasbourg, France, 67091
Hopital de Hautepierre CHRU de Strasbourg

Germany

Berlin, Germany, 10117

NeuroCure Clinical Research Center (NCRC)

Bochum, Germany, 44791
St. Josef-Hospital, Klinik für Neurologie

Düsseldorf, Germany, 40225
Heinrich-Heine Universitätsklinik Düsseldorf

Hungary

Budapest, Hungary, 1204
Jahn Ferenc Dél-Pesti Kórház

Italy
Lazio Locations

Roma, Lazio, Italy, 189
Azienda Ospedaliera Sant'Andrea-Universitr di Roma La Sapien

Lombardia Locations

Milano, Lombardia, Italy, 20132
Ospedale San Raffaele

Sicilia Locations

Catania, Sicilia, Italy, 95123
PO G.Rodolico, AOU Policlinico-Vittorio Emanuele Catania

Cefalu, Sicilia, Italy, 90015
Fond. Ist. S. Raffaele – giglio

Japan

Bunkyo-ku, Japan, 113-8431
Juntendo University Hospital; Neurology

Fukuoka, Japan, 812-8582
Kyushu University Hospital; Neurology

Fukushima, Japan, 960-1295
Fukushima Medical University Hospital; Neurology

Kagoshima, Japan, 890-8520
Kagoshima University Medical And Dental Hospital; Neurology and Geriatorics

Niigata, Japan, 951-8520
Niigata University Medical and Dental Hospital; Neurology

Osaka, Japan, 589-8511
Kindai University Hospital; Neurology

Sendai, Japan, 980-8574
Tohoku University Hospital; Neurology

Shinjuku-ku, Japan, 162-8666
Tokyo Women's Medical University Hospital; Neurology

Suita, Japan, 565-0871
Osaka University Hospital; Neurology

Tokyo, Japan, 187-8551
National Center of Neurology and Psychiatry

Poland

Katowice, Poland, 40-123
NZOZ Wielospecjalistyczna Poradnia Lekarska SYNAPSIS

Katowice, Poland, 40-571
M.A. - LEK A. M. Maciejowscy SC. Centrum Terapii SM

Katowice, Poland, 40-684
Centrum Medyczne Dendryt

Lublin, Poland, 20-954
Samodzielny Publiczny Szpital Kliniczny nr 4 w Lublinie

Pozna?, Poland, 60-355
Szpital Kliniczny im. H.Swiecickiego UM w Poznaniu

Warsaw, Poland
Instytut Psychiatrii i Neurologii

Warszawa, Poland, 02-097
Samodzielny Publiczny Centralny Szpital Klinicznyi

Spain

Barcelona, Spain, 08036
Hospital Clinic de Barcelona

Madrid, Spain, 28040
Hospital Clinico San Carlos; Servicio de Nefrologia

Taiwan

Kwei Shen, Taiwan, 33305
Chang Gung Medical Foundation - LinKou Chang Gung Memorial Hospital – Neurology

Taichung, Taiwan, 40447
China Medical University Hospital; Neurology – Taichung

Tainan, Taiwan, 704
National Cheng Kung University Hospital; Neurology

Taipei, Taiwan, 100
National Taiwan University Hospital; Neurology

Taipei, Taiwan, 11217
Taipei Veterans General Hospital-Neurology

Ukraine
Kharkiv Governorate Locations

Kharkiv, Kharkiv Governorate, Ukraine, 61000
Kharkivska miska dytiacha likarnia # 5

Tavria Okruha Locations

Dnipropetrovsk, Tavria Okruha, Ukraine, 49100
KZ "Dnipropetrovska oblasna dytiacha klinichna likarnia" DOR

United Kingdom

Cardiff, United Kingdom, CF14 4XW
University Hospital of Wales; Dept of Neurology

Chinnor, United Kingdom, OX3 9DU
John Radcliffe Hospital; Neurosciences

London, United Kingdom, WC1N 3BG
The National Hospital for Neurology & Neurosurgery

London, United Kingdom, WC1N 3JH
Great Ormond Street Hospital For Children; Neurology

Eligibility Criteria
Description

Inclusion Criteria

- Patients must be diagnosed as having either neuromyelitis optica (NMO) or NMO spectrum disorder (NMOSD), defined as the following:
  - NMO as defined by Wingerchuk et al. 2006 criteria (requires all of the following three criteria: (1) Optic neuritis, (2) Acute myelitis, (3) At least two of three supportive criteria: Contiguous spinal cord lesion identified on a magnetic resonance imaging (MRI) scan extending over three vertebral segments; Brain MRI not meeting diagnostic criteria for multiple sclerosis (MS); NMO-IgG seropositive status)
  - NMOSD as defined by either of the following Wingerchuk 2007 criteria with anti-AQP4 antibody (Ab) seropositive status at screening ((1) Idiopathic single or recurrent events of longitudinally extensive myelitis [$\geq$3 vertebral segment spinal cord MRI lesion]; (2) Optic neuritis: recurrent or simultaneous bilateral); For patients aged 12–17 years, a minimum of 4 patients should be positive for anti-AQP4Ab status at screening
- Clinical evidence of at least two documented relapses (including first attack) in the last 2 years prior to screening, at least one of which has occurred in the 12 months prior to screening

- EDSS score from 0 to 6.5 inclusive at screening
- Age 12–74 years, inclusive at the time of informed consent
- One of the following baseline treatments must be at a stable dose as a monotherapy for 8 weeks prior to baseline: Azathioprine; Mycophenolate mofetil; Oral corticosteroids. For participants aged 12–17 years, either of the following baseline treatments for relapse prevention can be allowed: Azathioprine + oral corticosteroids; Mycophenolate mofetil + oral corticosteroids
- Ability and willingness to provide written informed consent and to comply with the requirements of the protocol

For adolescents who may be enrolled after the end of the double-blind period, the inclusion criterion 2 is as follows (other criteria are same): Clinical evidence of at least two documented relapses (including the first attack) prior to screening.

Exclusion Criteria

Exclusion criteria related to previous or concomitant therapy:

- Any previous treatment with IL-6 inhibitory therapy (e.g. tocilizumab), alemtuzumab, total body irradiation, or bone marrow transplantation at any time
- Any previous treatment with anti-CD20, eculizumab, belimumab, interferon, natalizumab, glatiramer acetate, fingolimod, teriflunomide, or dimethyl fumarate within 6 months prior to baseline
- Any previous treatment with anti-CD4, cladribine, or mitoxantrone within 2 years prior to baseline
- Treatment with any investigational agent within 3 months prior to baseline

Exclusions for general safety:

- Pregnancy or lactation
- For patients of reproductive potential, a positive result from a serum pregnancy test at screening, or not willing to use reliable means of contraception (physical barrier [patient or partner] in conjunction with a spermicidal product, contraceptive pill, patch, injectables, intrauterine device, or intrauterine system) during the treatment period and for at least 3 months after the last dose of study drug
- Any surgical procedure (except for minor surgeries) within 4 weeks prior to baseline
- Evidence of other demyelinating disease or progressive multifocal leukoencephalopathy (PML)
- Evidence of serious uncontrolled concomitant diseases that may preclude patient participation, such as other nervous system disease, cardiovascular disease, hematologic/hematopoiesis disease, respiratory disease, muscular disease, endocrine disease, renal/urologic disease, digestive system disease, congenital or acquired severe immunodeficiency
- Known active infection (excluding fungal infections of nail beds or caries dentium) within 4 weeks prior to baseline
- Evidence of chronic active hepatitis B or C

- History of drug or alcohol abuse within 1 year prior to baseline
- History of diverticulitis that, in the Investigator's opinion, may lead to increased risk of complications such as lower gastrointestinal perforation
- Evidence of active tuberculosis (TB; excluding patients receiving chemoprophylaxis for latent TB infection)
- Evidence of active interstitial lung disease
- Receipt of any live or live attenuated vaccine within 6 weeks prior to baseline
- History of malignancy within the last 5 years, including solid tumors, hematologic malignancies, and in situ carcinoma (except basal cell and squamous cell carcinomas of the skin, or in situ carcinoma of the cervix uteri that have been completely excised and cured)
- History of severe allergic reaction to a biologic agent (e.g. shock, anaphylactic reactions)
- Active suicidal ideation within 6 months prior to screening, or history of suicide attempt within 3 years prior to screening
- Following laboratory abnormalities at screening*.
  - White blood cells (WBC) $<3.0 \times 10^3$/microliter (μL)
  - Absolute neutrophil count (ANC) $<2.0 \times 10^3/\mu L$
  - Absolute lymphocyte count $<0.5 \times 10^3/\mu L$
  - Platelet count $<10 \times 10^4/\mu L$
  - Aspartate aminotransferase (AST) or alanine aminotransferase (ALT) >1.5 times the upper limit of normal (ULN) * If retest is conducted, the last value of retest before randomization must meet study criteria.

For adolescents who may be enrolled after the end of the double-blind period, the annotation in the exclusion criterion 20 is as follows (other criteria are same): * If retest is conducted, the last value of retest before baseline must meet study criteria.

Ages Eligible for Study
12 Years to 74 Years (Child, Adult, Older Adult)

Sexes Eligible for Study
All

Accepts Healthy Volunteers
No

Design Details
Primary Purpose: Treatment
Allocation: Randomized
Interventional Model: Parallel Assignment
Masking: Double (Participant Investigator)

Arms and interventions

Participant group/arm	Intervention/treatment
Experimental: satralizumab + baseline treatment Participants randomized to this arm for the double-blind period will receive satralizumab in addition to baseline treatment. The double-blind period ends when either the participant has a treated relapse or the total number of protocol-defined relapses confirmed by the Clinical Endpoint Committee (CEC) reaches 26. In the open-label extension period, the participant will receive (with or without baseline treatment) an SC injection of satralizumab at Weeks 0, 2, and 4, and Q4W thereafter, with the last study drug administration on or before 31 December 2021	Drug: satralizumab • Satralizumab will be administered subcutaneously (SC) at Weeks 0, 2, and 4, and thereafter once every 4 weeks (Q4W) • Other names: – SA237 – RG6168 – RO5333787 Drug: baseline treatment • As specified in the protocol, one of the following drugs at a stable dose is required as monotherapy for baseline treatment during the double-blind period: azathioprine (AZA); mycophenolate mofetil (MMF); or oral corticosteroids (CS). For participants aged 12–17 years at the time of informed consent, baseline treatment with AZA or MMF in combination with oral CS is also permitted. Change or termination of baseline treatment is only permitted during the open-label extension period
Placebo comparator: placebo + baseline treatment Participants randomized to this arm for the double-blind period will receive placebo in addition to baseline treatment. The double-blind period ends when either the participant has a treated relapse or the total number of protocol-defined relapses confirmed by the Clinical Endpoint Committee (CEC) reaches 26. In the open-label extension period, the participant will receive (with or without baseline treatment) an SC injection of satralizumab at Weeks 0, 2, and 4, and Q4W thereafter, with the last study drug administration on or before 31 December 2021	Drug: placebo • Placebo will be administered subcutaneously (SC) at Weeks 0, 2, and 4, and thereafter once every 4 weeks (Q4W) Drug: baseline treatment • As specified in the protocol, one of the following drugs at a stable dose is required as monotherapy for baseline treatment during the double-blind period: azathioprine (AZA); mycophenolate mofetil (MMF); or oral corticosteroids (CS). For participants aged 12–17 years at the time of informed consent, baseline treatment with AZA or MMF in combination with oral CS is also permitted. Change or termination of baseline treatment is only permitted during the open-label extension period

Primary outcome measures

Outcome measure	Measure description	Time frame
Time to first protocol-defined relapse (TFR) in the double-blind period	TFR was defined as time from randomization to the first occurrence of relapse in the DB period. Protocol-defined relapse was occurrence of new or worsening neurological symptoms attributable to neurological neuromyelitis optica (NMO) or neuromyelitis optica spectrum disorder (NMOSD) as adjudicated by an independent clinical endpoint committee (CEC). Symptoms had to persist for >24 h and not be attributable to confounding clinical factors (e.g., fever, infection, injury, change in mood, adverse reactions to medications). New or worsening neurological symptoms that occurred <31 days following onset of a protocol-defined relapse were considered part of same relapse (i.e., if 2 relapses had onset days that were 30 days of one another, they were counted only as 1 relapse), and onset date used in the analysis was the date of first relapse	Up to Week 224

Secondary outcome measures

Outcome measure	Measure description	Time frame
Change from baseline at Week 24 in the visual analog scale (VAS) score for pain during the DB period	The VAS is a subjective measure of pain consisting of a 100 mm line with two endpoints representing 0 = "no pain" and 100 = "pain as bad as it could be". Participants rated their pain by placing a mark on the line corresponding to their current level of pain. The distance along the line from the "no pain" marker was measured with a ruler giving a pain score out of 100. A higher score indicated more pain and lower scores reflected a better health state. A negative change from baseline indicates an improvement. ANCOVA was used for analysis to report the adjusted mean and standard error (SE)	Baseline, Week 24
Change from baseline at Week 24 in the functional assessment of chronic illness therapy (FACIT) fatigue score during the DB Period	The FACIT Fatigue scale is a 13-item questionnaire that assesses self-reported fatigue and its impact on daily activities and function over the past 7 days. As each of the 13 items of the scale ranges from 0 to 4, the range of possible scores was computed using FACIT scoring algorithm as 0–52, where 0 is the worst possible score and 52 is the best which indicated less fatigue. A positive change from baseline indicates an improvement. ANCOVA was used for analysis to report the adjusted mean and SE	Baseline, Week 24

Outcome measure	Measure description	Time frame
Relapse-free rate during the DB period	Protocol-defined relapse was the occurrence of new or worsening neurological symptoms attributable to neurological neuromyelitis optica (NMO) or neuromyelitis optica spectrum disorder (NMOSD). Symptoms had to persist for >24 h and not be attributable to confounding clinical factors (e.g., fever, infection, injury, change in mood, adverse reactions to medications). New or worsening neurological symptoms that occurred <31 days following onset of a protocol-defined relapse were considered part of the same relapse (i.e., if 2 relapses had onsets within 30 days of one another, they were counted as 1), and onset date used in analysis was the date of first relapse	Up to Week 216
Annualized relapse rate (ARR) during the DB period	The ARR is calculated as the total number of participants with relapses experienced divided by the patient-years at risk. Protocol-defined relapse was the occurrence of new or worsening neurological symptoms attributable to neurological NMO or NMOSD. Symptoms had to persist for >24 h and not be attributable to confounding clinical factors (e.g., fever, infection, injury, change in mood, adverse reactions to medications). New or worsening neurological symptoms that occurred <31 days following the onset of a protocol-defined relapse were considered part of same relapse (2 relapses with onset days in 30 days of one another were counted as 1 relapse); the onset date used in the analysis was the date of first relapse	Up to Week 216
Change from baseline in modified Rankin scale (mRS) scores at 24-week intervals during the DB period	The mRS is a 7-point disability scale that assesses the degree of disability in participants with neurological impairment. Possible scores range from 0 (no symptoms at all) up to 6 (death). Higher scores reflect increased disability. A negative change from baseline indicates an improvement	Baseline up to Week 216
Change from baseline in Zarit Burden Interview (ZBI) scores at 24-week intervals during the DB period	The ZBI is the measurement to assess caregiver burden. The 22 items ask for the strain caregivers perceive. Responses range from 0 (never) to 4 (nearly always). The overall ZBI score ranges from 0 to 88. The higher the total score, the heavier the perceived burden. A negative change from baseline indicates an improvement	Baseline up to Week 168
Change from baseline in expanded disability status scale (EDSS) scores at 24-week intervals during the DB period	The EDSS is an ordinal scale with values from 0 points (normal neurological examination) to 10 points (death) increasing in half-point increments once an EDSS of 1.0 has been reached. Higher scores represent increased disability. A negative change from baseline indicates an improvement	Baseline up to Week 216

Outcome measure	Measure description	Time frame
Change from baseline in visual acuity (Snellen Chart) at 24-week intervals during the DB period	Visual acuity was measured using Snellen 20-foot wall chart and then converted to logMAR visual acuity scoring. Lower values indicate better visual acuity. Data are reported for right eye (OD) and left eye (OS). A negative change from baseline indicates an improvement	Baseline up to Week 216
Change from baseline in Short Form Generic Health Survey (SF-36) mental component summary scores at 24-week intervals during the DB period	The SF-36v2 is a multi-purpose, short-form health survey with 36 questions. It has 8 domains (vitality, physical functioning, bodily pain, general health, role-physical, role emotional, social role functioning, and mental health) of functional health and well-being scores as well as psychometrically based physical and mental health summary measures and a preference-based health utility index. The component scores were transformed to a 0–100 scale, where a higher score indicates a better quality of life. A positive change from baseline indicates an improvement	Baseline up to Week 216
Change from baseline in SF-36 physical component summary scores at 24-week intervals during the DB period	The SF-36v2 is a multi-purpose, short-form health survey with 36 questions. It has 8 domains (vitality, physical functioning, bodily pain, general health, role-physical, role emotional, social role functioning, and mental health) of functional health and well-being scores as well as psychometrically based physical and mental health summary measures and a preference-based health utility index. The component scores were transformed to a 0–100 scale, where a higher score indicates a better quality of life. A positive change from baseline indicates an improvement	Baseline up to Week 216
Change from baseline in SF-36 bodily pain domain scores at 24-week intervals during the DB period	The SF-36v2 is a multi-purpose, short-form health survey with 36 questions. It has 8 domains (vitality, physical functioning, bodily pain, general health, role-physical, role emotional, social role functioning, and mental health) of functional health and well-being scores as well as psychometrically based physical and mental health component summary measures and a preference-based health utility index. The domain scores were transformed to a 0–100 scale, where higher scores indicate better quality of life. A positive change from baseline indicates an improvement	Baseline up to Week 216
Change from baseline in SF-36 general health domain scores at 24-week intervals during the DB period	The SF-36v2 is a multi-purpose, short-form health survey with 36 questions. It has 8 domains (vitality, physical functioning, bodily pain, general health, role-physical, role emotional, social role functioning, and mental health) of functional health and well-being scores as well as psychometrically based physical and mental health component summary measures and a preference-based health utility index. The domain scores were transformed to a 0–100 scale, where higher scores indicate better quality of life. A positive change from baseline indicates an improvement	Baseline up to Week 216

Outcome measure	Measure description	Time frame
Change from baseline in SF-36 mental health domain scores at 24-week intervals during the DB period	The SF-36v2 is a multi-purpose, short-form health survey with 36 questions. It has 8 domains (vitality, physical functioning, bodily pain, general health, role-physical, role emotional, social role functioning, and mental health) of functional health and well-being scores as well as psychometrically based physical and mental health component summary measures and a preference-based health utility index. The domain scores were transformed to a 0–100 scale, where higher scores indicate better quality of life. A positive change from baseline indicates an improvement	Baseline up to Week 216
Change from baseline in SF-36 physical functioning domain scores at 24-week intervals during the DB period	The SF-36v2 is a multi-purpose, short-form health survey with 36 questions. It has 8 domains (vitality, physical functioning, bodily pain, general health, role-physical, role emotional, social role functioning, and mental health) of functional health and well-being scores as well as psychometrically based physical and mental health component summary measures and a preference-based health utility index. The domain scores were transformed to a 0–100 scale, where higher scores indicate better quality of life. A positive change from baseline indicates an improvement	Baseline up to Week 216
Change from baseline in SF-36 Role-emotional domain scores at 24- week intervals during the DB period	The SF-36v2 is a multi-purpose, short-form health survey with 36 questions. It has 8 domains (vitality, physical functioning, bodily pain, general health, role-physical, role emotional, social role functioning, and mental health) of functional health and well-being scores as well as psychometrically based physical and mental health component summary measures and a preference-based health utility index. The domain scores were transformed to a 0–100 scale, where higher scores indicate better quality of life. A positive change from baseline indicates an improvement	Baseline up to Week 216
Change from baseline in SF-36 role-physical domain scores at 24-week intervals during the DB period	The SF-36v2 is a multi-purpose, short-form health survey with 36 questions. It has 8 domains (vitality, physical functioning, bodily pain, general health, role-physical, role emotional, social role functioning, and mental health) of functional health and well-being scores as well as psychometrically based physical and mental health component summary measures and a preference-based health utility index. The domain scores were transformed to a 0–100 scale, where higher scores indicate better quality of life. A positive change from baseline indicates an improvement	Baseline up to Week 216

Outcome measure	Measure description	Time frame
Change from baseline in SF-36 social role functioning domain scores at 24-week intervals during the DB period	The SF-36v2 is a multi-purpose, short-form health survey with 36 questions. It has 8 domains (vitality, physical functioning, bodily pain, general health, role-physical, role emotional, social role functioning, and mental health) of functional health and well-being scores as well as psychometrically based physical and mental health component summary measures and a preference-based health utility index. The domain scores were transformed to a 0–100 scale, where higher scores indicate better quality of life. A positive change from baseline indicates an improvement	Baseline up to Week 216
Change from baseline in SF-36 vitality domain scores at 24-week intervals during the DB period	The SF-36v2 is a multi-purpose, short-form health survey with 36 questions. It has 8 domains (vitality, physical functioning, bodily pain, general health, role-physical, role emotional, social role functioning, and mental health) of functional health and well-being scores as well as psychometrically based physical and mental health component summary measures and a preference-based health utility index. The domain scores were transformed to a 0–100 scale, where higher scores indicate better quality of life. A positive change from baseline indicates an improvement	Baseline up to Week 216
Change from baseline in EuroQoL-5 Dimensions (EQ-5D) index scores at 24-week intervals during the DB period	The EQ-5D is a participant-answered questionnaire measuring 5 dimensions of mobility, self-care, usual activities, pain/discomfort, and anxiety/depression with 3 possible response categories: (1) no problems; (2) some problems; (3) severe problems. The scores from 5 dimensions are used as input to generate EQ-5D index score using scoring algorithm. The EQ-5D index score is scored on a scale of −0.2 to 1. A higher score reflects a better health state. A positive change from baseline indicates an improvement	Baseline up to Week 216
Serum satralizumab concentration during the DB period		Baseline, Weeks 2, 4, 5, 6, 8, and every 4 weeks thereafter up to Week 224
Serum soluble IL-6 receptor (sIL-6R) concentration during the DB period		Baseline, Weeks 2, 4, and every 4 weeks thereafter up to Week 224
Serum high sensitivity C-reactive protein (hsCRP) concentration during the DB period		Baseline, Weeks 2, 4, and every 4 weeks thereafter up to Week 224

Outcome measure	Measure description	Time frame
Serum interleukin-6 (IL-6) concentration during the DB period		Baseline, Weeks 2, 4, and every 4 weeks thereafter up to Week 224
Number of participants with at least one adverse event in the DB period	An adverse event is any untoward medical occurrence in a participant administered a pharmaceutical product which does not necessarily have to have a causal relationship with the treatment. An adverse event can therefore be any unfavorable and unintended sign (including an abnormal laboratory finding, for example), symptom, or disease temporally associated with the use of a pharmaceutical product, whether or not considered related to the pharmaceutical product. Pre-existing conditions which worsen during a study are also considered as adverse events	Up to Week 224
Number of participants with at least one serious adverse event in the DB period	A serious adverse event is defined as any untoward medical occurrence that, at any dose, results in death, is life-threatening, requires hospitalization or prolongation of existing hospitalization, results in disability/incapacity, is a congenital anomaly/birth defect, or is medically significant or requires intervention to prevent one or other of the outcomes listed above	Up to Week 224
Number of participants with non-serious adverse events of special interest in the DB period	Non-serious adverse events of special interest for this study included: (1) cases of an elevated alanine aminotransferase (ALT) or aspartate aminotransferase (AST) in combination with either an elevated bilirubin or clinical jaundice, (2) suspected transmission of an infectious agent by the study treatment	Up to Week 224
Number of participants with selected adverse events in the DB period	Selected adverse events for this study included: (1) non-serious infections that required treatments with intravenous (IV) antibiotic, antifungal, antiviral, (2) opportunistic infections that required treatments with oral antibiotics, antifungals, or antivirals, (3) injection-related reactions (IRRs; an AE which occurred within 24 h after study treatment injection except where the event was not considered an allergic reaction), and (4) anaphylaxis (an acute allergic/hypersensitivity reaction)	Up to Week 224

Outcome measure	Measure description	Time frame
Number of participants with suicidal behaviors and ideations collected by Columbia-suicide severity rating scale in the DB period	The Columbia-Suicide Severity Rating Scale (C-SSRS) is an assessment tool to evaluate suicidal ideation and behavior. Categories have binary responses (yes/no) and include Wish to be Dead; Non-specific Active Suicidal Thoughts; Active Suicidal Ideation with Any Methods (Not Plan) without Intent to Act; Active Suicidal Ideation with Some Intent to Act, without Specific Plan; Active Suicidal Ideation with Specific Plan and Intent, Preparatory Acts and Behavior; Aborted Attempt; Interrupted Attempt; Actual Attempt (non-fatal); Completed Suicide. Suicidal ideation or behavior is indicated by a "yes" answer to any of the listed categories. A score of 0 is assigned if no suicide risk is present. A score of 1 or higher indicates suicidal ideation or behavior	Baseline and post-baseline (up to Week 224)
Percentage of participants with anti-drug antibodies to satralizumab in the DB period	Reported here is the percentage of participants with at least one positive anti-drug antibody measurement during the DB period	Up to approximately Week 224
Percentage of participants with anti-drug antibodies to satralizumab overall S237 period	Reported here is the percentage of participants with at least one positive anti-drug antibody measurement during the overall S237 period	Up to approximately Week 368

Sponsor
Hoffmann-La Roche

Collaborators
- Chugai Pharmaceutical

Investigators
- Study Director: Clinical Trials, Hoffmann-La Roche

General Publications
No publications available

Results

Outcome Measures

1. Time to First Protocol-Defined Relapse (TFR) in the Double-Blind Period
   Type: Primary | Time Frame: up to Week 224

Description	TFR was defined as time from randomization to first occurrence of relapse in the DB period. Protocol-defined relapse was the occurrence of new or worsening neurological symptoms attributable to neurological neuromyelitis optica (NMO) or neuromyelitis optica spectrum disorder (NMOSD) as adjudicated by an independent clinical endpoint committee (CEC). Symptoms had to persist for >24 h and not be attributable to confounding clinical factors (e.g., fever, infection, injury, change in mood, adverse reactions to medications). New or worsening neurological symptoms that occurred <31 days following onset of a protocol-defined relapse were considered part of same relapse (i.e., if 2 relapses had onset days that were 30 days of one another, they were counted only as 1 relapse), and onset date used in the analysis was the date of first relapse
Time frame	Up to Week 224
Analysis population description	ITT population included all participants randomized to the treatment groups. For participants who had not relapsed, the TFR was censored on the date of end of the DB period

Arm/group title	Placebo + baseline treatment	Satralizumab + baseline treatment
Arm/group description	Participants received matching placebo, subcutaneous (SC) at Weeks 0, 2, and 4, and every 4 weeks (Q4W) thereafter throughout the double-blind (DB) period up to protocol-defined relapse or treated relapse in addition to baseline treatment. Following the DB period, all participants received satralizumab 120 mg SC injection (with or without baseline treatment) at Weeks 0, 2, and 4, and Q4W thereafter up to the clinical cut-off date (CCOD). At the CCOD, participants who had not experienced a relapse during the DB period were invited to initiate satralizumab 120 mg SC injection (with or without baseline treatment at Weeks 0, 2, and 4, and Q4W thereafter) after 4 weeks from their last study treatment dose in the DB period Show less	Participants received satralizumab 120 mg SC injection at Weeks 0, 2, and 4, and Q4W thereafter throughout the DB period up to protocol-defined relapse or treated relapse in addition to baseline treatment. Following the DB period, all participants received satralizumab 120 mg SC injection (with or without baseline treatment) at Weeks 0, 2, and 4, and Q4W thereafter up to the CCOD. At the CCOD, participants who had not experienced a relapse during the DB period were invited to continue satralizumab 120 mg SC injection (with or without baseline treatment at Weeks 0, 2, and 4, and Q4W thereafter) after 4 weeks from their last study treatment dose in the DB period Show less

Overall number of participants analyzed	42	41
Median (95% confidence interval) ǀ unit of measure: weeks	120.6[a] (37.0 to NA)	NA[b] (NA to NA)
Statistical analysis 1: placebo + baseline treatment, satralizumab + baseline treatment ǀ superiority ǀ log rank		

[a] Upper limit of confidence interval (CI) was not reached due to the low number of participants with events

[b] Median was not reached due to the low number of participants with events. Lower and upper limit of CI was not reached due to the low number of participants with events

2. Change from Baseline at Week 24 in the Visual Analog Scale (VAS) Score for Pain During the DB Period

   Type: Secondary ǀ Time Frame: Baseline, Week 24

Description	The VAS is a subjective measure of pain consisting of a 100 mm line with two endpoints representing 0 = "no pain" and 100 = "pain as bad as it could be". Participants rated their pain by placing a mark on the line corresponding to their current level of pain. The distance along the line from the "no pain" marker was measured with a ruler giving a pain score out of 100. A higher score indicated more pain and lower scores reflected a better health state. A negative change from baseline indicates an improvement. ANCOVA was used for analysis to report the adjusted mean and standard error (SE)
Time frame	Baseline, Week 24
Analysis population description	ITT population included all participants randomized to the treatment groups. Number analyzed is the number of participants with data available for analyses at the given timepoint. Missing data were imputed by baseline observation carried forward (BOCF) method

Arm/group title	Placebo + baseline treatment	Satralizumab + baseline treatment
Arm/group description	Participants received matching placebo, subcutaneous (SC) at Weeks 0, 2, and 4, and every 4 weeks (Q4W) thereafter throughout the double-blind (DB) period up to protocol-defined relapse or treated relapse in addition to baseline treatment. Following the DB period, all participants received satralizumab 120 mg SC injection (with or without baseline treatment) at Weeks 0, 2, and 4, and Q4W thereafter up to the clinical cut-off date (CCOD). At the CCOD, participants who had not experienced a relapse during the DB period were invited to initiate satralizumab 120 mg SC injection (with or without baseline treatment at Weeks 0, 2, and 4, and Q4W thereafter) after 4 weeks from their last study treatment dose in the DB period Show less	Participants received satralizumab 120 mg SC injection at Weeks 0, 2, and 4, and Q4W thereafter throughout the DB period up to protocol-defined relapse or treated relapse in addition to baseline treatment. Following the DB period, all participants received satralizumab 120 mg SC injection (with or without baseline treatment) at Weeks 0, 2, and 4, and Q4W thereafter up to the CCOD. At the CCOD, participants who had not experienced a relapse during the DB period were invited to continue satralizumab 120 mg SC injection (with or without baseline treatment at Weeks 0, 2, and 4, and Q4W thereafter) after 4 weeks from their last study treatment dose in the DB period Show less
Overall number of participants analyzed	42	41
Baseline [a]Mean (standard error) ǀ unit of measure: score on scale	34.619(4.026)	27.561(4.399)
Change from baseline at Week 24[a]	−3.505(2.357)	2.871(2.391)
Statistical analysis 1: placebo + baseline treatment, satralizumab + baseline treatment ǀ superiority ǀ ANCOVA		

[a] Mean (standard error) ǀ unit of measure: score on scale

3. Change from Baseline at Week 24 in the Functional Assessment of Chronic Illness Therapy (FACIT) Fatigue Score During the DB Period
Type: Secondary | Time Frame: Baseline, Week 24

Description	The FACIT Fatigue scale is a 13-item questionnaire that assesses self-reported fatigue and its impact on daily activities and function over the past 7 days. As each of the 13 items of the scale ranges from 0 to 4, the range of possible scores was computed using FACIT scoring algorithm as 0–52, where 0 is the worst possible score and 52 is the best which indicated less fatigue. A positive change from baseline indicates an improvement. ANCOVA was used for analysis to report the adjusted mean and SE
Time frame	Baseline, Week 24
Analysis population description	ITT population included all participants randomized to the treatment groups. Number analyzed is the number of participants with data available for analyses at the given timepoint. Missing data were imputed using BOCF method

Arm/group title	Placebo + baseline treatment	Satralizumab + baseline treatment
Arm/group description	Participants received matching placebo, subcutaneous (SC) at Weeks 0, 2, and 4, and every 4 weeks (Q4W) thereafter throughout the double-blind (DB) period up to protocol-defined relapse or treated relapse in addition to baseline treatment. Following the DB period, all participants received satralizumab 120 mg SC injection (with or without baseline treatment) at Weeks 0, 2, and 4, and Q4W thereafter up to the clinical cut-off date (CCOD). At the CCOD, participants who had not experienced a relapse during the DB period were invited to initiate satralizumab 120 mg SC injection (with or without baseline treatment at Weeks 0, 2, and 4, and Q4W thereafter) after 4 weeks from their last study treatment dose in the DB period Show less	Participants received satralizumab 120 mg SC injection at Weeks 0, 2, and 4, and Q4W thereafter throughout the DB period up to protocol-defined relapse or treated relapse in addition to baseline treatment. Following the DB period, all participants received satralizumab 120 mg SC injection (with or without baseline treatment) at Weeks 0, 2, and 4, and Q4W thereafter up to the CCOD. At the CCOD, participants who had not experienced a relapse during the DB period were invited to continue satralizumab 120 mg SC injection (with or without baseline treatment at Weeks 0, 2, and 4, and Q4W thereafter) after 4 weeks from their last study treatment dose in the DB period Show less
Overall number of participants analyzed	42	41
Baseline [a]Mean (standard error) | unit of measure: score on scale	33.857(1.746)	34.732(1.646)

Change from baseline at Week 24[a]	2.234(0.943)	0.145(0.963)
Statistical analysis 1: placebo + baseline treatment, satralizumab + baseline treatment | superiority | ANCOVA		

[a] Mean (standard error) | unit of measure: score on scale

4. Relapse-Free Rate During the DB Period
   Type: Secondary | Time Frame: up to Week 216

Description	Protocol-defined relapse was the occurrence of new or worsening neurological symptoms attributable to neurological neuromyelitis optica (NMO) or neuromyelitis optica spectrum disorder (NMOSD). Symptoms had to persist for >24 h and not be attributable to confounding clinical factors (e.g., fever, infection, injury, change in mood, adverse reactions to medications). New or worsening neurological symptoms that occurred <31 days following onset of a protocol-defined relapse were considered part of same relapse (i.e., if 2 relapses had onsets within 30 days of one another, they were counted as 1), and onset date used in the analysis was the date of first relapse
Time frame	Up to Week 216
Analysis population description	ITT population included all participants randomized to the treatment groups

Arm/group title	Placebo + baseline treatment	Satralizumab + baseline treatment
Arm/group description	Participants received matching placebo, subcutaneous (SC) at Weeks 0, 2, and 4, and every 4 weeks (Q4W) thereafter throughout the double-blind (DB) period up to protocol-defined relapse or treated relapse in addition to baseline treatment. Following the DB period, all participants received satralizumab 120 mg SC injection (with or without baseline treatment) at Weeks 0, 2, and 4, and Q4W thereafter up to the clinical cut-off date (CCOD). At the CCOD, participants who had not experienced a relapse during the DB period were invited to initiate satralizumab 120 mg SC injection (with or without baseline treatment at Weeks 0, 2, and 4, and Q4W thereafter) after 4 weeks from their last study treatment dose in the DB period Show more	Participants received satralizumab 120 mg SC injection at Weeks 0, 2, and 4, and Q4W thereafter throughout the DB period up to protocol-defined relapse or treated relapse in addition to baseline treatment. Following the DB period, all participants received satralizumab 120 mg SC injection (with or without baseline treatment) at Weeks 0, 2, and 4, and Q4W thereafter up to the CCOD. At the CCOD, participants who had not experienced a relapse during the DB period were invited to continue satralizumab 120 mg SC injection (with or without baseline treatment at Weeks 0, 2, and 4, and Q4W thereafter) after 4 weeks from their last study treatment dose in the DB period Show more

Overall number of participants analyzed	34	37
Week 12		
Number analyzed	34 participants	37 participants
[a]Measure type: number | unit of measure: percentage of participants	89.86	94.99
Week 24		
Number analyzed	34 participants	37 participants
[a]	84.41	88.86
Week 36		
Number analyzed	34 participants	37 participants
[a]	69.49	88.86
Week 48		
Number analyzed	34 participants	37 participants
[a]	66.02	88.86
Week 72		
Number analyzed	34 participants	37 participants
[a]	58.68	81.46
Week 96		
Number analyzed	34 participants	37 participants
[a]	58.68	77.58
Week 120		
Number analyzed	34 participants	37 participants
[a]	54.17	73.70
Week 144		
Number analyzed	34 participants	37 participants
[a]	49.24	73.70
Week 168		
Number analyzed	34 participants	37 participants
[a]	43.77	73.70
Week 192		
Number analyzed	0 participants	37 participants
[a]		73.70
Week 216		
Number analyzed	0 participants	37 participants
[a]		73.70

[a] Measure type: number | unit of measure: percentage of participants

5. Annualized Relapse Rate (ARR) During the DB Period

Type: Secondary | Time Frame: up to Week 216

Description	The ARR is calculated as the total number of participants with relapses experienced divided by the patient years at risk. Protocol-defined relapse was the occurrence of new or worsening neurological symptoms attributable to neurological NMO or NMOSD. Symptoms had to persist for >24 h and not be attributable to confounding clinical factors (e.g., fever, infection, injury, change in mood, adverse reactions to medications). New or worsening neurological symptoms that occurred <31 days following the onset of a protocol-defined relapse were considered part of same relapse (2 relapses with onset days in 30 days of one another were counted as 1 relapse), onset date used in the analysis was the date of first relapse
Time frame	Up to Week 216
Analysis population description	ITT population included all participants randomized to the treatment groups

Arm/group title	Placebo + baseline treatment	Satralizumab + baseline treatment
Arm/group description	Participants received matching placebo, subcutaneous (SC) at Weeks 0, 2, and 4, and every 4 weeks (Q4W) thereafter throughout the double-blind (DB) period up to protocol-defined relapse or treated relapse in addition to baseline treatment. Following the DB period, all participants received satralizumab 120 mg SC injection (with or without baseline treatment) at Weeks 0, 2, and 4, and Q4W thereafter up to the clinical cut-off date (CCOD). At the CCOD, participants who had not experienced a relapse during the DB period were invited to initiate satralizumab 120 mg SC injection (with or without baseline treatment at Weeks 0, 2, and 4, and Q4W thereafter) after 4 weeks from their last study treatment dose in the DB period Show less	Participants received satralizumab 120 mg SC injection at Weeks 0, 2, and 4, and Q4W thereafter throughout the DB period up to protocol-defined relapse or treated relapse in addition to baseline treatment. Following the DB period, all participants received satralizumab 120 mg SC injection (with or without baseline treatment) at Weeks 0, 2, and 4, and Q4W thereafter up to the CCOD. At the CCOD, participants who had not experienced a relapse during the DB period were invited to continue satralizumab 120 mg SC injection (with or without baseline treatment at Weeks 0, 2, and 4, and Q4W thereafter) after 4 weeks from their last study treatment dose in the DB period Show less
Overall number of participants analyzed	42	41
Measure type: number (95% confidence interval) | unit of measure: patients w relapse/ patient-years at risk	0.32(0.19–0.51)	0.11(0.05–0.21)

6. Change from baseline in Modified Rankin Scale (MRS) scores at 24-week intervals during the DB Period
   Type: Secondary | Time Frame: Baseline up to week 216

Description	The mRS is a 7-point disability scale that assesses the degree of disability in participants with neurological impairment. Possible scores range from 0 (no symptoms at all) up to 6 (death). Higher scores reflect increased disability. A negative change from baseline indicates an improvement
Time frame	Baseline up to Week 216
Analysis population description	ITT population included all participants randomized to the treatment groups. Number analyzed is the number of participants with data available for analyses at the given timepoint

Arm/group title	Placebo + baseline treatment	Satralizumab + baseline treatment
Arm/group description	Participants received matching placebo, subcutaneous (SC) at Weeks 0, 2, and 4, and every 4 weeks (Q4W) thereafter throughout the double-blind (DB) period up to protocol-defined relapse or treated relapse in addition to baseline treatment. Following the DB period, all participants received satralizumab 120 mg SC injection (with or without baseline treatment) at Weeks 0, 2, and 4, and Q4W thereafter up to the clinical cut-off date (CCOD). At the CCOD, participants who had not experienced a relapse during the DB period were invited to initiate satralizumab 120 mg SC injection (with or without baseline treatment at Weeks 0, 2, and 4, and Q4W thereafter) after 4 weeks from their last study treatment dose in the DB period Show more	Participants received satralizumab 120 mg SC injection at Weeks 0, 2, and 4, and Q4W thereafter throughout the DB period up to protocol-defined relapse or treated relapse in addition to baseline treatment. Following the DB period, all participants received satralizumab 120 mg SC injection (with or without baseline treatment) at Weeks 0, 2, and 4, and Q4W thereafter up to the CCOD. At the CCOD, participants who had not experienced a relapse during the DB period were invited to continue satralizumab 120 mg SC injection (with or without baseline treatment at Weeks 0, 2, and 4, and Q4W thereafter) after 4 weeks from their last study treatment dose in the DB period Show more
Overall number of participants analyzed	42	41
Baseline		
Number analyzed	42 participants	41 participants
[a]Mean (standard deviation) | unit of measure: score on scale	1.55(0.97)	1.90(1.14)

Change from baseline at Week 24		
Number analyzed	29 participants	29 participants
[a]	−0.03(0.42)	−0.03(0.50)
Change from baseline at Week 48		
Number analyzed	17 participants	24 participants
[a]	−0.18(0.53)	−0.13(0.45)
Change from baseline at Week 72		
Number analyzed	15 participants	23 participants
[a]	0.07(0.70)	0.00(0.52)
Change from baseline at Week 96		
Number analyzed	16 participants	21 participants
[a]	0.13(0.62)	−0.19(0.51)
Change from baseline at Week 120		
Number analyzed	10 participants	20 participants
[a]	−0.10(0.74)	−0.05(0.51)
Change from baseline at Week 144		
Number analyzed	9 participants	15 participants
[a]	−0.11(0.93)	−0.20(0.41)
Change from baseline at Week 168		
Number analyzed	3 participants	9 participants
[a]	−0.67(0.58)	−0.11(0.33)
Change from baseline at Week 192		
Number analyzed	0 participants	2 participants
[a]		−0.50(0.71)

Change from baseline at Week 216		
Number analyzed	0 participants	1 participants
a		0.00[b](NA)

[a] Mean (standard deviation) | unit of measure: score on scale
[b] Standard deviation (SD) was not calculable for 1 participant

Additional Results Available

Completed

Ampyra for Optic Neuritis in Multiple Sclerosis

ClinicalTrials.gov ID NCT01337986

Sponsor Washington University School of Medicine
Information provided by Washington University School of Medicine (Responsible Party)
Last Update Posted 2020-01-30

Brief Summary
Fifty subjects will be enrolled in this Phase II, investigator-initiated, randomized, and blinded cross-over trial of dalfampridine of 8 weeks of duration The study will test the hypothesis that dalfampridine, when administered to subjects with incomplete visual recovery after optic neuritis from MS, will result in symptomatic improvement in visual function. The study will consist of one screening/baseline visit, one visit during treatment with active drug, and one visit on placebo. After the baseline visit, subjects will be randomly assigned to receive study medication or placebo for the first 3 weeks, followed by a 2-week wash-out and then treatment reallocation for the latter 3 weeks.

Detailed Description
Optic neuritis (ON) is the presenting feature of multiple sclerosis (MS) in 15% of cases and occurs over the disease course in 50% of patients. (1–3) Vision remains a major concern for MS patients, as visual dysfunction leads to lower quality of life. (4–6) Despite the high prevalence of ON in MS, treatment and management options remain limited. Although intravenous glucocorticoids are employed to aid recovery of an acute episode of ON, no convincing evidence supports their efficacy in altering the degree of long-term recovery. (7) Although some individuals with ON can have a dramatic recovery from blindness, ON often impairs visual function permanently. In the Optic Neuritis Treatment Trial, 63% reported that vision had not returned to normal after 6 months, and 20% had vision worse than 20/20 after 5 years of follow-up (8, 9).

Visual impairment creates difficulties at home and work, leading to decreased independence and impaired mobility within the community. Visual dysfunction in combination with MS impairments within cerebellar and proprioceptive systems can be particularly disabling.

Optic neuritis classically impairs one's ability to read print or a computer screen, to drive in bright or low light, and to appreciate colors and contrasts. Unfortunately, when optic neuritis results in lasting impairment, there are no pharmacologic therapies to restore vision. Low vision specialists may provide magnifying glasses, brighter lights, and advice to optimize the position of objects at home and in the workplace. Better treatment options are needed to improve visual function.

Ampyra (dalfampridine) is a potassium-channel antagonist, with a mechanism of action to improve nerve conduction in demyelinated axons, resulting in an electrophysiologic and clinical benefit. 10–22 Demyelinated axons within the anterior visual pathway would be a prime and ideal target to study the effects of Ampyra. In fact, Stefoski et al. demonstrated visual function benefit in an open-label study of IV 4-aminopyridine in 12 subjects. 21 The optic nerves are a well-defined white-matter tract, commonly affected in MS, and with clear clinical outcome measures.

In addition, visual evoked potentials (VEPs) can be included within the study design as a secondary endpoint, to confirm improved nerve conduction. Because VEPs are such a precise, reliable, and accepted measure of demyelination, the anterior visual pathway is ideal in vivo human system to study the electro-physiologic effects of a therapeutic such as Ampyra.

Hypothesis 1: Dalfampridine treatment will improve visual function, measured by the 5% ETDRS contrast sensitivity chart, in subjects with long-term visual impairment secondary to optic neuritis from MS.

Hypothesis 2: Dalfampridine treatment will reduce visually evoked potential P100 latency following remote optic neuritis.

Hypothesis 3: Dalfampridine treatment will result in an improvement in secondary endpoints, including visual fields, high contrast visual acuity, color vision, and quality of life.

The study will be conducted at the Department of Neurology and Neurosurgery, Washington University School of Medicine, St. Louis, the institution at which Dr. Naismith is based. The MS patients will come from the 1800 active MS patients in our clinic and the 3500 in the St. Louis area.

Fifty subjects will be enrolled in this Phase II, investigator-initiated, randomized, and blinded cross-over trial of dalfampridine of 8-week duration. The study will test the hypothesis that dalfampridine, when administered to subjects with incomplete visual recovery after optic neuritis from MS, will result in symptomatic improvement in visual function. The study will consist of one screening/baseline visit, one visit during treatment with active drug, and one visit on placebo. After the baseline visit, subjects will be randomly assigned to receive study medication or placebo for the first 3 weeks, followed by a 2-week wash-out, and then treatment reallocation for the latter 3 weeks.

Official Title
Dalfampridine After Optic Neuritis to Improve Visual Function in Multiple Sclerosis

Conditions
Multiple Sclerosis
Optic Neuritis

Intervention/Treatment
- Drug: Dalfampridine/Placebo
- Drug: Placebo/Dalfampridine

Other Study ID Numbers
- Ampyra Vision 2011 RTN
- WU HRPO#: 201104126 (Other Identifier) (Other: Washington University HRPO)

Study Start
2011-05

Primary Completion (Actual)
2013-12

Study Completion (Actual)
2013-12

Enrollment (Actual)
53

Study Type
Interventional

Phase
Phase 2 Phase 3

MedlinePlus Genetics related topics: Multiple sclerosis
MedlinePlus related topics: Multiple Sclerosis
Genetic and Rare Diseases Information Center resources: Optic Neuritis
Drug Information available for: Dalfampridine

United States
Missouri Locations

Saint Louis, Missouri, United States, 63110
Washington University (John L. Trotter MS Center)

Eligibility Criteria
Description

Inclusion criteria are as follows:

- At least one previous clinical episode of optic neuritis,
- The last episode of ON must have occurred at least 12 months prior to study entry,
- Clinically definite MS, defined by the revised McDonald criteria, 23
- Ages 18–70,
- Visual acuity greater than or equal to 20/30,
- Must be able to read at least 2 of the 5 letters on the top line of the 5% ETDRS chart (logMAR 0.96) at 3, 2, or 1 m, and
- Must have sufficient cognitive function to understand the consent process and to reliably perform all clinical assessments.

Exclusion criteria are as follows:

- Any ophthalmologic condition, other than ON, which can affect vision, including nystagmus in the primary position of gaze,
- History of seizures or spells with altered level of consciousness,
- Pregnancy or breastfeeding,
- An MS exacerbation or use of glucocorticoids within 3 months of entry,
- A history of moderate to severe renal insufficiency,
- Previous use of 4-aminopyridine, in any formulation, in the prior 4 weeks.

Ages Eligible for Study
18 Years to 55 Years (Adult)

Sexes Eligible for Study
- All

Accepts Healthy Volunteers
- No

Design Details
Primary Purpose: Treatment
Allocation: Randomized
Interventional Model: Crossover Assignment
Masking: Single (Participant)

Arms and interventions

Participant group/arm	Intervention/treatment
Active comparator: group B: dalfampridine first Dalfampridine/placebo: Weeks 1–3: dalfampridine 10 mg (1 tablet) every 12 h for 3 weeks. Weeks 4–5: 2 weeks of wash-out. Weeks 5–8: placebo (sugar pill) 1 tablet every 12 h for 3 weeks	Drug: dalfampridine/placebo • Weeks 1–3: dalfampridine 10 mg (1 tablet) every 12 h for 3 weeks. Weeks 4–5: 2 weeks of wash-out. Weeks 5–8: Placebo (sugar pill) 1 tablet every 12 h for 3 weeks • Other names: – Ampyra (R) – Fampridine
Active comparator: group A: dalfampridine second Placebo/dalfampridine: Weeks 1–3: placebo (sugar pill) 1 tablet every 12 h for 3 weeks. Weeks 4–5: 2 weeks of wash-out. Weeks 6–8: dalfampridine 10 mg (1 tablet) every 12 h for 3 weeks	Drug: placebo/dalfampridine • Weeks 1–3: placebo (sugar pill) 1 tablet every 12 h for 3 weeks. Weeks 4–5: 2 weeks of wash-out. Weeks 6–8: Dalfampridine 10 mg (1 tablet) every 12 h for 3 weeks • Other names: – Ampyra (R) – Fampridine

Primary outcome measures

Outcome measure	Measure description	Time frame
Efficacy of dalfampridine on visual function by early diabetic treatment retinopathy study (EDTRS) 5% contrast sensitivity scores	Per protocol analysis to assess differences in EDTRS 5% contrast sensitivity (LogMAR) scores at visits 2 and 3 Relative to Visit 1 on patients taking dalfampridine vs. placebo	Visit 1 (Week 0), Visit 2 (Week 3), and Visit 3 (Week 8)
Efficacy of dalfampridine on visual function assessed by change from baseline in raw letters by EDTRS 5% contrast sensitivity	Per protocol analysis to assess the difference in number of letters on the EDTRS 5% contrast sensitivity (LogMAR) chart scores at visits 2 and 3 Relative to Visit 1	Visit 1 (Week 0), Visit 2 (Week 3), and Visit 3 (Week 8)
Difference in EDTRS 5% contrast sensitivity (LogMAR score) at Visits 2 and 3 Relative to Visit 1	Intent to treat analysis of treatment effect in primary endpoint EDTRS 5% contrast sensitivity. Improvement from baseline scores	Visit 1 (Week 0), Visit 2 (Week 3), and Visit 3 (Week 8)
Change from baseline in raw letters by EDTRS 5% contrast sensitivity	Intent to treat analysis of treatment effect in primary endpoint EDTRS 5% contrast sensitivity. Change in the number of letters able to read while on dalfampridine and placebo relative to their baseline scores	Visit 1 (Week 0), Visit 2 (Week 3), and Visit 3 (Week 8)

Secondary outcome measures

Outcome measure	Measure description	Time frame
Percentage of eyes that improved by 2 lines (10 letters) on the sloan 5% contrast sensitivity chart		Visit 1 (Week 0), Visit 2 (Week 3), and Visit 3 (Week 8)
Percentage of eyes that improved by one line (5 letters)	Percentage of eyes that improved by one line (5 letters) on the 5% contrast sensitivity chart	Visit 1 (Week 0), Visit 2 (Week 3), and Visit 3 (Week 8)
Visual evoked potential P100 latency per treatment arm	Visual evoked potential 60 min P100 latency on dalfampridine vs. placebo	Visit 1 (Week 0), Visit 2 (Week 3), and Visit 3 (Week 8)
Odds ratio quartile of visual field index	The Visual Field Index (VFI) is a global index that assigns a number between 1 and 100% based on an aggregate percentage of visual function, with 100% being a perfect age-adjusted visual field Probability of falling in the best quartile for visual field (VFI) measures (Q1), relative to the three next quartiles for worse VFIs (Q2-4), while on Dalfampridine vs. Placebo. Due to the clustered observations at different times in a cross-over design, the visual field data are not suited to a normal theory model and should not be expressed as a continuous variable. Thus, a categorical model that uses a multinomial distribution for the measurement of 4 categories was selected for proper statistical modeling, with results expressed as odds ratios	Visit 1 (Week 0—baseline), Visit 2 (Week 3—post intervention 1), and Visit 3 (Week 8—post intervention 2)
Changes in color vision total error score from baseline based upon the Farnsworth Munsell Hue 100 Sort Test (FM100)	Dalfampridine will change color vision Total Error Scores from baseline on the Farnsworth Munsell 100 Hue Sort Test. Farnsworth Munsell 100 Hue Test requires placing 100 color palettes in the correct order based upon color hue. Scores are determined by the frequency and severity of any displacement in the correct order. One error equates to one misplaced hue, by one step or position. An error score greater than 500 indicates virtually no color discrimination. An error score of 0 indicates no errors in ordering the hues. A Total Error Score of 0–128 could be seen in a normal population	Visit 1 (Week 0—baseline), Visit 2 (Week 3—postintervention 1), and Visit 3 (Week 8—postintervention 2)

Outcome measure	Measure description	Time frame
Dalfampridine effect on quality of life change from baseline	Dalfampridine treatment will result in a change in quality of life. The National Eye Institute Visual Function Questionnaire consists of 25 questions characterizing visual function at home and in the community. Score ranges from 100 (best) to 0 (worst)	Visit 1 (Week 0), Visit 2 (Week 3), and Visit 3 (Week 8)
Difference in Pelli-Robson Score at Visits 2 and 3 Relative to Visit 1	Difference in Pelli-Robson Score at Visits 2 and 3 Relative to Visit 1 on Dalfampridine vs. Placebo. Pelli-Robson is scored based on the numbers read on the chart converted to LogMAR units. The scale is 0.00 (worst) to 2.35 (best)	Visit 1 (Week 0), Visit 2 (Week 3), and Visit 3 (Week 8)

Sponsor
Washington University School of Medicine

Collaborators
- Acorda Therapeutics

Investigators
- Principal Investigator: Robert T Naismith, MD, Washington University School of Medicine

General Publications

- Frohman EM, Frohman TC, Zee DS, McColl R, Galetta S. The neuro-ophthalmology of multiple sclerosis. Lancet Neurol. 2005 Feb;4(2):111–21. https://doi.org/10.1016/S1474-4422(05)00992-0
- Arnold AC. Evolving management of optic neuritis and multiple sclerosis. Am J Ophthalmol. 2005 Jun;139(6):1101–8. https://doi.org/10.1016/j.ajo.2005.01.031.
- Balcer LJ. Clinical practice. Optic neuritis. N Engl J Med. 2006 Mar 23;354(12):1273–80. https://doi.org/10.1056/NEJMcp053247. No abstract available.
- Ma SL, Shea JA, Galetta SL, Jacobs DA, Markowitz CE, Maguire MG, Balcer LJ. Self-reported visual dysfunction in multiple sclerosis: new data from the VFQ-25 and development of an MS-specific vision questionnaire. Am J Ophthalmol. 2002 May;133(5):686–92. https://doi.org/10.1016/s0002-9394(02)01337-5.
- Noble J, Forooghian F, Sproule M, Westall C, O'Connor P. Utility of the National Eye Institute VFQ-25 questionnaire in a heterogeneous group of multiple sclerosis patients. Am J Ophthalmol. 2006 Sep;142(3):464–8. https://doi.org/10.1016/j.ajo.2006.04.051.
- Mowry EM, Loguidice MJ, Daniels AB, Jacobs DA, Markowitz CE, Galetta SL, Nano-Schiavi ML, Cutter GR, Maguire MG, Balcer LJ. Vision related quality of life in multiple sclerosis: correlation with new measures of low and high contrast letter acuity. J Neurol Neurosurg Psychiatry. 2009 Jul;80(7):767–72. https://doi.org/10.1136/jnnp.2008.165449. Epub 2009 Feb 23.

- Beck RW, Cleary PA, Anderson MM Jr., Keltner JL, Shults WT, Kaufman DI, Buckley EG, Corbett JJ, Kupersmith MJ, Miller NR, et al. A randomized, controlled trial of corticosteroids in the treatment of acute optic neuritis. The Optic Neuritis Study Group. N Engl J Med. 1992 Feb 27;326(9):581–8. https://doi.org/10.1056/NEJM199202273260901.
- Visual function 5 years after optic neuritis: experience of the Optic Neuritis Treatment Trial. The Optic Neuritis Study Group. Arch Ophthalmol. 1997 Dec;115(12):1545–52.
- Cleary PA, Beck RW, Bourque LB, Backlund JC, Miskala PH. Visual symptoms after optic neuritis. Results from the Optic Neuritis Treatment Trial. J Neuroophthalmol. 1997 Mar;17(1):18–23; quiz 24–8. https://doi.org/10.1016/s0002-9394(14)70814-1.
- Goodman AD, Brown TR, Krupp LB, Schapiro RT, Schwid SR, Cohen R, Marinucci LN, Blight AR; Fampridine MS-F203 Investigators. Sustained-release oral fampridine in multiple sclerosis: a randomised, double-blind, controlled trial. Lancet. 2009 Feb 28;373(9665):732–8. https://doi.org/10.1016/S0140-6736(09)60442-6.
- Fujihara K, Miyoshi T. The effects of 4-aminopyridine on motor evoked potentials in multiple sclerosis. J Neurol Sci. 1998 Jul 15;159(1):102–6. https://doi.org/10.1016/s0022-510x(98)00143-9.
- Schwid SR, Petrie MD, McDermott MP, Tierney DS, Mason DH, Goodman AD. Quantitative assessment of sustained-release 4-aminopyridine for symptomatic treatment of multiple sclerosis. Neurology. 1997 Apr;48(4):817–21. https://doi.org/10.1212/wnl.48.4.817.
- Davis FA, Stefoski D, Quandt FN. Mechanism of action of 4-aminopyridine in the symptomatic treatment of multiple sclerosis. Ann Neurol. 1995 May;37(5):684. https://doi.org/10.1002/ana.410370524. No abstract available.
- Bever CT Jr., Young D, Anderson PA, Krumholz A, Conway K, Leslie J, Eddington N, Plaisance KI, Panitch HS, Dhib-Jalbut S, et al. The effects of 4-aminopyridine in multiple sclerosis patients: results of a randomized, placebo-controlled, double-blind, concentration-controlled, crossover trial. Neurology. 1994 Jun;44(6):1054–9. https://doi.org/10.1212/wnl.44.6.1054.
- Polman CH, Bertelsmann FW, van Loenen AC, Koetsier JC. 4-aminopyridine in the treatment of patients with multiple sclerosis. Long-term efficacy and safety. Arch Neurol. 1994 Mar;51(3):292–6. https://doi.org/10.1001/archneur.1994.00540150090022.
- van Diemen HA, Polman CH, van Dongen MM, Nauta JJ, Strijers RL, van Loenen AC, Bertelsmann FW, Koetsier JC. 4-Aminopyridine induces functional improvement in multiple sclerosis patients: a neurophysiological study. J Neurol Sci. 1993 Jun;116(2):220–6. https://doi.org/10.1016/0022-510x(93)90329-w.
- van Diemen HA, Polman CH, van Dongen TM, van Loenen AC, Nauta JJ, Taphoorn MJ, van Walbeek HK, Koetsier JC. The effect of 4-aminopyridine on clinical signs in multiple sclerosis: a randomized, placebo-controlled, double-blind, cross-over study. Ann Neurol. 1992 Aug;32(2):123–30. https://doi.org/10.1002/ana.410320203.

- Stefoski D, Davis FA, Fitzsimmons WE, Luskin SS, Rush J, Parkhurst GW. 4-Aminopyridine in multiple sclerosis: prolonged administration. Neurology. 1991 Sep;41(9):1344–8. https://doi.org/10.1212/wnl.41.9.1344.
- Polman CH, van Diemen HA, van Dongen MM, Koetsier JC, van Loenen AC, van Walbeek HK. 4-Aminopyridine in multiple sclerosis. Ann Neurol. 1990 Oct;28(4):589. https://doi.org/10.1002/ana.410280421. No abstract available.
- Davis FA, Stefoski D, Rush J. Orally administered 4-aminopyridine improves clinical signs in multiple sclerosis. Ann Neurol. 1990 Feb;27(2):186–92. https://doi.org/10.1002/ana.410270215.
- Polman CH, Reingold SC, Edan G, Filippi M, Hartung HP, Kappos L, Lublin FD, Metz LM, McFarland HF, O'Connor PW, Sandberg-Wollheim M, Thompson AJ, Weinshenker BG, Wolinsky JS. Diagnostic criteria for multiple sclerosis: 2005 revisions to the "McDonald Criteria". Ann Neurol. 2005 Dec;58(6):840–6. https://doi.org/10.1002/ana.20703.
- Jones RE, Heron JR, Foster DH, Snelgar RS, Mason RJ. Effects of 4-aminopyridine in patients with multiple sclerosis. J Neurol Sci. 1983 Aug-Sep;60(3):353–62. https://doi.org/10.1016/0022-510x(83)90145-4.
- Vollmer T, Henney HR 3rd. Pharmacokinetics and tolerability of single escalating doses of fampridine sustained-release tablets in patients with multiple sclerosis: a Phase I-II, open-label trial. Clin Ther. 2009 Oct;31(10):2206–14. https://doi.org/10.1016/j.clinthera.2009.10.008.
- Vollmer T, Blight AR, Henney HR 3rd. Steady-state pharmacokinetics and tolerability of orally administered fampridine sustained-release 10-mg tablets in patients with multiple sclerosis: a 2-week, open-label, follow-up study. Clin Ther. 2009 Oct;31(10):2215–23. https://doi.org/10.1016/j.clinthera.2009.10.007.
- Beck RW, Ruchman MC, Savino PJ, Schatz NJ. Contrast sensitivity measurements in acute and resolved optic neuritis. Br J Ophthalmol. 1984 Oct;68(10):756–9. https://doi.org/10.1136/bjo.68.10.756.
- Trobe JD, Beck RW, Moke PS, Cleary PA. Contrast sensitivity and other vision tests in the optic neuritis treatment trial. Am J Ophthalmol. 1996 May;121(5):547–53. https://doi.org/10.1016/s0002-9394(14)75429-7.
- Farnsworth D. The Farnsworth-Munsell 100-hue and dichotomous tests for color vision. J Opt Soc Am 1943;33:568–574.
- Naismith RT, Tutlam NT, Xu J, Klawiter EC, Shepherd J, Trinkaus K, Song SK, Cross AH. Optical coherence tomography differs in neuromyelitis optica compared with multiple sclerosis. Neurology. 2009 Mar 24;72(12):1077–82. https://doi.org/10.1212/01.wnl.0000345042.53843.d5.
- Naismith RT, Tutlam NT, Xu J, Shepherd JB, Klawiter EC, Song SK, Cross AH. Optical coherence tomography is less sensitive than visual evoked potentials in optic neuritis. Neurology. 2009 Jul 7;73(1):46–52. https://doi.org/10.1212/WNL.0b013e3181aaea32.
- Naismith RT, Xu J, Tutlam NT, Trinkaus K, Cross AH, Song SK. Radial diffusivity in remote optic neuritis discriminates visual outcomes. Neurology. 2010 May 25;74(21):1702–10. https://doi.org/10.1212/WNL.0b013e3181e0434d.

- Naismith RT, Xu J, Tutlam NT, Scully PT, Trinkaus K, Snyder AZ, Song SK, Cross AH. Increased diffusivity in acute multiple sclerosis lesions predicts risk of black hole. Neurology. 2010 May 25;74(21):1694–701. https://doi.org/10.1212/WNL.0b013e3181e042c4. Erratum In: Neurology. 2010 Sep 7;75(10):938.
- Naismith RT, Xu J, Tutlam NT, Snyder A, Benzinger T, Shimony J, Shepherd J, Trinkaus K, Cross AH, Song SK. Disability in optic neuritis correlates with diffusion tensor-derived directional diffusivities. Neurology. 2009 Feb 17;72(7):589–94. https://doi.org/10.1212/01.wnl.0000335766.22758.cd. Epub 2008 Dec 10.
- Naismith RT, Shepherd JB, Weihl CC, Tutlam NT, Cross AH. Acute and bilateral blindness due to optic neuropathy associated with copper deficiency. Arch Neurol. 2009 Aug;66(8):1025–7. https://doi.org/10.1001/archneurol.2009.70.
- Vanden Bosch ME, Wall M. Visual acuity scored by the letter-by-letter or probit methods has lower retest variability than the line assignment method. Eye (Lond). 1997;11 (Pt 3):411–7. https://doi.org/10.1038/eye.1997.87.
- Acorda Therapeutics. AMPRYA package insert (2010).

Results

Outcome Measures

1. Efficacy of Dalfampridine on Visual Function by Early Diabetic Treatment Retinopathy Study (EDTRS) 5% Contrast Sensitivity Scores

   Type: Primary | Time Frame: Visit 1 (Week 0), Visit 2 (Week 3), and Visit 3 (Week 8)

Description	Per protocol analysis to assess differences in EDTRS 5% contrast sensitivity (LogMAR) scores at visits 2 and 3 relative to Visit 1 on patients taking dalfampridine vs. placebo
Time frame	Visit 1 (Week 0), Visit 2 (Week 3), and Visit 3 (Week 8)
Analysis population description	Per protocol analysis

Arm/group title	Group B: dalfampridine	Group B: placebo	Group A: placebo	Group A: dalfampridine
Arm/group description	Dalfampridine/placebo: Weeks 1–3: dalfampridine 10 mg (1 tablet) every 12 h for 3 weeks. Weeks 4–5: 2 weeks of wash-out. Weeks 5–8: placebo (sugar pill) 1 tablet every 12 h for 3 weeks Show less	Dalfampridine/placebo: Weeks 1–3: dalfampridine 10 mg (1 tablet) every 12 h for 3 weeks. Weeks 4–5: 2 weeks of wash-out. Weeks 5–8: placebo (sugar pill) 1 tablet every 12 h for 3 weeks Show less	Placebo/dalfampridine: Weeks 1–3: placebo (sugar pill) 1 tablet every 12 h for 3 weeks. Weeks 4–5: 2 weeks of wash-out. Weeks 6–8: dalfampridine 10 mg (1 tablet) every 12 h for 3 weeks Show less	Placebo/dalfampridine: Weeks 1–3: placebo (sugar pill) 1 tablet every 12 h for 3 weeks. Weeks 4–5: 2 weeks of wash-out. Weeks 6–8: dalfampridine 10 mg (1 tablet) every 12 h for 3 weeks Show less

Overall number of participants analyzed	20	20	18	18
Overall number of units analyzed Type of units analyzed: eligible eyes	30	30	29	29
Mean (standard deviation) I unit of measure: LogMAR score	−0.04(0.02)	−0.06(0.02)	−0.08(0.02)	−0.06(0.02)

Statistical analysis 1: group B: dalfampridine, group B: placebo, group A: placebo, group A: dalfampridine I superiority or other (legacy) I mixed models analysis
Statistical analysis 2: group B: dalfampridine, group B: placebo, group A: placebo, group A: dalfampridine I superiority or other (legacy) I mixed models analysis

2. Efficacy of Dalfampridine on Visual Function Assessed by Change from Baseline in Raw Letters by EDTRS 5% Contrast Sensitivity
   Type: Primary I Time Frame: Visit 1 (Week 0), Visit 2 (Week 3), and Visit 3 (Week 8)

Description	Per protocol analysis to assess the difference in number of letters on the EDTRS 5% contrast sensitivity (LogMAR) chart scores at visits 2 and 3 relative to Visit 1
Time frame	Visit 1 (Week 0), Visit 2 (Week 3), and Visit 3 (Week 8)
Analysis population description	Per protocol analysis

Arm/group title	Group B: dalfampridine	Group B: placebo	Group A: placebo	Group A: dalfampridine
Arm/group description	Dalfampridine/ placebo: Weeks 1–3: dalfampridine 10 mg (1 tablet) every 12 h for 3 weeks. Weeks 4–5: 2 weeks of wash-out. Weeks 5–8: placebo (sugar pill) 1 tablet every 12 h for 3 weeks Show less	Dalfampridine/ placebo: Weeks 1–3: dalfampridine 10 mg (1 tablet) every 12 h for 3 weeks. Weeks 4–5: 2 weeks of wash-out. Weeks 5–8: placebo (sugar pill) 1 tablet every 12 h for 3 weeks Show less	Placebo/ dalfampridine: Weeks 1–3: placebo (sugar pill) 1 tablet every 12 h for 3 weeks. Weeks 4–5: 2 weeks of wash-out. Weeks 6–8: dalfampridine 10 mg (1 tablet) every 12 h for 3 weeks Show less	Placebo/ dalfampridine: Weeks 1–3: Placebo (sugar pill) 1 tablet every 12 h for 3 weeks. Weeks 4–5: 2 weeks of wash-out. Weeks 6–8: dalfampridine 10 mg (1 tablet) every 12 h for 3 weeks Show less
Overall number of participants analyzed	20	20	18	18
Overall number of units analyzed Type of units analyzed: eligible eyes	30	30	29	29
Mean (standard deviation) ǀ unit of measure: letters	2(1)	2(1)	4(1)	3(1)

3. Difference in EDTRS 5% Contrast Sensitivity (LOGMAR Score) at Visits 2 and 3 Relative to Visit 1

   Type: Primary ǀ Time Frame: Visit 1 (Week 0), Visit 2 (Week 3), and Visit 3 (Week 8)

Description	Intent to treat analysis of treatment effect in primary endpoint EDTRS 5% contrast sensitivity. Improvement from baseline scores
Time frame	Visit 1 (Week 0), Visit 2 (Week 3), and Visit 3 (Week 8)
Analysis population description	Intent to treat population, scores from morning and afternoon were averaged

Arm/group title	Dalfampridine	Placebo
Arm/group description	Patient assessments while on dalfampridine	Patient assessments while on dalfampridine
Overall number of participants analyzed	46	46
Mean (standard deviation) ǀ unit of measure: 5% Contrast LogMAR score	0.06(0.02)	0.05(0.02)

Statistical analysis 1: dalfampridine, placebo ǀ superiority or Other (legacy) ǀ mixed models analysis
Statistical analysis 2: dalfampridine, placebo ǀ superiority or other (legacy) ǀ mixed models analysis

4. Change from Baseline in RAW Letters by EDTRS 5% Contrast Sensitivity
   Type: Primary ǀ Time Frame: Visit 1 (Week 0), Visit 2 (Week 3), and Visit 3 (Week 8)

Description	Intent to treat analysis of treatment effect in primary endpoint EDTRS 5% contrast sensitivity. Change in the number of letters able to read while on dalfampridine and placebo relative to their baseline scores
Time frame	Visit 1 (Week 0), Visit 2 (Week 3), and Visit 3 (Week 8)
Analysis population description	Intent to treat population, scores from morning and afternoon were averaged

Arm/group title	Dalfampridine	Placebo
Arm/group description	Patient assessments while on dalfampridine	Patient assessments while on dalfampridine
Overall number of participants analyzed	46	46
Mean (standard deviation) ǀ unit of measure: letters	3(1)	2.5(1)

5. Percentage of Eyes That Improved by 2 Lines (10 Letters) On the Sloan 5% Contrast Sensitivity Chart
   Type: Secondary ǀ Time Frame: Visit 1 (Week 0), Visit 2 (Week 3), and Visit 3 (Week 8)

Description	[Not specified]
Time frame	Visit 1 (Week 0), Visit 2 (Week 3), and Visit 3 (Week 8)
Analysis population description	[Not specified]

Arm/group title	Dalfampridine	Placebo	Both	None
Arm/group description	Improvement while on dalfampridine (not placebo)	Improvement while on placebo (not dalfampridine)	Improvement when taking dalfampridine or placebo (improvement with any treatment)	No improvement on dalfampridine/placebo
Overall number of participants analyzed	46	46	46	46
Overall number of units analyzed Type of units analyzed: number of eyes	72	72	72	72
Measure type: number (95% confidence interval) ǀ unit of measure: percentages of eyes that improved	9.7(4.0–19.0)	11.1(4.9–20.7)	11.1(4.9–20.7)	68.1(56.0–78.6)
Statistical analysis 1: dalfampridine, placebo, both, none ǀ superiority or other (legacy) ǀ regression, logistic				

6. Percentage of Eyes That Improved by One-Line (5 Letters)
   Type: Secondary ǀ Time Frame: Visit 1 (Week 0), Visit 2 (Week 3), and Visit 3 (Week 8)

Description	Percentage of eyes that improved by one-line (5 letters) on the 5% contrast sensitivity chart
Time frame	Visit 1 (Week 0), Visit 2 (Week 3), and Visit 3 (Week 8)
Analysis population description	Proportion as the percent of eyes improved by 1 line

Arm/group title	Dalfampridine	Placebo	Both	Neither
Arm/group description	Improvement while on dalfampridine	Improvement while on placebo	Improvement on dalfampridine and placebo	No improvement on dalfampridine or placebo

Overall number of participants analyzed	38	38	38	38
Overall number of units analyzed Type of units analyzed: number of eyes	72	72	72	72
Measure type: number (95% confidence interval) | unit of measure: percent of eyes	11.1(4.9–20.7)	15.3(7.9–25.7)	37.5(26.4–49.7)	36.1(25.1–48.3)
Statistical analysis 1: dalfampridine, placebo, both | superiority or other (legacy) | regression, logistic				

Additional results available

Completed

Efficacy and Safety Study of Satralizumab (SA237) as Monotherapy to Treat Participants with Neuromyelitis Optica (NMO) and Neuromyelitis Optica Spectrum Disorder (NMOSD)

ClinicalTrials.gov ID NCT02073279

Sponsor Hoffmann-La Roche
Information provided by Hoffmann-La Roche (Responsible Party)
Last Update Posted 2023-03-01

Brief Summary
The objectives of this study are to evaluate the efficacy, safety, pharmacodynamic, pharmacokinetic, and immunogenic profiles of satralizumab in participants with NMO and NMOSD.

Official Title
A Multicenter, Randomized, Double-Blind, Placebo-Controlled, Phase 3 Study to Evaluate the Efficacy and Safety of Satralizumab (SA237) as Monotherapy in Patients With Neuromyelitis Optica (NMO) and Neuromyelitis Optica Spectrum Disorder (NMOSD)

Conditions
Multiple Sclerosis
Optic Neuritis

Intervention/Treatment
- Drug: Dalfampridine/Placebo
- Drug: Placebo/Dalfampridine

Other Study ID Numbers
- Ampyra Vision 2011 RTN
- WU HRPO#: 201104126 (Other Identifier) (Other: Washington University HRPO)

Study Start
2011-05

Primary Completion (Actual)
2013-12

Study Completion (Actual)
2013-12

Enrollment (Actual)
53

Study Type
Interventional

Phase
Phase 2 Phase 3

United States
Missouri Locations

Saint Louis, Missouri, United States, 63110
Washington University (John L. Trotter MS Center)

Eligibility Criteria
Description

Inclusion criteria are:

- At least one previous clinical episode of optic neuritis,
- The last episode of ON must have occurred at least 12 months prior to study entry,
- Clinically definite MS, defined by the revised McDonald criteria, 23
- Ages 18–70,
- Visual acuity greater than or equal to 20/30
- Must be able to read at least 2 of the 5 letters on the top line of the 5% ETDRS chart (logMAR 0.96) at 3, 2, or 1 m, and
- Must have sufficient cognitive function to understand the consent process and to reliably perform all clinical assessments.

Exclusion criteria are as follows:

- Any ophthalmologic condition, other than ON, which can affect vision, including nystagmus in the primary position of gaze,
- History of seizures or spells with altered level of consciousness,

- Pregnancy or breastfeeding,
- An MS exacerbation or use of glucocorticoids within 3 months of entry,
- A history of moderate to severe renal insufficiency,
- Previous use of 4-aminopyridine, in any formulation, in the prior 4 weeks.

Ages Eligible for Study
18 Years to 55 Years (Adult)

Sexes Eligible for Study
All

Accepts Healthy Volunteers
No

Design Details
Primary Purpose: Treatment
Allocation: Randomized
Interventional Model: Crossover Assignment
Masking: Single (Participant)

Arms and interventions

Participant group/arm	Intervention/treatment
Active comparator: group B: dalfampridine first Dalfampridine/placebo: Weeks 1–3: dalfampridine 10 mg (1 tablet) every 12 h for 3 weeks. Weeks 4–5: 2 weeks of wash-out. Weeks 5–8: placebo (sugar pill) 1 tablet every 12 h for 3 weeks	Drug: dalfampridine/placebo • Weeks 1–3: dalfampridine 10 mg (1 tablet) every 12 h for 3 weeks. Weeks 4–5: 2 weeks of wash-out. Weeks 5–8: placebo (sugar pill) 1 tablet every 12 h for 3 weeks • Other names: – Ampyra (R) – Fampridine
Active comparator: group A: dalfampridine second Placebo/dalfampridine: Weeks 1–3: placebo (sugar pill) 1 tablet every 12 h for 3 weeks. Weeks 4–5: 2 weeks of wash-out. Weeks 6–8: dalfampridine 10 mg (1 tablet) every 12 h for 3 weeks	Drug: placebo/dalfampridine • Weeks 1–3: placebo (sugar pill) 1 tablet every 12 h for 3 weeks. Weeks 4–5: 2 weeks of wash-out. Weeks 6–8: dalfampridine 10 mg (1 tablet) every 12 h for 3 weeks • Other names: – Ampyra (R) – Fampridine

Primary outcome measures

Outcome measure	Measure description	Time frame
Efficacy of dalfampridine on visual function by early diabetic treatment retinopathy study (EDTRS) 5% contrast sensitivity scores	Per protocol analysis to assess differences in EDTRS 5% contrast sensitivity (LogMAR) scores at visits 2 and 3 relative to Visit 1 on patients taking dalfampridine vs. placebo	Visit 1 (Week 0), Visit 2 (Week 3), and Visit 3 (Week 8)
Efficacy of dalfampridine on visual function assessed by change from baseline in raw letters by EDTRS 5% contrast sensitivity	Per protocol analysis to assess the difference in number of letters on the EDTRS 5% contrast sensitivity (LogMAR) chart scores at visits 2 and 3 relative to Visit 1	Visit 1 (Week 0), Visit 2 (Week 3), and Visit 3 (Week 8)

Outcome measure	Measure description	Time frame
Difference in EDTRS 5% contrast sensitivity (LogMAR Score) at Visits 2 and 3 relative to Visit 1	Intent to treat analysis of treatment effect in primary endpoint EDTRS 5% contrast sensitivity. Improvement from baseline scores	Visit 1 (Week 0), Visit 2 (Week 3), and Visit 3 (Week 8)
Change from baseline in raw letters by EDTRS 5% contrast sensitivity	Intent to treat analysis of treatment effect in primary endpoint EDTRS 5% contrast sensitivity. Change in the number of letters able to read while on dalfampridine and placebo relative to their baseline scores	Visit 1 (Week 0), Visit 2 (Week 3), and Visit 3 (Week 8)

Secondary outcome measures

Outcome measure	Measure description	Time frame
Percentage of eyes that improved by 2 lines (10 letters) on the sloan 5% contrast sensitivity chart		Visit 1 (Week 0), Visit 2 (Week 3) and Visit 3 (Week 8)
Percentage of eyes that improved by one line (5 letters)	Percentage of eyes that improved by one line (5 letters) on the 5% contrast sensitivity chart	Visit 1 (Week 0), Visit 2 (Week 3), and Visit 3 (Week 8)
Visual evoked potential P100 latency per treatment arm	Visual evoked potential 60 min P100 latency on dalfampridine vs. placebo	Visit 1 (Week 0), Visit 2 (Week 3), and Visit 3 (Week 8)
Odds ratio quartile of visual field index	The visual field index (VFI) is a global index that assigns a number between 1% and 100% based on an aggregate percentage of visual function, with 100% being a perfect age-adjusted visual field Probability of falling in the best quartile for visual field (VFI) measures (Q1), relative to the three next quartiles for worse VFIs (Q2-4), while on Dalfampridine vs. Placebo. Due to the clustered observations at different times in a cross-over design, the visual field data are not suited to a normal theory model and should not be expressed as a continuous variable. Thus, a categorical model that uses a multinomial distribution for the measurement of 4 categories was selected for proper statistical modeling, with results expressed as odds ratios	Visit 1 (Week 0—baseline), Visit 2 (Week 3—post intervention 1), and Visit 3 (Week 8—post intervention 2)

Outcome measure	Measure description	Time frame
Changes in color vision total error score from baseline based upon the Farnsworth Munsell Hue 100 Sort Test (FM100)	Dalfampridine will change color vision total error scores from baseline on the Farnsworth Munsell 100 Hue Sort Test. Farnsworth Munsell 100 Hue Test requires placing 100 color palettes in the correct order based upon color hue. Scores are determined by the frequency and severity of any displacement in the correct order. One error equates to one misplaced hue, by one step or position. An error score greater than 500 indicates virtually no color discrimination. An error score of 0 indicates no errors in ordering the hues. A Total Error Score of 0–128 could be seen in a normal population	Visit 1 (Week 0—baseline), Visit 2 (Week 3—postintervention 1), and Visit 3 (Week 8—post intervention 2)
Dalfampridine effect on quality of life change from baseline	Dalfampridine treatment will result in a change in quality of life. The National Eye Institute Visual Function Questionnaire consists of 25 questions characterizing visual function at home and in the community. Score ranges from 100 (best) to 0 (worst)	Visit 1 (Week 0), Visit 2 (Week 3), and Visit 3 (Week 8)
Difference in Pelli-Robson Score at Visits 2 and 3 relative to Visit 1	Difference in Pelli-Robson Score at Visits 2 and 3 relative to Visit 1 on dalfampridine vs. placebo. Pelli-Robson is scored based on the numbers read on the chart converted to LogMAR units. The scale is 0.00 (worst) to 2.35 (best)	Visit 1 (Week 0), Visit 2 (Week 3), and Visit 3 (Week 8)

Sponsor

Washington University School of Medicine

Collaborators

- Acorda Therapeutics

Investigators

- Principal Investigator: Robert T Naismith, MD, Washington University School of Medicine

General Publications

- Frohman EM, Frohman TC, Zee DS, McColl R, Galetta S. The neuro-ophthalmology of multiple sclerosis. Lancet Neurol. 2005 Feb;4(2):111–21. https://doi.org/10.1016/S1474-4422(05)00992-0.
- Arnold AC. Evolving management of optic neuritis and multiple sclerosis. Am J Ophthalmol. 2005 Jun;139(6):1101–8. https://doi.org/10.1016/j.ajo.2005.01.031.
- Balcer LJ. Clinical practice. Optic neuritis. N Engl J Med. 2006 Mar 23;354(12):1273–80. https://doi.org/10.1056/NEJMcp053247. No abstract available.
- Ma SL, Shea JA, Galetta SL, Jacobs DA, Markowitz CE, Maguire MG, Balcer LJ. Self-reported visual dysfunction in multiple sclerosis: new data from the

VFQ-25 and development of an MS-specific vision questionnaire. Am J Ophthalmol. 2002 May;133(5):686–92. https://doi.org/10.1016/s0002-9394(02)01337-5.

- Noble J, Forooghian F, Sproule M, Westall C, O'Connor P. Utility of the National Eye Institute VFQ-25 questionnaire in a heterogeneous group of multiple sclerosis patients. Am J Ophthalmol. 2006 Sep;142(3):464–8. https://doi.org/10.1016/j.ajo.2006.04.051.
- Mowry EM, Loguidice MJ, Daniels AB, Jacobs DA, Markowitz CE, Galetta SL, Nano-Schiavi ML, Cutter GR, Maguire MG, Balcer LJ. Vision related quality of life in multiple sclerosis: correlation with new measures of low and high contrast letter acuity. J Neurol Neurosurg Psychiatry. 2009 Jul;80(7):767–72. https://doi.org/10.1136/jnnp.2008.165449. Epub 2009 Feb 23.
- Beck RW, Cleary PA, Anderson MM Jr., Keltner JL, Shults WT, Kaufman DI, Buckley EG, Corbett JJ, Kupersmith MJ, Miller NR, et al. A randomized, controlled trial of corticosteroids in the treatment of acute optic neuritis. The Optic Neuritis Study Group. N Engl J Med. 1992 Feb 27;326(9):581–8. https://doi.org/10.1056/NEJM199202273260901.
- Visual function 5 years after optic neuritis: experience of the Optic Neuritis Treatment Trial. The Optic Neuritis Study Group. Arch Ophthalmol. 1997 Dec;115(12):1545–52.
- Cleary PA, Beck RW, Bourque LB, Backlund JC, Miskala PH. Visual symptoms after optic neuritis. Results from the Optic Neuritis Treatment Trial. J Neuroophthalmol. 1997 Mar;17(1):18–23; quiz 24–8. https://doi.org/10.1016/s0002-9394(14)70814-1.
- Goodman AD, Brown TR, Krupp LB, Schapiro RT, Schwid SR, Cohen R, Marinucci LN, Blight AR; Fampridine MS-F203 Investigators. Sustained-release oral fampridine in multiple sclerosis: a randomised, double-blind, controlled trial. Lancet. 2009 Feb 28;373(9665):732–8. https://doi.org/10.1016/S0140-6736(09)60442-6.
- Fujihara K, Miyoshi T. The effects of 4-aminopyridine on motor evoked potentials in multiple sclerosis. J Neurol Sci. 1998 Jul 15;159(1):102–6. https://doi.org/10.1016/s0022-510x(98)00143-9.
- Schwid SR, Petrie MD, McDermott MP, Tierney DS, Mason DH, Goodman AD. Quantitative assessment of sustained-release 4-aminopyridine for symptomatic treatment of multiple sclerosis. Neurology. 1997 Apr;48(4):817–21. https://doi.org/10.1212/wnl.48.4.817.
- Davis FA, Stefoski D, Quandt FN. Mechanism of action of 4-aminopyridine in the symptomatic treatment of multiple sclerosis. Ann Neurol. 1995 May;37(5):684. https://doi.org/10.1002/ana.410370524. No abstract available.
- Bever CT Jr., Young D, Anderson PA, Krumholz A, Conway K, Leslie J, Eddington N, Plaisance KI, Panitch HS, Dhib-Jalbut S, et al. The effects of 4-aminopyridine in multiple sclerosis patients: results of a randomized, placebo-controlled, double-blind, concentration-controlled, crossover trial. Neurology. 1994 Jun;44(6):1054–9. https://doi.org/10.1212/wnl.44.6.1054.

- Polman CH, Bertelsmann FW, van Loenen AC, Koetsier JC. 4-aminopyridine in the treatment of patients with multiple sclerosis. Long-term efficacy and safety. Arch Neurol. 1994 Mar;51(3):292–6. https://doi.org/10.1001/archneur.1994.00540150090022.
- van Diemen HA, Polman CH, van Dongen MM, Nauta JJ, Strijers RL, van Loenen AC, Bertelsmann FW, Koetsier JC. 4-Aminopyridine induces functional improvement in multiple sclerosis patients: a neurophysiological study. J Neurol Sci. 1993 Jun;116(2):220–6. https://doi.org/10.1016/0022-510x(93)90329-w.
- van Diemen HA, Polman CH, van Dongen TM, van Loenen AC, Nauta JJ, Taphoorn MJ, van Walbeek HK, Koetsier JC. The effect of 4-aminopyridine on clinical signs in multiple sclerosis: a randomized, placebo-controlled, double-blind, cross-over study. Ann Neurol. 1992 Aug;32(2):123–30. https://doi.org/10.1002/ana.410320203.
- Stefoski D, Davis FA, Fitzsimmons WE, Luskin SS, Rush J, Parkhurst GW. 4-Aminopyridine in multiple sclerosis: prolonged administration. Neurology. 1991 Sep;41(9):1344–8. https://doi.org/10.1212/wnl.41.9.1344.
- Polman CH, van Diemen HA, van Dongen MM, Koetsier JC, van Loenen AC, van Walbeek HK. 4-Aminopyridine in multiple sclerosis. Ann Neurol. 1990 Oct;28(4):589. https://doi.org/10.1002/ana.410280421. No abstract available.
- Davis FA, Stefoski D, Rush J. Orally administered 4-aminopyridine improves clinical signs in multiple sclerosis. Ann Neurol. 1990 Feb;27(2):186–92. https://doi.org/10.1002/ana.410270215.
- Polman CH, Reingold SC, Edan G, Filippi M, Hartung HP, Kappos L, Lublin FD, Metz LM, McFarland HF, O'Connor PW, Sandberg-Wollheim M, Thompson AJ, Weinshenker BG, Wolinsky JS. Diagnostic criteria for multiple sclerosis: 2005 revisions to the "McDonald Criteria". Ann Neurol. 2005 Dec;58(6):840–6. https://doi.org/10.1002/ana.20703.
- Jones RE, Heron JR, Foster DH, Snelgar RS, Mason RJ. Effects of 4-aminopyridine in patients with multiple sclerosis. J Neurol Sci. 1983 Aug-Sep;60(3):353–62. https://doi.org/10.1016/0022-510x(83)90145-4.
- Vollmer T, Henney HR 3rd. Pharmacokinetics and tolerability of single escalating doses of fampridine sustained-release tablets in patients with multiple sclerosis: a Phase I-II, open-label trial. Clin Ther. 2009 Oct;31(10):2206–14. https://doi.org/10.1016/j.clinthera.2009.10.008.
- Vollmer T, Blight AR, Henney HR 3rd. Steady-state pharmacokinetics and tolerability of orally administered fampridine sustained-release 10-mg tablets in patients with multiple sclerosis: a 2-week, open-label, follow-up study. Clin Ther. 2009 Oct;31(10):2215–23. https://doi.org/10.1016/j.clinthera.2009.10.007.
- Beck RW, Ruchman MC, Savino PJ, Schatz NJ. Contrast sensitivity measurements in acute and resolved optic neuritis. Br J Ophthalmol. 1984 Oct;68(10):756–9. https://doi.org/10.1136/bjo.68.10.756.
- Trobe JD, Beck RW, Moke PS, Cleary PA. Contrast sensitivity and other vision tests in the optic neuritis treatment trial. Am J Ophthalmol. 1996 May;121(5):547–53. https://doi.org/10.1016/s0002-9394(14)75429-7.

- Farnsworth D. The Farnsworth-Munsell 100-hue and dichotomous tests for color vision. J Opt Soc Am 1943;33:568–574.
- Naismith RT, Tutlam NT, Xu J, Klawiter EC, Shepherd J, Trinkaus K, Song SK, Cross AH. Optical coherence tomography differs in neuromyelitis optica compared with multiple sclerosis. Neurology. 2009 Mar 24;72(12):1077–82. https://doi.org/10.1212/01.wnl.0000345042.53843.d5.
- Naismith RT, Tutlam NT, Xu J, Shepherd JB, Klawiter EC, Song SK, Cross AH. Optical coherence tomography is less sensitive than visual evoked potentials in optic neuritis. Neurology. 2009 Jul 7;73(1):46–52. https://doi.org/10.1212/WNL.0b013e3181aaea32.
- Naismith RT, Xu J, Tutlam NT, Trinkaus K, Cross AH, Song SK. Radial diffusivity in remote optic neuritis discriminates visual outcomes. Neurology. 2010 May 25;74(21):1702–10. https://doi.org/10.1212/WNL.0b013e3181e0434d.
- Naismith RT, Xu J, Tutlam NT, Scully PT, Trinkaus K, Snyder AZ, Song SK, Cross AH. Increased diffusivity in acute multiple sclerosis lesions predicts risk of black hole. Neurology. 2010 May 25;74(21):1694–701. https://doi.org/10.1212/WNL.0b013e3181e042c4. Erratum In: Neurology. 2010 Sep 7;75(10):938.
- Naismith RT, Xu J, Tutlam NT, Snyder A, Benzinger T, Shimony J, Shepherd J, Trinkaus K, Cross AH, Song SK. Disability in optic neuritis correlates with diffusion tensor-derived directional diffusivities. Neurology. 2009 Feb 17;72(7):589–94. https://doi.org/10.1212/01.wnl.0000335766.22758.cd. Epub 2008 Dec 10.
- Naismith RT, Shepherd JB, Weihl CC, Tutlam NT, Cross AH. Acute and bilateral blindness due to optic neuropathy associated with copper deficiency. Arch Neurol. 2009 Aug;66(8):1025–7. https://doi.org/10.1001/archneurol.2009.70.
- Vanden Bosch ME, Wall M. Visual acuity scored by the letter-by-letter or probit methods has lower retest variability than the line assignment method. Eye (Lond). 1997;11 (Pt 3):411–7. https://doi.org/10.1038/eye.1997.87.
- Acorda Therapeutics. AMPRYA package insert (2010).

Results

Outcome Measures

1. Time to First Protocol-Defined Relapse (TFR) During the Double-Blind (DB) Period
   Type: Primary | Time Frame: Up to Week 216

Description	TFR was defined as time from randomization to first occurrence of relapse in the DB period. Protocol-defined relapse was the occurrence of new or worsening neurological symptoms attributable to neurological neuromyelitis optica (NMO) or neuromyelitis optica spectrum disorder (NMOSD). Symptoms had to persist for >24 h and not be attributable to confounding clinical factors (e.g., fever, infection, injury, change in mood, adverse reactions to medications). New or worsening neurological symptoms that occurred <31 days following onset of a protocol-defined relapse were considered part of same relapse (i.e., if 2 relapses had onset days that were 30 days of one another, they were counted only as 1 relapse), and onset date used in the analysis was the date of first relapse
Time frame	Up to Week 216
Analysis population description	ITT population included all participants randomized to the treatment groups. For participants who had not relapsed, the TFR was censored on the date of end of the DB period

Arm/group title	Placebo, then satralizumab	Satralizumab, then satralizumab
Arm/group description	Participants received matching placebo, subcutaneous (SC) injection at Weeks 0, 2, and 4, and every 4 weeks (Q4W) thereafter throughout the double-blind (DB) period up to protocol-defined relapse. Following the DB period, all participants received satralizumab 120 mg SC injection at Weeks 0, 2, and 4, and Q4W thereafter up to the clinical cut-off date (CCOD). At the CCOD, participants who had not experienced a relapse during the DB period were invited to initiate satralizumab 120 mg SC injection (at Weeks 0, 2, and 4, and Q4W thereafter) after 4 weeks from their last study treatment dose in the DB period Show less	Participants received satralizumab 120 mg subcutaneous (SC) injection at Weeks 0, 2, and 4, and every 4 weeks (Q4W) thereafter throughout the double-blind (DB) period. Participants who experienced a protocol-defined relapse could continue in the Open-Label Extension (OLE) period 31 days after relapse. Participants who completed the DB period without relapse could participate in the OLE period 4 weeks after receiving their last dose in the DB period. All OLE participants received satralizumab 120 mg SC injection at Weeks 0, 2, and 4, and Q4W thereafter Show less
Overall number of participants analyzed	32	63
Median (95% confidence interval) | unit of measure: weeks	128.3[a] (29.9 to NA)	NA[b] (135.7 to NA)

Statistical analysis 1: placebo, then satralizumab, satralizumab, then satralizumab I superiority I log rank

[a] Upper limit of CI was not reached due to low number of participants with events
[b] Median was not reached due to the low number of participants with events. Upper limit of CI was not reached due to the low number of participants with events

2. Change from Baseline to Week 24 in Visual Analog Scale (VAS) for Pain During the DB Period

   Type: Secondary I Time Frame: Baseline, Week 24

Description	The VAS is a subjective measure of pain consisting of a 100 mm line with two endpoints representing 0 = "no pain" and 100 = "pain as bad as it could be". Participants rated their pain by placing a mark on the line corresponding to their current level of pain. The distance along the line from the "no pain" marker was measured with a ruler giving a pain score out of 100. A higher score indicated more pain and lower scores reflected a better health state. A negative change from baseline indicates an improvement. ANCOVA was used for analysis to report the adjusted mean and standard error (SE)
Time frame	Baseline, Week 24
Analysis population description	ITT population included all participants randomized to the treatment groups. Number analyzed is the number of participants with data available for analyses at the given timepoint. Missing data were imputed by BOCF method

Arm/group title	Placebo, then satralizumab	Satralizumab, then satralizumab
Arm/group description	Participants received matching placebo, subcutaneous (SC) injection at Weeks 0, 2, and 4, and every 4 weeks (Q4W) thereafter throughout the double-blind (DB) period up to protocol-defined relapse. Following the DB period, all participants received satralizumab 120 mg SC injection at Weeks 0, 2, and 4, and Q4W thereafter up to the clinical cut-off date (CCOD). At the CCOD, participants who had not experienced a relapse during the DB period were invited to initiate satralizumab 120 mg SC injection (at Weeks 0, 2, and 4, and Q4W thereafter) after 4 weeks from their last study treatment dose in the DB period Show less	Participants received satralizumab 120 mg subcutaneous (SC) injection at Weeks 0, 2, and 4, and every 4 weeks (Q4W) thereafter throughout the double-blind (DB) period. Participants who experienced a protocol defined relapse could continue in the Open-Label Extension (OLE) period 31 days after relapse. Participants who completed the DB period without relapse could participate in the OLE period 4 weeks after receiving their last dose in the DB period. All OLE participants received satralizumab 120 mg SC injection at Weeks 0, 2, and 4, and Q4W thereafter Show less
Overall number of participants analyzed	32	62

Baseline [a]Mean (standard error) ǀ unit of measure: score on scale	27.563(5.438)	31.661(3.665)
Change from baseline to Week 24[a]	−5.949(4.832)	−2.735(4.260)
Statistical analysis 1: placebo, then satralizumab, satralizumab, then satralizumab ǀ superiority ǀ ANCOVA		

[a] Mean (standard error) ǀ unit of measure: score on scale

3. Change from Baseline to Week 24 in Functional Assessment of Chronic Illness Therapy (FACIT) Fatigue Scale During the DB Period
   Type: Secondary ǀ Time Frame: Baseline, Week 24

Description	The FACIT Fatigue scale is a 13-item questionnaire that assesses self-reported fatigue and its impact on daily activities and function over the past 7 days. As each of the 13 items of the scale ranges from 0 to 4, the range of possible scores was computed using FACIT scoring algorithm as 0–52, where 0 is the worst possible score and 52 is the best which indicated less fatigue. A positive change from baseline indicates an improvement
Time frame	Baseline, Week 24
Analysis population description	ITT population included all participants randomized to the treatment groups. Number analyzed is the number of participants with data available for analyses at the given timepoint. Missing data were imputed using BOCF method

Arm/group title	Placebo, then satralizumab	Satralizumab, then satralizumab

Arm/group description	Participants received matching placebo, subcutaneous (SC) injection at Weeks 0, 2, and 4, and every 4 weeks (Q4W) thereafter throughout the double-blind (DB) period up to protocol-defined relapse. Following the DB period, all participants received satralizumab 120 mg SC injection at Weeks 0, 2, and 4, and Q4W thereafter up to the clinical cut-off date (CCOD). At the CCOD, participants who had not experienced a relapse during the DB period were invited to initiate satralizumab 120 mg SC injection (at Weeks 0, 2, and 4, and Q4W thereafter) after 4 weeks from their last study treatment dose in the DB period Show less	Participants received satralizumab 120 mg subcutaneous (SC) injection at Weeks 0, 2, and 4, and every 4 weeks (Q4W) thereafter throughout the double-blind (DB) period. Participants who experienced a protocol-defined relapse could continue in the Open-Label Extension (OLE) period 31 days after relapse. Participants who completed the DB period without relapse could participate in the OLE period 4 weeks after receiving their last dose in the DB period. All OLE participants received satralizumab 120 mg SC injection at Weeks 0, 2, and 4, and Q4W thereafter Show less
Overall number of participants analyzed	32	62
Baseline [a]Mean (standard error) I unit of measure: score on scale	29.656(2.280)	30.590(1.492)
Change from baseline to Week 24[a]	3.602(1.820)	5.709(1.610)
Statistical analysis 1: placebo, then satralizumab, satralizumab, then satralizumab I superiority I ANCOVA		

[a] Mean (standard error) I unit of measure: score on scale

4. Relapse-Free Rate During the DB Period
   Type: Secondary I Time Frame: Up to Week 216

Description	Protocol-defined relapse was the occurrence of new or worsening neurological symptoms attributable to neurological neuromyelitis optica (NMO) or neuromyelitis optica spectrum disorder (NMOSD). Symptoms had to persist for >24 h and not be attributable to confounding clinical factors (e.g., fever, infection, injury, change in mood, adverse reactions to medications). New or worsening neurological symptoms that occurred <31 days following onset of a protocol-defined relapse were considered part of same relapse (i.e., if 2 relapses had onsets within 30 days of one another, they were counted as 1), and onset date used in the analysis was the date of first relapse
Time frame	Up to Week 216
Analysis population description	ITT population included all participants randomized to the treatment groups

Arm/group title	Placebo, then satralizumab	Satralizumab, then satralizumab
Arm/group description	Participants received matching placebo, subcutaneous (SC) injection at Weeks 0, 2, and 4, and every 4 weeks (Q4W) thereafter throughout the double-blind (DB) period up to protocol-defined relapse. Following the DB period, all participants received satralizumab 120 mg SC injection at Weeks 0, 2, and 4, and Q4W thereafter up to the clinical cut-off date (CCOD). At the CCOD, participants who had not experienced a relapse during the DB period were invited to initiate satralizumab 120 mg SC injection (at Weeks 0, 2, and 4, and Q4W thereafter) after 4 weeks from their last study treatment dose in the DB period Show more	Participants received satralizumab 120 mg subcutaneous (SC) injection at Weeks 0, 2, and 4, and every 4 weeks (Q4W) thereafter throughout the double-blind (DB) period. Participants who experienced a protocol-defined relapse could continue in the Open-Label Extension (OLE) period 31 days after relapse. Participants who completed the DB period without relapse could participate in the OLE period 4 weeks after receiving their last dose in the DB period. All OLE participants received satralizumab 120 mg SC injection at Weeks 0, 2, and 4, and Q4W thereafter Show more
Overall number of participants analyzed	23	56
Week 12		
Number analyzed	23 participants	56 participants
[a]Measure type: number I unit of measure: percentage of participants	74.87	88.89
Week 24		
Number analyzed	23 participants	56 participants
[a]	71.61	85.71
Week 36		
Number analyzed	23 participants	56 participants
[a]	61.85	79.37
Week 48		
Number analyzed	23 participants	56 participants
[a]	61.85	76.13
Week 72		
Number analyzed	23 participants	56 participants
[a]	51.21	74.40
Week 96		

Number analyzed	23 participants	56 participants
[a]	51.21	72.14
Week 120		
Number analyzed	23 participants	56 participants
[a]	51.21	72.14
Week 144		
Number analyzed	23 participants	56 participants
[a]	34.14	62.80
Week 168		
Number analyzed	23 participants	56 participants
[a]	34.14	62.80
Week 192		
Number analyzed	23 participants	56 participants
[a]	34.14	62.80
Week 216		
Number analyzed	23 participants	0 participants
[a]	34.14	

[a] Measure type: number | unit of measure: percentage of participants

5. Annualized Relapse Rate (ARR) During the DB Period
   Type: Secondary | Time Frame: Up to Week 216

Description	The ARR is calculated as the total number of participants with adjudicated PDRs experienced divided by the patient years at risk. Protocol-defined relapse was the occurrence of new or worsening neurological symptoms attributable to neurological NMO or NMOSD. Symptoms had to persist for >24 h and not be attributable to confounding clinical factors (e.g., fever, infection, injury, change in mood, adverse reactions to medications). New or worsening neurological symptoms that occurred <31 days following the onset of a protocol-defined relapse were considered part of same relapse (2 relapses with onset days in 30 days of one another were counted as 1 relapse), onset date used in the analysis was the date of first relapse
Time frame	Up to Week 216
Analysis population description	ITT population included all participants randomized to the treatment groups

Arm/group title	Placebo, then satralizumab	Satralizumab, then satralizumab
Arm/group description	Participants received matching placebo, subcutaneous (SC) injection at Weeks 0, 2, and 4, and every 4 weeks (Q4W) thereafter throughout the double-blind (DB) period up to protocol-defined relapse. Following the DB period, all participants received satralizumab 120 mg SC injection at Weeks 0, 2, and 4, and Q4W thereafter up to the clinical cut-off date (CCOD). At the CCOD, participants who had not experienced a relapse during the DB period were invited to initiate satralizumab 120 mg SC injection (at Weeks 0, 2, and 4, and Q4W thereafter) after 4 weeks from their last study treatment dose in the DB period Show less	Participants received satralizumab 120 mg subcutaneous (SC) injection at Weeks 0, 2, and 4, and every 4 weeks (Q4W) thereafter throughout the double-blind (DB) period. Participants who experienced a protocol-defined relapse could continue in the Open-Label Extension (OLE) period 31 days after relapse. Participants who completed the DB period without relapse could participate in the OLE period 4 weeks after receiving their last dose in the DB period. All OLE participants received satralizumab 120 mg SC injection at Weeks 0, 2, and 4, and Q4W thereafter Show less
Overall number of participants analyzed	32	63
Measure type: number (95% confidence interval) | unit of measure: patients w PDRs/ patient-years at risk	0.41(0.24–0.67)	0.17(0.10–0.26)

6. Change from baseline in Short Form Generic Health Survey (SF-36) Bodily Pain Domain scores at 24-week intervals during the DB period
   Type: Secondary | Time Frame: Baseline up to Week 216

Description	The SF-36v2 is a multi-purpose, short-form health survey with 36 questions. It has 8 domains (vitality, physical functioning, bodily pain, general health, role-physical, role emotional, social role functioning, and mental health) of functional health and well-being scores as well as psychometrically based physical and mental health component summary measures and a preference-based health utility index. The domain scores were transformed to a 0–100 scale, where higher scores indicate better quality of life. A positive change from baseline indicates an improvement
Time frame	Baseline up to Week 216
Analysis population description	ITT population included all participants randomized to the treatment groups. Number analyzed is the number of participants with data available for analyses at the given timepoint

Arm/group title	Placebo, then satralizumab	Satralizumab, then satralizumab
Arm/group description	Participants received matching placebo, subcutaneous (SC) injection at Weeks 0, 2, and 4, and every 4 weeks (Q4W) thereafter throughout the double-blind (DB) period up to protocol-defined relapse. Following the DB period, all participants received satralizumab 120 mg SC injection at Weeks 0, 2, and 4, and Q4W thereafter up to the clinical cut-off date (CCOD). At the CCOD, participants who had not experienced a relapse during the DB period were invited to initiate satralizumab 120 mg SC injection (at Weeks 0, 2, and 4, and Q4W thereafter) after 4 weeks from their last study treatment dose in the DB period Show more	Participants received satralizumab 120 mg subcutaneous (SC) injection at Weeks 0, 2, and 4, and every 4 weeks (Q4W) thereafter throughout the double-blind (DB) period. Participants who experienced a protocol-defined relapse could continue in the Open-Label Extension (OLE) period 31 days after relapse. Participants who completed the DB period without relapse could participate in the OLE period 4 weeks after receiving their last dose in the DB period. All OLE participants received satralizumab 120 mg SC injection at Weeks 0, 2, and 4, and Q4W thereafter Show more
Overall number of participants analyzed	32	62
Baseline		
Number analyzed	32 participants	62 participants
[a]Mean (standard deviation) | unit of measure: score on scale	42.86(11.28)	43.20(11.08)
Change from baseline at Week 24		
Number analyzed	20 participants	54 participants
[a]	−0.89(8.35)	−0.13(8.09)
Change from baseline at Week 48		
Number analyzed	18 participants	46 participants
[a]	1.75(5.42)	1.36(8.89)
Change from baseline at Week 72		
Number analyzed	13 participants	43 participants

[a]	3.19(8.04)	0.91(9.23)
Change from baseline at Week 96		
Number analyzed	8 participants	31 participants
[a]	3.43(5.60)	2.38(7.82)
Change from baseline at Week 120		
Number analyzed	3 participants	16 participants
[a]	0.00(8.07)	0.53(6.21)
Change from baseline at Week 144		
Number analyzed	2 participants	12 participants
[a]	−2.22(8.84)	2.59(6.66)
Change from baseline at Week 168		
Number analyzed	1 participant	10 participants
[a]	0.80[b] (NA)	4.19 (7.01)
Change from baseline at Week 192		
Number analyzed	1 participant	2 participants
[a]	−8.47[c](NA)	0(0)
Change from baseline at Week 216		
Number analyzed	1 participant	0 participants
[a]	−12.50[c] (NA)	

[a] Mean (standard deviation) | unit of measure: score on scale

[b] Standard deviation (SD) was not calculable for 1 participant

[c] SD was not calculable for 1 participant

Additional Results Available

Completed

Europe

Paraorbital-Occipital Alternating Current Stimulation Therapy for Optic Neuropathy (MCT optnerve)

ClinicalTrials.gov ID NCT01280877

Sponsor University of Magdeburg
Information provided by Bernhard A. Sabel, University of Magdeburg (Responsible Party)
Last Update Posted 2017-01-30

Brief Summary
The aim is to validate that non-invasive brain stimulation can increase cortical excitability in the visual system. The investigators assess if transcranial alternating current stimulation (tACS) can improve visual field size in patients with optic nerve damage. Hypothesis: tACS would improve visual functions within the defective visual field (primary outcome measure).

Detailed Description
In addition, the correlation between the brain-derived neurotrophic factor (BDNF) or other plasticity markers is correlated to the improvement of the visual field after stimulation.

Official Title
Multicenter Study of Paraorbital-Occipital Alternating Current Stimulation Therapy in Patients With Optic Neuropathy

Conditions
Optic Nerve Diseases
Optic Nerve Injuries
Optic Neuropathies

Intervention/Treatment
- Device: tACS
- Device: Sham stimulation

Other Study ID Numbers
- EBS-PP-2010-08-10-001

Study Start
2010-12

Primary Completion (Actual)
2012-02

Study Completion (Actual)
2012-02

Enrollment (Actual)
90

Study Type
Interventional

Phase
Not Applicable

Germany

Berlin, Germany, 10117
Klinik für Neurologie, Charité Campus Mitte, Universitätsmedizin Berlin

Göttingen, Germany, 37075
Klinische Neurophysiologie & Abteilung Augenheilkunde, Universitätsmedizin Göttingen

Kassel, Germany, 34125
Augenklinik Kassel am Klinikum Kassel GmbH

Magdeburg, Germany, 39120
Inst. f. Medizinische Psychologie, Universitätsklinikum Magdeburg

Eligibility Criteria
Description

Inclusion Criteria
- Patients with optic nerve lesion
- Stable visual field defect with residual vision
- Lesion age at least 6 months
- Age at least 18 years
- No completely blindness, residual vision still existent

Exclusion Criteria
- Electric or electronic implants, e.g. heart pacemaker
- Any metal artifacts in head and truncus
- Epilepsy
- Auto-immune diseases in acute stage
- Mental diseases, e.g. schizophrenia etc.
- Unstable diabetes, diabetes causing diabetic retinopathy
- Addiction
- High blood pressure (max. 160/100 mmHg)
- Instable or high level of intraocular pressure (i.e. >27 mmHg)
- Retinitis pigmentosa
- Pathological nystagmus

- Presence of an un-operated tumor anywhere in the body
- Pregnant or breastfeeding women
- Photo sensibility
- Fundus hypertonicus
- Acute conjunctivitis

Ages Eligible for Study
18 Years and older (Adult, Older Adult)

Sexes Eligible for Study
All

Accepts Healthy Volunteers
No

Study Plan

Design Details
Primary Purpose: Treatment
Allocation: Randomized
Interventional Model: Parallel Assignment
Masking: Double (Participant Outcomes Assessor)

Arms and interventions

Participant group/arm	Intervention/treatment
Experimental: verum stimulation Complete treatment with transorbital alternating current stimulation (tACS)	Device: tACS • Transorbital alternating current stimulation (tACS) is applied with a multi-channel device with paraorbital montage of 4 stimulation electrodes generating weak current pulses in predetermined firing bursts of 8–14 pulses. The amplitude of each current pulse was below 1000 μA. Current intensity was individually adjusted according to how well patients perceived phosphenes, i.e. any sensation of flickering light in response to the rtACS stimulation
Sham comparator: sham stimulation Same electrode montage set-up is used during tACS- and placebo-stimulation. Sham stimulation condition consists of minimal treatment with low intensity/few impulses tACS	Device: sham stimulation • tACS is applied with the same device with equal electrode set-up procedures but only one of four channels actually delivers current. The current intensity of this channel is individually adjusted (preselected on the side of lesioned eye) according to the patient ability to clearly perceive single phosphenes or any skin irritation phenomena (like weak sense of needles or vibration) whenever a single pulse is applied. The amplitude of pulses is always below 1000 μA. Current pulses are given as 1 pulse per minute during 25–35 min of session time. Session duration is equal for verum and sham patients. The perception of the single pulses leaves sham patients at the impression that they might receive the verum intervention, but the total number of pulses is less than 0.5% of verum tACS

Primary outcome measures

Outcome measure	Measure description	Time frame
Detection accuracy (DA) change in percent over baseline within defective visual field	Central visual fields are assessed with computer-based high-resolution perimetry (HRP). Based on such plots, areas of the visual field are characterized as intact, partially damaged, or absolutely impaired (blind). Detection accuracy (DA) change in percent above baseline within defective visual field sectors is defined as the primary outcome criterion	Baseline—8 weeks after stimulation; first follow-up 2 days after treatment course; second follow-up 8 weeks after treatment course

Secondary outcome measures

Outcome measure	Measure description	Time frame
DA change in percent over baseline regarding the damage region of the tested visual field (computer-based high-resolution perimetry)	This parameter includes also intact sectors that are tested with HRP. It is hypothesized that improvements of the primary outcome criterion will outweigh the relative change in intact sectors as measured with HRP	Baseline—8 weeks after stimulation; first follow-up 2 days after treatment course; second follow-up 8 weeks after treatment course
EEG parameters	EEG power spectra	Baseline—8 weeks after stimulation; first follow-up 2 days after treatment course; second follow-up 8 weeks after treatment course
Reaction time change in ms	Reaction time (RT) in HRP	Baseline—8 weeks after stimulation; first follow-up 2 days after treatment course; second follow-up 8 weeks after treatment course
Visual acuity (VA)		Baseline—8 weeks after stimulation; first follow-up 2 days after treatment course; second follow-up 8 weeks after treatment course
DA in static and kinetic conventional perimetry		Baseline—8 weeks after stimulation; first follow-up 2 days after treatment course; second follow-up 8 weeks after treatment course

Sponsor

University of Magdeburg

Collaborators

- EBS Technologies GmbH

Investigators

- Principal Investigator: Bernhard A Sabel, Prof. Dr., Direktor, Institut für Medizinische Psychologie, Leipziger Str. 44, D-39120 Magdeburg, Germany

General Publications

No publications available

No Results Posted

Completed

Trial of Alternating Current Stimulation in Optic Neuropathy (SCT Optnerve)

ClinicalTrials.gov ID NCT01270126

Sponsor University of Magdeburg
Information provided by Bernhard A. Sabel, University of Magdeburg (Responsible Party)
Last Update Posted 2020-11-09

Brief Summary

Non-invasive brain stimulation can increase cortical excitability in the visual system, but it is not known if this is of clinical value. The investigators now assessed if repetitive, transcranial alternating current stimulation (rtACS) can improve visual field size in patients with optic nerve damage. The investigators hypothesized that rtACS would improve visual functions within the defective visual field sectors of the visual field (primary outcome measure).

Detailed Description

In a prospective, double-blind, randomized, placebo-controlled clinical trial, 22 patients with optic nerve damage were randomly assigned to a rtACS- ($n = 12$) or placebo-group ($n = 10$). Visual field measures, visual acuity, and EEG recordings were collected before and after a daily 20–40 min treatment for 10-days and at a 2-month follow-up. Primary outcome measure was detection accuracy (DA) in defective visual field sectors of computer-based high-resolution perimetry (HRP). Secondary outcome parameters included DA in static and kinetic perimetry, reaction time (RT) in HRP, visual acuity (VA), contrast vision, and EEG power spectra.

Official Title

Treatment of Patients With Optic Neuropathy Using Transorbital Alternating Current Stimulation—a Randomized Trial

Conditions
Optic Nerve Diseases
Optic Nerve Injuries
Optic Neuropathies

Intervention/Treatment
- Device: Repetitive transorbital alternating current stimulation

Other Study ID Numbers
- EBS_optnerve_SCT

Study Start
2006-11

Primary Completion (Actual)
2010-12

Study Completion (Actual)
2010-12

Enrollment (Actual)
22

Study Type
Interventional

Phase
Not Applicable

Germany

Magdeburg, Germany, 39120
Institute of Medical Psychology

Description

Inclusion Criteria
- Patients with optic nerve lesion
- Stable visual field defect with residual vision
- Lesion age at least 6 months

Exclusion Criteria
- Heart pacemakers and any metal artifacts in head and truncus
- Epileptic seizure within the last 3 years
- Photosensitive epilepsy as determined by EEG
- Mental diseases (schizophrenia etc.)
- Unstable diabetes, diabetes causing diabetic retinopathy
- Macular degeneration, maculopathy with decimal visual acuity below 0.4
- High blood pressure

- Instable or high level of intraocular pressure (i.e. >27 mmHg)
- Presence of an un-operated tumor anywhere in the body
- Total blindness
- Primary or secondary glaucoma
- Pathological nystagmus

Ages Eligible for Study
18 Years to 70 Years (Adult, Older Adult)

Sexes Eligible for Study
All

Accepts Healthy Volunteers
No

Design Details
Primary Purpose: Treatment
Allocation: Randomized
Interventional Model: Parallel Assignment
Masking: Double (Participant Outcomes Assessor)

Arms and interventions

Participant group/arm	Intervention/treatment
Experimental: rtACS (verum condition) Repetitive transorbital alternating current stimulation (rtACS)	Device: repetitive transorbital alternating current stimulation • Repetitive, transorbital alternating current stimulation (rtACS) was applied with a multi-channel device generating weak current pulses in predetermined firing bursts of 2–9 pulses. The amplitude of each current pulse was below 1000 μA. Current intensity was individually adjusted according to how well patients perceived phosphenes, i.e. any sensation of flickering light in response to the rtACS stimulation • Other names: – EBS Alpha Synch
No Intervention: sham stimulation (placebo condition) A clicking sound was presented, and the same electrode montage set-up was used during rtACS- and placebo stimulation, except that placebo patients received no current (stimulator turned off)	

Primary outcome measures

Outcome measure	Measure description	Time frame
Detection accuracy (DA) change in percent over baseline within defective visual field sectors	Central visual fields were assessed with computer-based high-resolution perimetry (HRP). Based on such plots, areas of the visual field were characterized as intact, partially damaged, or absolutely impaired (blind). Detection accuracy (DA) change in percent above baseline within defective visual field sectors was defined as the primary outcome criterion	Outcome measures were assessed at initial diagnostics (baseline) and after 10 days stimulation at postdiagnostics

Secondary outcome measures

Outcome measure	Measure description	Time frame
Other visual and EEG parameters	Secondary outcome parameters included DA in static and kinetic perimetry, reaction time (RT) in HRP, visual acuity (VA), contrast vision, and EEG power spectra	Nov 2006–Dec 2010

Sponsor
University of Magdeburg

Collaborators
- EBS Technologies GmbH

Investigators
- Principal Investigator: Bernhard A Sabel, PhD, University of Magdeburg

General Publications
No publications available

Results
Outcome Measures

1. Detection Accuracy (DA) Change in Percent Over Baseline Within Defective Visual Field Sectors

   Type: Primary | Time Frame: Outcome measures were assessed at initial diagnostics (baseline) and after 10 days of stimulation at postdiagnostics

Description	Central visual fields were assessed with computer-based high-resolution perimetry (HRP). Based on such plots, areas of the visual field were characterized as intact, partially damaged, or absolutely impaired (blind). Detection accuracy (DA) change in percent above baseline within defective visual field sectors was defined as the primary outcome criterion
Time frame	Outcome measures were assessed at initial diagnostics (baseline) and after 10 days of stimulation at postdiagnostics
Analysis population description	[Not specified]

Arm/group title	rtACS (verum condition)	Sham stimulation (placebo condition)
Arm/group description	Repetitive transorbital alternating current stimulation (rtACS) Repetitive transorbital alternating current stimulation: repetitive, transorbital alternating current stimulation (rtACS) was applied with a multi-channel device generating weak current pulses in predetermined firing bursts of 2–9 pulses. The amplitude of each current pulse was below 1000 μA. Current intensity was individually adjusted according to how well patients perceived phosphenes, i.e. any sensation of flickering light in response to the rtACS stimulation Show more	A clicking sound was presented and the same electrode montage set-up was used during rtACS- and placebo stimulation, except that placebo patients received no current (stimulator turned off) Show more
Overall number of participants analyzed	12	10
Mean (standard deviation) I unit of measure: percent change	24.75(22.40)	39.16(25.26)

2. Other Visual and EEG Parameters
Type: Secondary I Time Frame: Nov 2006–Dec 2010

Outcome Measure Data Not Reported

Description	Secondary outcome parameters included DA in static and kinetic perimetry, reaction time (RT) in HRP, visual acuity (VA), contrast vision, and EEG power spectra
Time frame	Nov 2006–Dec 2010
Analysis population description	[Not specified]

Completed

Citicoline in Non-arteritic Ischemic Optic Neuropathy

ClinicalTrials.gov ID NCT03758118

Sponsor Fondazione G.B. Bietti, IRCCS
Information provided by Fondazione G.B. Bietti, IRCCS (Responsible Party)
Last Update Posted 2018-11-29

Brief Summary

The investigators tested the hypothesis whether the treatment with Citicoline in oral solution (OS-Citicoline) would increase or stabilize visual acuity, retinal ganglion cells (RGCs) function, and neural conduction along the visual pathways (neuroenhancement), and/or induce preservation of RGCs fibers' loss (neuroprotection) in a human model of neurodegeneration: non-arteritic ischemic optic neuropathy (NAION).

Detailed Description

The investigators enrolled 36 patients with bilateral or monolateral NAION and 20 age-similar controls. Nineteen NAION patients received 500 mg/day of OS-Citicoline for a 6-month period followed by 3 months of wash-out (NC Group); 17 NAION patients were not treated (NN Group) from baseline up to 9 months. We assessed all subjects at baseline, at 6 and 9 months of follow-up: Visual acuity (VA), Pattern Electroretinogram (PERG), Visual Evoked Potentials (VEP), retinal nerve fiber layer thickness (RNFL-T), and Humphrey 24-2 visual field mean deviation (HFA MD). Mean differences were statistically evaluated by ANOVA between Groups, and correlations were verified by Pearson's test.

Official Title

Neuroprotection and Neuroenhancement in a Model of Optic Nerve Neurodegeneration (Non Arteritic Ischemic OpticNeuropathy): Study of Morpho-functional Changes Related to Treatment With Citicoline Oral Solution

Conditions

Non-arteritic Ischemic Optic Neuropathy

Intervention/Treatment

- Dietary Supplement: Citicoline

Other Study ID Numbers

- 85356727

Study Start (Actual)

2017-02-20

Primary Completion (Actual)

2017-07-25

Study Completion (Actual)

2018-04-25

Enrollment (Actual)

40

Study Type

Interventional

Phase

Not Applicable

Italy

Roma, Italy, 00184
Britannico Hospital

Eligibility Criteria
Description

Inclusion Criteria

- Acute visual reduction episode from NAION occurring for more than 6 months
- Typical defects of the visual field evidenced with the Goldmann perimetry or with Humphrey perimetry 30-2
- Visual acuity not less than 1/10
- Having suspended any potential neuroprotective therapies (e.g., Coenzyme Q10) for at least 6 months.

Exclusion Criteria

- Ocular surgery in the 3 months preceding the study, including surgery for cataracts in the previous 3 months.
- Cataract or maculopathy
- Known hypersensitivity to the study product
- Positive history for diseases of the optic nerve (retrobulbar optic neuropathy, glaucoma) or systemic diseases which could preclude the enrolment in the study according to the investigators' judgment
- Pregnant or nursing women, or women of potential childbearing age not using adequate contraception.
- Diabetes, SLE, rheumatoid arthritis, mixed connective tissue disease

Ages Eligible for Study
45 Years to 80 Years (Adult, Older Adult)

Sexes Eligible for Study
All

Accepts Healthy Volunteers
Yes

Design Details
Primary Purpose: Treatment
Allocation: Randomized
Interventional Model: Parallel Assignment
Masking: Double (Investigator Outcomes Assessor)

Arms and interventions

Participant group/arm	Intervention/treatment
Active comparator: NAION patients OS-citicoline treated In a group of patients with NAION, OS-citicoline will be administered (500 mg/day) for 6 months followed by 3 months of suspension	Dietary supplement: citicoline • Citicoline administered in oral solution

Participant group/arm	Intervention/treatment
No intervention: NAION patients untreated In one group of patients with NAION no type of treatment will be performed during 9 months of observation	

Primary outcome measures

Outcome measure	Measure description	Time frame
Change from baseline in visual acuity at 9 month	Increase in visual acuity was evaluated by early treatment diabetic retinopathy study (ETDRS) charts and measured as a logarithm of the minimum angle of resolution (LogMAR)	9 months vs. baseline

Secondary outcome measures

Outcome measure	Measure description	Time frame
Change from baseline in retinal ganglion cells function at 9 month	Pattern-electroretinogram recordings. Increase of P50-N95 amplitude (measured in microvolt)	9 months vs. baseline
Change from baseline in optic nerve function at 9 months	Visual evoked potential recordings. Shortening of the main parameter P100 implicit time measured in milliseconds	9 months vs. baseline
Change from baseline in optic nerve morphology at 9 months	Reduction of overall retinal nerve fiber thickness by optical coherence tomography measured in micron	9 months vs. baseline
Change from baseline in visual field defects at 9 months	improvement of the visual field by static perimetry (increase of the main indexes mean deviation measured in dB)	9 months vs. baseline

Sponsor

Fondazione G.B. Bietti, IRCCS

Collaborators

No information provided

Investigators

- Principal Investigator: Vincenzo MF Parisi, MD, Fondazione Bietti - IRCCS

General Publications

- Carelli V, La Morgia C, Ross-Cisneros FN, Sadun AA. Optic neuropathies: the tip of the neurodegeneration iceberg. Hum Mol Genet. 2017 Oct 1;26(R2): R139–R150. https://doi.org/10.1093/hmg/ddx273.
- Cho YS. The role of necroptosis in the treatment of diseases. BMB Rep. 2018 May;51(5):219–224. https://doi.org/10.5483/bmbrep.2018.51.5.074.
- Hayreh SS, Zimmerman B. Visual field abnormalities in nonarteritic anterior ischemic optic neuropathy: their pattern and prevalence at initial examination. Arch Ophthalmol. 2005 Nov;123(11):1554–62. https://doi.org/10.1001/archopht.123.11.1554.

- Patel HR, Margo CE. Pathology of Ischemic Optic Neuropathy. Arch Pathol Lab Med. 2017 Jan;141(1):162–166. https://doi.org/10.5858/arpa.2016-0027-RS.
- Parisi V, Gallinaro G, Ziccardi L, Coppola G. Electrophysiological assessment of visual function in patients with non-arteritic ischaemic optic neuropathy. Eur J Neurol. 2008 Aug;15(8):839–45. https://doi.org/10.1111/j.1468-1331.2008.02200.x. Epub 2008 Jun 28.
- Balducci N, Morara M, Veronese C, Barboni P, Casadei NL, Savini G, Parisi V, Sadun AA, Ciardella A. Optical coherence tomography angiography in acute arteritic and non-arteritic anterior ischemic optic neuropathy. Graefes Arch Clin Exp Ophthalmol. 2017 Nov;255(11):2255–2261. https://doi.org/10.1007/s00417-017-3774-y. Epub 2017 Aug 31.
- Khalilpour S, Latifi S, Behnammanesh G, Majid AMSA, Majid ASA, Tamayol A. Ischemic optic neuropathy as a model of neurodegenerative disorder: A review of pathogenic mechanism of axonal degeneration and the role of neuroprotection. J Neurol Sci. 2017 Apr 15;375:430–441. https://doi.org/10.1016/j.jns.2016.12.044. Epub 2016 Dec 26.

Results Not Posted

Completed

Middle East

Traumatic Optic Neuropathy Treatment Trial 2 (TONTT-2)

ClinicalTrials.gov ID NCT03308448

Sponsor Iran University of Medical Sciences
Information provided by Iran University of Medical Sciences (Responsible Party)
Last Update Posted 2023-04-03

Brief Summary
After introducing intravenous erythropoietin (EPO) as an option for the treatment of patients with indirect traumatic optic neuropathy in 2011 and publishing noninferiority trial in Oct. 2017, TONTT2 is aiming to find out the best dose and timing of EPO administration in this group of patients.

Detailed Description
Patients with TON will be visited. After being eligible to enter the study and obtaining informed consent, they will be randomly assigned into three groups of different total doses of intravenous administration of EPO to which patients and outcome assessors will be masked. They will be assessed at different follow-up time periods with the last follow-up of at least 3 months.

Official Title
Traumatic Optic Neuropathy Treatment Trial 2; Efficacy of Different Doses of Erythropoietin. A Multicenter, Double Blind RCT

Conditions
Traumatic Optic Neuropathy

Intervention/Treatment
- Drug: Recombinant human erythropoietin

Other Study ID Numbers
- IUMS 96-03-124-31806

Study Start (Actual)
2018-01-06

Primary Completion (Actual)
2022-08-06

Study Completion (Actual)
2023-03-02

Enrollment (Actual)
93

Study Type
Interventional

Phase
Phase 3

Iran, Islamic Republic of

Mashhad, Iran, Islamic Republic of
Mashhad University of Medical Sciences

Tehran, Iran, Islamic Republic of
Tehran University of Medical Sciences

Tehran Locations

Tehrān, Tehran, Iran, Islamic Republic of
Iran University of Medical Sciences

Eligibility Criteria
Description

Inclusion Criteria
- Having indirect traumatic optic neuropathy (with normal eye and fundus exam)
- Trauma to treatment interval of 3 weeks and less
- Age of 7 years and more

Exclusion Criteria

- Direct optic neuropathy,
- Glaucoma,
- Any retinopathy
- Globe laceration
- Age under 7
- Hypertension,
- Polycythemia,
- Creatine more than 3 mg/dL,
- Sensitivity to EPO
- Patients who have received any other form of treatment for their traumatic optic neuropathy

Ages Eligible for Study

7 Years and older (Child, Adult, Older Adult)

Sexes Eligible for Study

All

Accepts Healthy Volunteers

No

Design Details

Primary Purpose: Treatment

Allocation: Randomized

Interventional Model: Parallel Assignment

Interventional Model Description: three treatment groups of patients with TON will receive different total dose of EPO.

Masking: Double (Participant Outcomes Assessor)

Masking Description: Participants are unaware of the dose of EPO. Outcome assessors are masked to the dose of EPO

Arms and interventions

Participant group/arm	Intervention/treatment
Active comparator: group 1 Intervention is intra-venous injection of Eprex or EPO [recombinant human erythropoietin, Pooyesh Darou Biopharmaceuticals CO., Tehran, Iran, 4000 unit/mL solution in prefilled syringe], 300 units/kg/day for 3 consecutive days (total: 900/kg in 3 days)	Drug: recombinant human erythropoietin • Intravenous administration of recombinant human erythropoietin (4000 u/vial) with different dosage for each group • Other names: – EPO, Eprex
Active comparator: group 2 Intervention is an intra-venous injection of Eprex or EPO [recombinant human erythropoietin, Pooyesh Darou Biopharmaceuticals CO., Tehran, Iran, 4000 unit/mL solution in prefilled syringe], 600 units/kg/day for 3 consecutive days (total: 1800/kg in 3 days)	Drug: recombinant human erythropoietin • Intravenous administration of recombinant human erythropoietin (4000 u/vial) with different dosage for each group • Other names: – EPO, Eprex

Participant group/arm	Intervention/treatment
Active comparator: group 3 Intervention is an intra-venous injection of Eprex or EPO [recombinant human erythropoietin, Pooyesh Darou Biopharmaceuticals CO., Tehran, Iran, 4000 unit/mL solution in prefilled syringe], 600 units/kg/day for 3 consecutive days then repetition of the same treatment in month 1 (Total: 3600/kg in 2 sets of 3-day treatment, 1 month apart)	Drug: recombinant human erythropoietin • Intravenous administration of recombinant human erythropoietin (4000 u/vial) with different dosages for each group • Other names: – EPO, Eprex

Primary outcome measures

Outcome measure	Measure description	Time frame
Change in mean LogMAR best corrected visual acuity (BCVA) from 20/20 to no light perception (NLP) as assessed by Snellen visual acuity chart and analyzed based on mean LogMAR change	Best corrected visual acuity is measured (Snellen eye chart) and recorded as 20/20-20/25, 20/30, 20/40, 20, 50, 20/70, 20/100, 20/200 and then counting finger (CF), hand motion (HM), light perception (LP), and no light perception (NLP)	Before treatment and on day 1, 2, 3, 7, 30, and 90 days after the treatment and through study completion, an average of 24 months

Secondary outcome measures

Outcome measure	Measure description	Time frame
Change in mean log unit of relative afferent pupillary defect (RAPD) from 0.3 to 1.8 log unit as assessed by neutral density filter	RAPD will be measured based on six log units of 0.3, 0.6, 0.9, 1.2, 1.5, and 1.8 in which the higher the number the higher the severity score of RAPD	Before treatment and on day 1, 2, 3, 7, 30, and 90 days after the treatment and through study completion, an average of 24 months
Change in mean number of visible color plates in color vision test book. It is from 14/14 to 0/14 as assessed by Ishihara 14-plate color test book	Using Ishihara 14-plate color vision test book, the color vision will be recorded as a fraction of 14 plates; e.g. 10/14. Patients with lower than 20/200 vision will have 0/14 since they cannot read the color plates	Before treatment and on day 1, 2, 3, 7, 30, and 90 days after the treatment and through study completion, an average of 24 months
Number of patients with treatment-related adverse effects as assessed by history taking (change in mood, vertigo, faint), examination (blood pressure), and blood tests (CBC, BUN, Cr., K, Na, PT, PTT, INR, Ca., Ph)	History taking (change in mood, vertigo, faint), examination (blood pressure) and blood tests (CBC, BUN, Cr., K, Na, PT, PTT, INR, Ca., Ph) will be performed before treatment and on days 1, 2, and 3 after treatment	Before treatment and on day 1, 2 and 3 after treatment

Sponsor
Iran University of Medical Sciences

Collaborators
- Mashhad University of Medical Sciences
- Tehran University of Medical Sciences

Investigators
- Study Chair: Mohsen B Kashkouli, MD, Iran University of Medical Sciences

General Publications
- Kashkouli MB, Pakdel F, Sanjari MS, Haghighi A, Nojomi M, Homaee MH, Heirati A. Erythropoietin: a novel treatment for traumatic optic neuropathy-a pilot study. Graefes Arch Clin Exp Ophthalmol. 2011 May;249(5):731–6. https://doi.org/10.1007/s00417-010-1534-3. Epub 2010 Oct 2.
- Entezari M, Esmaeili M, Yaseri M. A pilot study of the effect of intravenous erythropoetin on improvement of visual function in patients with recent indirect traumatic optic neuropathy. Graefes Arch Clin Exp Ophthalmol. 2014 Aug;252(8):1309–13. https://doi.org/10.1007/s00417-014-2691-6. Epub 2014 Jul 2.
- Kashkouli MB, Yousefi S, Nojomi M, Sanjari MS, Pakdel F, Entezari M, Etezad-Razavi M, Razeghinejad MR, Esmaeli M, Shafiee M, Bagheri M. Traumatic optic neuropathy treatment trial (TONTT): open label, phase 3, multicenter, semi-experimental trial. Graefes Arch Clin Exp Ophthalmol. 2018 Jan;256(1):209–218. https://doi.org/10.1007/s00417-017-3816-5. Epub 2017 Oct 6.

No Results Posted

Terminated

United States

Reason: Unable to record n95 pERG Peak (Primary Measure), as LHON subjects are unable to focus on target

Near-Infrared Light-Emitting Diode (NIR-LED) Therapy for Leber's

Hereditary Opticneuropathy (LHON) (LHON)

ClinicalTrials.gov ID NCT01389817

Sponsor Medical College of Wisconsin
Information provided by Harry T Whelan, MD, Medical College of Wisconsin (Responsible Party)
Last Update Posted 2014-09-29

Brief Summary
The overall objective of the proposed research is to test the hypothesis that Near-infrared Light-emitting Diode (NIR-LED) therapy will stimulate mitochondrial function, attenuate oxidative stress, and improve cell survival and vision in subjects with Leber's Hereditary Optic Neuropathy (LHON).

Detailed Description
To determine the effects of short-term (3 month) near-infrared light NIR-LED therapy on anatomic and functional abnormalities of LHON as assessed by a wide variety of ophthalmologic tests, including visual acuity, optical coherence tomography, pattern electroretinography (pERG) N95 retinal ganglion cell peak, fERG-PhNR (flash ERG-Photopic Negative Response), and fundus photography.

Official Title
Near-infrared Light-emitting Diode (NIR-LED) Therapy for Leber's Hereditary Optic Neuropathy (LHON)

Conditions
Leber's Hereditary Optic Neuropathy (LHON)

Intervention/Treatment
- Device: Near-infrared light-emitting diode (NIR-LED) therapy (Med Light 630 PRO (Medical Devices Inc.))

Other Study ID Numbers
- PRO14842

Study Start
2011-07

Primary Completion (Actual)
2013-05

Study Completion (Actual)
2013-05

Enrollment (Actual)
4

Study Type
Interventional

Phase
Phase 1 Phase 2

United States
Wisconsin Locations

Milwaukee, Wisconsin, United States, 53226
Froedtert Memorial Lutheran Hospital

Milwaukee, Wisconsin, United States, 53226
Medical College of Wisconsin

Milwaukee, Wisconsin, United States, 53226
The Eye Institute

Eligibility Criteria
Description

Inclusion Criteria

- Sex—male and female. Men are affected with visual loss more frequently than women, with a male predominance of ~85%. A minimum of 25% of men and 5% of women at risk for LHON experience visual loss.
- Age—18 years or older. The onset of visual loss typically occurs between the ages of 15 and 35 years, but otherwise, classic LHON has been reported in many individuals both younger and older, with a range of age at onset from 2 to 80 years.
- Diagnosis of LHON or a carrier of the gene mutation. Patient must be evaluated by molecular confirmation, with the 11,778 and other mutations of Leber's Hereditary Optic Neuropathy stratified in later data analysis.
- Able and willing to provide informed consent.

Exclusion Criteria

- Has an optic nerve disease other than LHON.
- Significant renal disease, defined as a history of chronic renal failure requiring dialysis or kidney transplant.
- Participation in an investigational trial within 30 days of NIR-LED treatment that involved treatment with any drug that has not received regulatory approval at the time of study entry. (Note: subjects cannot receive another investigational drug while participating in the study during the first 6 months.)
- Major surgery within 28 days prior to participation or major surgery planned during the next 6 months. Major surgery is defined as a surgical procedure that is more extensive than fine needle biopsy/aspiration, placement of a central venous access device, removal/biopsy of a skin lesion, or placement of a peripheral venous catheter.

Ages Eligible for Study
18 Years and older (Adult, Older Adult)

Sexes Eligible for Study
All

Accepts Healthy Volunteers
Yes

Design Details
Primary Purpose: Treatment
Allocation: Non-Randomized
Interventional Model: Parallel Assignment
Masking: None (Open Label)

Arms and interventions

Participant group/arm	Intervention/treatment
Experimental: symptomatic LHON patients Study Arm 1 symptomatic LHON patients. Male and female LHON patients with treatable bilateral optic atrophy. Treat the worst of the 2 eyes if there is a measurable difference in subjective visual functions (visual acuity, peripheral vision)	Device: near-infrared light-emitting diode (NIR-LED) therapy (Med Light 630 PRO (Medical Devices Inc.)) • Subjects will be exposed to light emitted from a Med Light 630 PRO (Medical Devices Inc.) at a wavelength of 630 nm (+/−15 nm) with an exposure of 4 J/cm^2. This is accomplished by applying the 50 mW/cm^2 LED-generated light to the closed study eye for 80 s. Treatments involve application of the LED-generated light for 80 s, twice daily • Other names: – Med Light 630 PRO (Medical Devices Inc.)
No intervention: asymptomatic LHON mutation carriers Study Arm 2 asymptomatic LHON mutation carriers. Can be male or female; have some dysfunction, with changes occurring over months. Patients in study arm 2 will not be exposed to NIR-LED, but only undergo diagnostic studies	

Primary outcome measures

Outcome measure	Measure description	Time frame
N95 Peak Via pERG and fERG-PhNR	The primary comparison will be a paired comparison of pre- and post-treatment retinal ganglion cell N95 pattern electroretinogram (pERG) peaks and fERG-Photopic Negative Response (PhNR). Pairing will be done between a subject's treatment and control eye	12 months

Sponsor
Medical College of Wisconsin

Collaborators
No information provided

Investigators
- Principal Investigator: Harry T Whelan, MD, Medical College of Wisconsin

General Publications
No publications available

Unknown Status

Middle East

NAION Treatment with Oral Prednisolone and Erythropoietin Injection (NAION)

ClinicalTrials.gov ID NCT03715881

Sponsor Shahid Beheshti University of Medical Sciences
Information provided by Zahra Rabbani Khah, Shahid Beheshti University of Medical Sciences (Responsible Party)
Last Update Posted 2018-10-23

Brief Summary
This randomized double-blind clinical trial is performed on all recent (within the last 5 days) NAION patients referred to hospitals affiliated with the Shahid Beheshti University of Medical Sciences, Iran. The patients will be equally and randomly assigned into two experimental groups and a control group. The first experimental group will receive 1000 units of erythropoietin every 12 h for 3 days. The second experimental group will receive 50 mg of oral prednisolone from the onset of the disease for 1 week, with the dose gradually reduced within 2 weeks and then discontinued. In addition, the subjects in the second experimental group will receive 300 mg of ranitidine daily. The third group will receive placebo. Eye examination with color vision, perimetry, and peripapillary optical coherence tomography (to measure the thickness of the retinal nerve fiber layer) will be performed before the intervention, and 1, 3, and 6 months after the intervention. SITA standard visual field testing will be done using the Visual Field Analyzer Humphrey 750 Field (Carl Zeiss, USA). The thickness of the retinal nerve fiber layer will be measured by optical coherence tomography (Cirrus Zeiss Cirrus HD-OCT, Carl Zeiss, USA).

The q-q plot and Kolmogorov-Smirnov tests will be performed to test the normal distribution of data. Descriptive statistics including frequency, percentages, standard deviation, median, and range will be used. Other statistical tests including ANOVA, Kruskal-Wallis, Chi-Square, and Fischer's exact tests will be performed. All statistical analyses will be performed in SPSS (version 20) at significance level of 0.05.

Official Title
Scientific Title: Efficacy of Oral Prednisolone and Erythropoietin Injection in Treatment of Acute Non-Arteritic Anterior Ischemic Optic Neuropathy (NAION)

Conditions
Non-Arteritic Anterior Ischemic Optic Neuropathy (NAION)

Intervention/Treatment
- Drug: Oral prednisolone administration 50 mg
- Drug: Intravenous Erythropoietin injection

Other Study ID Numbers
- 95275

Study Start (Estimated)
2018-12-01

Primary Completion (Estimated)
2018-12-01

Study Completion (Estimated)
2019-03-01

Enrollment (Estimated)
99

Study Type
Interventional

Phase
Phase 2

Study Contact
Name: Homayon Nickkhah, MD
Phone Number: 009822591616
Email: labbafi@hotmail.com
Iran, Islamic Republic of

Tehran, Iran, Islamic Republic of
Recruiting
Ophthalmic Research Center

Contact
Homayon Nikkhah, MD
009822591616 labbafi@hotmail.com

Description

Inclusion Criteria
- All NAION patients (maximum time of disease occurrence: 5 days) referred to emergency department of Labbafinejad, Torfeh and Imam Hossein hospitals

Exclusion Criteria
- Glaucoma or any ocular, neurologic or systemic disease affecting the vision
- Abnormal laboratory test results such as ESR and CRP
- History of ocular surgery
- History of receiving medication for NAION
- Uncontrolled systemic disease such as diabetes or hypertension
- Contraindications of systemic steroids including active infection, active gastric ulcer, immunosuppression
- Contraindications of erythropoietin administration, such as polycythemia
- Unwillingness to participate in the study

Ages Eligible for Study
(Child, Adult, Older Adult)

Sexes Eligible for Study
All

Accepts Healthy Volunteers
Yes

Design Details
Primary Purpose: Treatment
Allocation: Randomized
Interventional Model: Parallel Assignment
Masking: Double (Participant Care Provider)

Arms and interventions

Participant group/arm	Intervention/treatment
Active comparator: oral prednisolone administration 50 mg oral prednisolone from the onset of the disease for 1 week, with the dose gradually reduced within 2 weeks and then discontinued	Drug: oral prednisolone administration 50 mg • 50 mg oral prednisolone from the onset of the disease for 1 week, with the dose gradually reduced within 2 weeks and then discontinued
Active comparator: intravenous erythropoietin injection 2. 1000 units of erythropoietin every 12 h for 3 days	Drug: intravenous erythropoietin injection • 1000 units of erythropoietin every 12 h for 3 days

Primary outcome measures

Outcome measure	Measure description	Time frame
Improvement in indices of visual acuity compared to normal course of the disease	Snellen visual acuity chart	6 months after the intervention
Improvement in indices visual field	Mean deviation and pattern standard deviation	6 months after the intervention
Improvement in indices of retinal nerve fiber thickness	Peripapillary optical coherence tomography	6 months after the intervention

Sponsor
Shahid Beheshti University of Medical Sciences

Collaborators
No information provided

Investigators
No information provided

General Publications
No publications available

No Results Posted

Unknown Status

Spain

Intravenous Infusion of Prostaglandins as Therapy in Patients with Anterior Non-arteritic Ischemic Optic Neuropathy (PG-NAION)

ClinicalTrials.gov ID NCT03851562

Sponsor Fundacion para la Formacion e Investigacion Sanitarias de la Region de Murcia
Information provided by Fundacion para la Formacion e Investigacion Sanitarias de la Region de Murcia (Responsible Party)
Last Update Posted 2019-02-25

Brief Summary
Correction of the deficit in the perfusion pressure of the microcirculation that supplies the nerve by intravenous infusion of Prostaglandin E1 (PGE1) (Alprostadil), expected to improve visual function in patients with ischemic optic neuropathy previous non-arteritic (NOIANA).

Official Title
Prospective, Unicentric, Randomized, Parallel, Double-blind, Placebo-controlled Phase II Clinical Trial to Evaluate Intravenous Infusion of Prostaglandins as Therapy in Patients With Anterior Non-arteritic Ischemic Optic Neuropathy

Conditions
Ischemic Optic Neuropathy

Intervention/Treatment
- Drug: Alprostadil 20 μg
- Drug: Placebo

Other Study ID Numbers
- FFIS/PG/2017/03

Study Start (Actual)
2018-06-13

Primary Completion (Estimated)
2019-06-13

Study Completion (Estimated)
2019-10-31

Enrollment (Estimated)
24

Study Type
Interventional

Phase
Phase 2

Study Contact
Name: Rocio Hernandez Clares, MD
Phone Number: 968369473.
Email: rociohclares@hotmail.com

Spain

Murcia, Spain, 30120
Recruiting
Hospital Clínico Universitario Virgen de la Arrixaca

Contact
Servicio de Neurología.
968369473

Principal Investigator
Rocio Hernandez Clares, MD

Eligibility Criteria
Description

Inclusion Criteria
- Patients of both sexes between the ages of 50 and 80, both inclusive. Patients with the first episode of ischemic optic neuropathy previous non-arteritic/NOIANA. Patients with NOIANA with an evolution time from the beginning of the clinic less than or equal to 15 days.
- Potentially fertile patients should have a negative pregnancy test in serum (beta-HCG/human chorionic gonadotropin) or urine.
- Patients who offer sufficient guarantees of adherence to the protocol.
- Patients who give written informed consent to participate in the study.

Exclusion Criteria
- Patients with previous optic of any etiology in the affected eye.
- Patients with previous diagnosis or symptoms at the time of arteritis of the temporal artery.
- Patients with optic neuropathy with bilateral clinical presentation of any etiology.
- Patients with loss of vision due to acute hypotension in the context of a surgical intervention, acute hemorrhage, or hemodynamic shock.
- Patients with severe loss of previous vision in the eye affected by ophthalmologic causes: severe cataract, glaucoma or intraocular pressure greater than 30 mm of mercury, severe diabetic retinopathy, macular degeneration associated with severe age.

- Patients with clinical onset in the month following major non-ocular or intraocular surgery
- Patients with abnormal elevation of CRP/C-reactive protein (>2 times the upper limit of normal)
- Patients with creatinine levels above 1.5 mg/dL.
- Patients on steroid treatment in the month prior to the episode.
- Patients under treatment with oral anticoagulants.
- Patients on treatment with hydroxychloroquine, ethambutol, and vigabatrin at any time before the episode.
- Patients in whom the use of PGE1 (Alprostadil) is contraindicated:
- Patients with participation in a clinical trial in the last 6 months.
- Patients with an inability to understand informed consent.
- Pregnant patients, in the postpartum period or during the active lactation period.
- Physically fertile patients

Ages Eligible for Study
50 Years to 80 Years (Adult, Older Adult)

Sexes Eligible for Study
All

Accepts Healthy Volunteers
No

Design Details
Primary Purpose: Treatment
Allocation: Randomized
Interventional Model: Parallel Assignment
Masking: Double (Participant Investigator)

Arms and interventions

Participant group/arm	Intervention/treatment
Experimental: alprostadil 20 μg 1 μg/kg patient weight up to a maximum of 60 μg	Drug: alprostadil 20 μg • Intravenous infusion of PGE1 (Days 0, +1 and +2)
Placebo comparator: placebo (physiological saline solution) Placebo (physiological saline solution)	Drug: placebo • Intravenous infusion of physiological saline solution

Primary outcome measures

Outcome measure	Measure description	Time frame
Determination of visual acuity	Test ETDRS (early treatment diabetic retinopathy study)	Change from baseline visual acuity at 90 days

Secondary outcome measures

Outcome measure	Measure description	Time frame
Number of serious adverse events	Adverse event	Day 1, day +4, day +30, day +90
Intraocular pressure	Intraocular pressure	Day 1, day +30, day +90
Visual field	Humphrey field analyzer (HFA)	Day 1, day +30, day +90
Thickness of the layer of nerve fibers and ganglion cells in the retina	Cirrus, Carl Zeiss Meditec, Dublin, California, ver: 6.0.2.81	Day 1, day +30, day +90
Fundoscopic evaluation	Biomicroscopy	Day 1, day +30, day +90
Hemodynamic indices of the ocular arteries	Doppler SIEMENS Antares™ System	Day 1, day +30, day +90
Optical disc area and cup/disc	Cirrus, Carl Zeiss Meditec, Dublin, California, ver: 6.0.2.81	Day 1, day +30, day +90

Sponsor
Fundacion para la Formacion e Investigacion Sanitarias de la Region de Murcia

Collaborators
No information provided

Investigators
No information provided

General Publications
No publications available

No Results Posted

Chapter 5
Addendum: Hereditary Optic Neuropathies

Leber's Hereditary Optic Neuropathy

Leber's hereditary optic neuropathy (LHON) is a mitochondrial disorder leading to the death of the retinal ganglion cells and is the most common primary mitochondrial disorder. Visual loss typically occurs in early adulthood although with ready availability of genetic testing, patients are being identified as LHON even into the seventh decade of life. Decreased vision in one or both eyes is an early symptom with the interval between visual loss occurrences ranging from days to months. According to Moster et al. (2016), the degree of visual loss correlates with the loss of ganglion cells and inner plexiform layer thickness on optical coherence tomography (OCT).

There are several mitochondrial DNA (mtDNA) mutations correlated with the development of LHON. The three most common ("primary") LHON mutations are: G11778A nucleotide change within the MT-ND4 gene, G3460A in MT-ND1 gene, and 14484T > C in the MT-ND6 gene. There are at least 13 more "secondary" LHON mutations, such as the mutation at position 4917 which codes for a part of the MT-ND2 subunit. These four mutations lead to a reduction of Nicotinamide Adenine Dinucleotide Coenzyme Q (NADH-CoQ) reductase activity, an enzyme crucial for oxidative phosphorylation, present in the inner membrane of the mitochondria which are located in the cytoplasm of human cells (Wallace et al. 1988; Howell et al. 1991; Brown et al. 2000; Man et al. 2002; Chinnery et al. 2011). There is variability in clinical severity due to mtDNA heteroplasmy in the retinal ganglion cell mitochondria. Increased oxidative stress and apoptosis within the optic nerve system have also been proposed as an instigating factor in the development of LHON as reported by Koilkonda and Guy (2011).

There are no proven treatments for this condition. Therapy has centered on reducing oxidative stress, leading to free radical formation and possible apoptosis, and increasing mitochondrial respiration. These treatments include vitamins and

J. N. Weiss, *Clinical Trials in Optic Nerve Disease Treatment*,
https://doi.org/10.1007/978-3-031-58815-0_5

cofactors such as coenzyme Q10, folic acid, vitamin B12, riboflavin, L-carnitine, and creatine, electron acceptors including vitamin C, free radical scavengers like idebenone, EPI-743, alpha lipoic acid, curcumin, and vitamin E, inhibitors of toxic metabolites like dichloroacetate and customized treatment for the individual patient (DiMauro and Mancuso 2007; Parikh et al. 2009). Idebenone has been used since 1992 and may increase mitochondrial complex 1 activity, but may produce variable effects on respiration (Angebabault et al. 2011).

RHODOS, the Rescue of Hereditary Optic Disease Outpatient Study, was a placebo-controlled trial that utilized idebenone, a free radical scavenger, to treat LHON. Angebabault et al. (2011) reported that 20% of treated patients demonstrated an improvement in vision. However, the European Medicines Agency and the Committee for Medicinal Products for Human Use refused to approve idebenone for LHON because of the lack of benefit in patients having vision loss for more than 5 years and because of, in their view, the questionable benefit in patients with vision loss of less than 1 year. EPI-743, an FDA-approved drug similar to coenzyme Q10 and idebenone, was used to treat five patients with different mtDNA mutations. Four of five patients demonstrated an improvement in visual function (Klopstock et al. 2011).

General Publications

- Ahmad T, Mukherjee S, Pattnaik B, Kumar M, Singh S, Kumar M, Rehman R, Tiwari BK, Jha KA, Barhanpurkar AP, Wani MR, Roy SS, Mabalirajan U, Ghosh B, Agrawal A. Miro1 regulates intercellular mitochondrial transport & enhances mesenchymal stem cell rescue efficacy. EMBO J. 2014;33:994–1010.
- Angebabault C, Gueguen N, Desquiret-Dumas V, Chevrollier A, Guillet V, Verny C, Cassereau J, Ferre M, Milea D, Amati-Bonneau P, Bonneau D, Procaccio V, Reynier P, Loiseau D. Idebenone increases mitochondrial complex I activity in fibroblasts from LHON patients while producing contradictory effects on respiration. BMC Res Notes. 2011;4:557.
- Arnhold S, Absenger Y, Klein H, Addicks K, Schraemeyer U. Transplantation of bone marrow-derived mesenchymal stem cells rescue photoreceptor cells in the dystrophic retina of the rhodopsin knockout mouse. Graefes Arch Clin Exp Ophthalmol. 2007;245:414–422.
- Avraham-Lubin BC, Goldenberg-Cohen N, Sadikov T, Askenasy N. VEGF induces neuroglial differentiation in bone marrow-derived stem cells and promotes microglia conversion following mobilization with GM-CSF. Stem Cell Rev. 2012;8:1199–1210.
- Brown MD, Trounce IA, Jun AS, Allen JC, Wallace DC. Functional analysis of lymphoblast and cybrid mitochondria containing the 3460, 11778, or 14484 Leber's hereditary optic neuropathy mitochondrial DNA mutation. J Biol Chem. 2000;275:39831–39836.
- Carelli V, La Morgia C, Sadun AA. Mitochondrial dysfunction in optic neuropathies: animal models and therapeutic options. Curr Opin Neurol. 2013;26:52–58.
- Chen Q, Long Y, Yuan X, Zou L, Sun J, Chen S, Perez-Polo JR, Yang K. Protective effects of bone marrow stromal cell transplantation in injured rodent brain: synthesis of neurotrophic factors. J Neurosci Res. 2005;80:611–619.

- Chinnery PF, Brown DT, Andrews RM, Singh-Kler R, Riordan-Eva P, Lindley J, Applegarth DA, Turnbull DM, Howell N. The mitochondrial ND6 gene is a hot spot for mutations that cause Leber's hereditary optic neuropathy. Brain. 2011;124(Pt 1):209–218.
- Dezawa M, Takahashi I, Esaki M, Takano M, Sawada H. Sciatic nerve regeneration in rats induced by transplantation of in vitro differentiate bone marrow stromal cells. Eur J Neurosci. 2001;14:1771–1776.
- DiMauro S, Mancuso M. Mitochondrial diseases: therapeutic approaches. Biosci Rep. 2007;27:125–137.
- Fernández-Messina L, Gutiérrez-Vázquez C, Rivas-García E, Sánchez-Madrid F, de la Fuente H. Immunomodulatory role of microRNAs transferred by extracellular vesicles. Biol Cell. 2015;107:61–77.
- Howell N, Bindoff LA, McCullough DA, Kubacka I, Poulton J, Mackey D, Taylor L, Turnbull DM. Leber's hereditary optic neuropathy: identification of the same mitochondrial ND1 mutation in six pedigrees. Am J Hum Genet. 1991;49:939–950.
- Huang W, Lv B, Zeng H, Shi D, Liu Y, Chen F, Li F, Liu X, Zhu R, Yu L, Jiang X. Paracrine factors secreted by MSCs promote astrocyte survival associated with GFAP downregulation after ischemic stroke via p38 MAPK and JNK. J Cell Physiol. 2015;230:2461–2475.
- Islam MN, Das SR, Emin MT, Wei M, Sun L, Westphalen K, Rowlands DJ, Quadri SK, Bhattacharya S, Bhattacharya J. Mitochondrial transfer from bone-marrow-derived stromal cells to pulmonary alveoli protects against acute lung injury. Nat Med. 2012;18:759–765
- Johnson TV, Bull ND, Martin KR. Identification of barriers to retinal engraftment of transplanted stem cells. Invest Ophthalmol Vis Sci. 2010;51:960–970.
- Johnson TV, Bull ND, Hunt DP, Marina N, Tomarev SI, Martin KR. Neuroprotective effects of intravitreal mesenchymal stem cell transplantation in experimental glaucoma. Invest Ophthalmol Vis Sci. 2010;51:2051–2059.
- Klopstock T, Yu-Wai-Man P, Dimitriadis K, Rouleau J, Heck S, Bailie M, Atawan A, Chattopadhyay S, Schubert M, Garip A, Kernt M, Petraki D, Rummey C, Leinonen M, Metz G, Griffiths PG, Meier T, Chinnery PF. A randomized placebo-controlled trial of idebenone in Leber's's hereditary optic neuropathy. Brain. 2011;134(Pt 9):2677–2686.
- Koilkonda RD, Guy J. Leber's hereditary optic neuropathy-gene therapy: from benchtop to bedside. J Ophthalmol. 2011;2011:179412.
- Kordelas L, Rebmann V, Ludwig AK, Radtke S, Ruesing J, Doeppner TR, Epple M, Horn PA, Beelen DW, Giebel B. MSC-derived exosomes: a novel tool to treat therapy-refractory graft-versus-host disease. Leukemia. 2014;28:970–973
- Las G, Shirihai OS. Miro1: new wheels for transferring mitochondria. EMBO J. 2014;33:939–941.
- Levkovitch-Verbin H, Sadan O, Vander S, Rosner M, Barhum Y, Melamed E, Offen D, Melamed S. Intravitreal injections of neurotrophic factors secreting

mesenchymal stem cells are neuroprotective in rat eyes following optic nerve transection. Invest Ophthalmol Vis Sci. 2010;51:6394–6400.

- Li X, Zhang Y, Yeung SC, Liang Y, Liang X, Ding Y, Ip MS, Tse HF, Mak JC, Lian Q. Mitochondrial transfer of induced pluripotent stem cell-derived mesenchymal stem cells to airway epithelial cells attenuates cigarette smoke-induced damage. Am J Respir Cell Mol Biol. 2014;51:455–465.
- Liu K, Ji K, Guo L, Wu W, Lu H, Shan P, Yan C. Mesenchymal stem cells rescue injured endothelial cells in an in vitro ischemia-reperfusion model via tunneling nanotube like structure-mediated mitochondrial transfer. Microvasc Res. 2014;92:10–18.
- Man PY, Turnbull DM, Chinnery PF. Leber's hereditary optic neuropathy. J Med Genet. 2002;39:162–169.
- Mansergh FC, Chadderton N, Kenna PF, Gobbo OL, Farrar GJ. Cell therapy using retinal progenitor cells shows therapeutic effect in a chemically-induced rotenone mouse model of Leber's hereditary optic neuropathy. Eur J Hum Genet. 2014;22:1314–1320.
- Mead B, Scheven BA. Mesenchymal stem cell therapy for retinal ganglion cell neuroprotection and axon regeneration. Neural Regen Res. 2015;10(3):371–373.
- Mead B, Logan A, Berry M, Leadbeater W, Scheven BA. Paracrine-mediated neuroprotection and neuritogenesis of axotomised retinal ganglion cells by human dental pulp stem cells: comparison with human bone marrow and adipose-derived mesenchymal stem cells. PLoS One. 2014;9:e109305.
- Mead B, Logan A, Berry M, Leadbeater W, Scheven BA. Intravitreally transplanted dental pulp stem cells promote neuroprotection and axon regeneration of retinal ganglion cells after optic nerve injury. Invest Ophthalmol Vis Sci. 2013;54:7544–7556.
- Mead B, Berry M, Logan A, Scott RA, Leadbeater W, Scheven BA. Stem cell treatment of degenerative eye disease. Stem Cell Res. 2015;14:243–257.
- Mesentier-Louro LA, Zaverucha-do-Valle C, da Silva-Junior AJ, Nascimento-Dos-Santos G, Gubert F, de Figueirêdo AB, Torres AL, Paredes BD, Teixeira C, Tovar-Moll F, Mendez-Otero R, Santiago MF. Distribution of mesenchymal stem cells and effects on neuronal survival and axon regeneration after optic nerve crush and cell therapy. PLoS One. 2014;9:e110722.
- Montzka K, Lassonczyk N, Tschöke B, Neuss S, Führmann T, Franzen R, Smeets R, Brook GA, Wöltje M. Neural differentiation potential of human bone marrow-derived mesenchymal stromal cells: misleading marker gene expression. BMC Neurosci. 2009;10:16.
- Moore AT. Cone and cone-rod dystrophies. J Med Genet. 1992;29:289–290.
- Moster SJ, Moster ML, Scannell BM, Sergott RC. Retinal ganglion cell and inner plexiform layer loss correlate with visual acuity loss in LHON: a longitudinal, segmentation OCT analysis. Invest Ophthalmol Vis Sci. 2016;57:3872–3883.
- Otani A, Dorrell MI, Kinder K, Moreno SK, Nusinowitz S, Banin E, Heckenlively J, Friedlander M. Rescue of retinal degeneration by intravitreally injected adult bone marrow-derived lineage-negative hematopoietic stem cells. J Clin Invest. 2004;114:765–774.

- Parikh S, Saneto R, Falk MJ, Anselm I, Cohen BH, Haas R, Medicine Society TM. A modern approach to the treatment of mitochondrial disease. Curr Treat Options Neurol. 2009;11:414–430.
- Sadun AA, Chicani CF, Ross-Cisneros FN, Barboni P, Thoolen M, Shrader WD, Kubis K, Carelli V, Miller G. Effect of EPI-743 on the clinical course of the mitochondrial disease Leber's hereditary optic neuropathy. Arch Neurol. 2012;69:331–338.
- Siqueria RC, Messias A, Voltarelli JC, Scott IU, Jorge R. Intravitreal injection of autologous bone marrow-derived mononuclear cells for hereditary retinal dystrophy: a Phase I trial. Retina. 2011;31:1207–1214.
- Wallace DC, Singh G, Lott MT, Hodge JA, Schurr TG, Lezza AM, Elsas LJ, Nikoskelainen EK. Mitochondrial DNA mutation associated with Leber's hereditary optic neuropathy. Science. 1988;242:1427–1430.
- Weiss JN, Benes SC, Levy S. Stem Cell Ophthalmology Treatment Study (SCOTS): improvement in serpiginous choroidopathy following autologous bone marrow-derived stem cell treatment. Neural Regen Res. 2016;11:1512–1516.
- Weiss JN, Levy S, Malkin A. Stem Cell Ophthalmology Treatment Study (SCOTS) for retinal and optic nerve diseases: a preliminary report. Neural Regen Res. 2015a;10:982–988.
- Weiss JN, Levy S, Benes SC. Stem Cell Ophthalmology Treatment Study (SCOTS) for retinal and optic nerve diseases: a case report of improvement in relapsing auto-immune optic neuropathy. Neural Regen Res. 2015b;10:1507–1515.
- Wilkins A, Kemp K, Ginty M, Hares K, Mallam E, Scolding N. Human bone marrow-derived mesenchymal stem cells secrete brain-derived neurotrophic factor which promotes neuronal survival in vitro. Stem Cell Res. 2009;3:63–70.
- Yu S, Tanabe T, Dezawa M, Ishikawa H, Yoshimura N. Effects of bone marrow stromal cell injection in an experimental glaucoma model. Biochem Biophys Res Commun. 2006;344:1071–1079.
- Zarzeczny A, Caulfield T. Emerging ethical, legal and social issues associated with stem cell research and the current role of the moral status of the embryo. Stem Cell Rev. 2009;5:96–101.

Nonarteritic Ischemic Optic Neuropathy (NAION)

Nonarteritic Ischemic Optic Neuropathy (NAION) (Walsh and Hoyt's Clinical Neuro-Ophthalmology: The Essentials, 2008, Bernstein et al. 2011; Atkins 2011; Mercado et al. 2012; Chen et al. 2013; Kernstock et al. 2014; Dickersin et al. 2012; Katz and Trobe 2015; Parsa and Hoyt 2015; Miller and Arnold 2015) is an ischemic, noninflammatory process involving the prelaminar, laminar, and retrolaminar optic nerve. In the United States, the annual incidence of NAION is 2.3–10.2 per 100,000 population. There is no gender predilection, the mean age of occurrence is from 57 to 65 years, and the condition occurs with a significantly higher frequency in the white population than in Hispanic or black individuals.

NAION typically presents with painless visual loss occurring over hours to days. The visual loss is generally static though a progressive form is noted in 22–37% of nonarteritic cases. Most cases of NAION are idiopathic, but specific causes such as hypotension and radiation injury have been identified. About 55–80% of the visual field defects demonstrate an altitudinal, generally inferior, loss.

The visual loss from NAION generally remains stable after 2 months following the initial incident. Within 4–6 weeks following NAION, the optic disc becomes atrophic, either in a sectoral or diffuse pattern. Involvement of the contralateral eye occurs in 14.7% of patients with a median follow-up of 5 years. Risk factors for second eye involvement were baseline visual acuity of 20/200 or worse and diabetes. Thrombosis has been implicated but not proven as a cause of NAION. If a decrease in perfusion secondary to an obstruction and not a complete occlusion is the instigating factor then pathologic confirmation will be elusive. Structurally small "crowded" optic discs, the "disc at risk" has been associated with the development of NAION. If a decrease in perfusion leads to axonal swelling, then a compartment syndrome may result leading to further ischemia and the development of NAION.

Histologic human studies support the concept that compromise of the posterior ciliary circulation plays a role in the development of NAION. Though the experimental development of NAION has been seen in monkeys by occluding the posterior ciliary arteries, not all nonhuman demonstrates permanent or transient damage following this procedure. It has been hypothesized that central retinal artery and pial arterioles anastomoses may prevent ischemia. This supportive mechanism may be absent through normal aging or from systemic diseases including hypertension or atherosclerosis.

Optic atrophy represents the morphologic consequence of multiple diseases that damage the ganglion cells and axons. Though inner retinal layer atrophy is seen in eyes with NAION (Rebolleda et al. 2015), a considerable portion of the retinal nerve fiber layer (RNFL) and the ganglion cell layer (GCC) remains in patients even with no light perception (NLP) vision (Miki et al. 2015).

Optic disc pallor cannot be directly equated with visual function. Optic disc measurement by ocular coherence tomography (OCT) is an anatomic, not functional test. Visual field testing is a subjective test reflecting visual function.

Treatments for NAION have included anticoagulants, diphenylhydantoin, atropine sulfate, steroids, and subtenons injections of vasodilators. None have been proven to be beneficial. The Ischemic Optic Neuropathy Decompression Trial demonstrated that optic nerve sheet decompression was potentially harmful (Dickersin and Li 2015).

General Publications

NAION

- Walsh and Hoyt's Clinical Neuro-Ophthalmology: The Essentials, Second Edition. Philadelphia: Lippincott Williams & Wilkins, 2008.
- Bernstein SL, Johnson MA, Miller NR. Nonarteritic anterior optic neuropathy (NAION) and its experimental models. Prog Retin Eye Res 2011;30:167–87. https://doi.org/10.1016/j.preteyeres.2011.02.003

- Atkins EJ. Nonarteritic anterior ischemic optic neuropathy. Curr Treat Options Neurol 2011;13:92–100. https://doi.org/10.1007/s11940-010-0099-0
- Mercado JL, Purvin VA, Kawasaki A, et al. Bilateral sequential non-arteritic anterior ischemic optic neuropathy: a comparison of visual outcomes in fellow eyes using quantitative analysis of gold man visual fields. Arch Ophthalmol 2012;130:863–7. https://doi.org/10.1001/archophthalmol.2012.581
- Chen T, Song D, Shan G, et al. The association between diabetes mellitus and non-arteritic anterior ischemic optic neuropathy: a systematic review and meta-analysis. PLoS One 2013;8:e76653. https://doi.org/10.1371/journal.pone.0076653.
- Kernstock C, Beisse F, Wiethoff S, et al. Assessment of functional and morphometric endpoints in patients with non-arteritic anterior ischemic optic neuropathy (NAION). Graefes Arch Clin Exp Ophthalmol 2014;252:515–21. https://doi.org/10.1007/s00417-014-2572-z.
- Dickersin K, Manheimer E, Li T. Surgery for nonarteritic anterior ischemic optic neuropathy. Cochrane Database Syst Rev 2012;1:CD001538.
- Katz DM, Trobe JD. Is there treatment for nonarteritic anterior ischemic optic neuropathy. Curr Opin Ophthalmol 2015;26:458–63. https://doi.org/10.1097/ICU.0000000000000199
- Parsa CF, Hoyt WF. Nonarteritic anterior ischemic optic neuropathy (NAION): a misnomer. Rearranging pieces of a puzzle to reveal a nonischemic papillopathy caused by vitreous separation. Ophthalmology 2015;122:439–42. https://doi.org/10.1016/j.ophtha.2014.11.011
- Miller NR, Arnold AC. Current concepts in the diagnosis, pathogenesis and management of nonarteritic anterior ischemic optic neuropathy. Eye (Lond) 2015;29:65–79. https://doi.org/10.1038/eye.2014.144
- Rebolleda G, Sanchez-Sanchez C, Gonzalez-Lopez JJ, et al. Papillomacular bundle and inner retinal thicknesses correlate with visual acuity in nonarteritic anterior ischemic optic neuropathy. Invest Ophthal Vis Sci 2015;56:682–92. https://doi.org/10.1167/iovs.14-15314
- Miki A, Endo T, Morimoto T, et al. Retinal nerve fiber layer and ganglion cell complex thicknesses measured with spectral-domain optical coherence tomography in eyes with no light perception due to nonglaucomatous optic neuropathy. Jpn J Ophthalmol 2015;59:230–5. https://doi.org/10.1007/s10384-015-0386-0
- Dickersin K, Li T. Surgery for nonarteritic anterior ischemic optic neuropathy. Cochrane Database Syst Rev2015;12:CD001538.
- Weiss JN, Levy S, Malkin A. Stem cell ophthalmology treatment trial (SCOTS) for retina and optic nerve disease: a preliminary report. Neural Regen Res 2015;10:982–8. https://doi.org/10.4103/1673-5374.158365
- Weiss JN, Levy S, Benes SC. Stem cell ophthalmology treatment trial (SCOTS) for retina and optic nerve disease: case report of improvement in relapsing auto-immune optic neuropathy. Neural Regen Res 2015;10:1507–15. https://doi.org/10.4103/1673-5374.165525
- Weiss JN, Levy S, Benes SC. Stem Cell Ophthalmology Treatment Study: bone marrow derived stem cells in the treatment of non-arteritic ischemic optic neuropathy (NAION). Stem Cell Investig 2017; 4:94. http://sci.amegroups.com/article/view/17421/17703

- Holladay JT. Proper Method for Calculating Average Visual Acuity. J Refract Surg 1997;13:388–91.
- Dezawa M, Takahashi I, Esaki M, et al. Sciatic nerve regeneration in rats induced by transplantation of in vitro differentiate bone marrow stromal cells. Eur J Neurosci 2001;14:1771–6. https://doi.org/10.1046/j.0953-816x.2001.01814.x
- Montzka K, Lassonczyk L, Tschoke B, et al. Neural differentiation potential of human bone marrow-derived mesenchymal stromal cells: misleading marker gene expression. BMC Neurosci 2009;10:16. https://doi.org/10.1186/1471-2202-10-16
- Wilkins A, Kemp K, Ginty M, et al. Human bone marrow-derived mesenchymal stem cells secrete brain-derived neurotrophic factor which promotes neuronal survival in vitro. Stem Cell Res 2009;3:63–70. https://doi.org/10.1016/j.scr.2009.02.006
- Zarzeczny A, Caulfield T. Emerging ethical, legal and social issues associated with stem cell research and the current role of the moral status of the embryo. Stem Cell Rev 2009;5:96–101. https://doi.org/10.1007/s12015-009-9062-4s
- Yu S, Tanabe T, Dezawa M, et al. Effects of bone marrow stromal cell injection in an experimental glaucoma model. Biochem Biophys Res Commun 2006;344:1071–9. https://doi.org/10.1016/j.bbrc.2006.03.231
- Johnson TV, Bull ND, Hunt DP, et al. Neuroprotective effects of intravitreal mesenchymal stem cell transplantation in experimental glaucoma. Invest Ophthalmol Vis Sci 2010;51:2051–9. https://doi.org/10.1167/iovs.09-4509
- Levkovitch-Verbin H, Sadan O, Vander S, et al. Intravitreal injections of neurotrophic factors secreting mesenchymal stem cells are neuroprotective in rat eyes following optic nerve transection. Invest Ophthalmol Vis Sci 2010;51:6394–400. https://doi.org/10.1167/iovs.09-4310
- Mead B, Logan A, Berry M, et al. Paracrine-mediated neuroprotection and neuritogenesis of axotomised retinal ganglion cells by human dental pulp stem cells: comparison with human bone marrow and adipose-derived mesenchymal stem cells. PLoS One 2014;9:e109305. https://doi.org/10.1371/journal.pone.0109305
- Mesentier-Louro LA, Zaverucha-do-Valle C, da Silva-Junior AJ, et al. Distribution of mesenchymal stem cells and effects on neuronal survival and axon regeneration after optic nerve crush and cell therapy. PLoS One 2014;9:e110722. https://doi.org/10.1371/journal.pone.0110722
- Mead B, Logan A, Berry M, et al. Intravitreally transplanted dental pulp stem cells promote neuroprotection and axon regeneration of retinal ganglion cells after optic nerve injury. Invest Ophthalmol Vis Sci 2013;54:7544–56. https://doi.org/10.1167/iovs.13-13045
- Johnson TV, Bull ND, Martin KR. Identification of barriers to retinal engraftment of transplanted stem cells. Invest Ophthalmol Vis Sci 2010;51:960–70. https://doi.org/10.1167/iovs.09-3884
- Mead B, Scheven BA. Mesenchymal stem cell therapy for retinal ganglion cell neuroprotection and axon regeneration. Neural Regen Res 2015;10:371–3. https://doi.org/10.4103/1673-5374.153681

- Mansergh FC, Chadderton N, Kenna PF, et al. Cell therapy using retinal progenitor cells shows therapeutic effect in a chemically-induced rotenone mouse model of Leber's hereditary optic neuropathy. Eur J Hum Genet 2014;22:1314–20. https://doi.org/10.1038/ejhg.2014.26
- Kordelas L, Rebmann V, Ludwig AK, et al. MSC-derived exosomes: a novel tool to treat therapy refractory graft-versus-host disease. Leukemia 2014;28:970–3.
- Fernández-Messina L, Gutiérrez-Vázquez C, Rivas-García E, et al. Immunomodulatory role of microRNAs transferred by extracellular vesicles. Biol Cell 2015;107:61–77. https://doi.org/10.1111/boc.201400081
- Wilkins A, Kemp K, Ginty M, et al. Human bone marrow-derived mesenchymal stem cells secrete brain-derived neurotrophic factor which promotes neuronal survival in vitro. Stem Cell Res 2009;3:63–70. https://doi.org/10.1016/j.scr.2009.02.006
- Chen Q, Long Y, Yuan X, et al. Protective effects of bone marrow stromal cell transplantation in injured rodent brain: synthesis of neurotrophic factors. J Neurosci Res 2005;80:611–9. https://doi.org/10.1002/jnr.20494
- Mead B, Berry M, Logan A, et al. Stem cell treatment of degenerative eye disease. Stem Cell Res 2015;14:243–57. https://doi.org/10.1016/j.scr.2015.02.003
- Huang W, Lv B, Zeng H, et al. Paracrine Factors Secreted by MSCs Promote Astrocyte Survival Associated with GFAP Downregulation After Ischemic Stroke Via p38MAPK and JNK. J Cell Physiol 2015;230:2461–75. https://doi.org/10.1002/jcp.24981
- Nagra PK, Foroozan R, Savino PJ, et al. Amiodarone induced optic neuropathy. Br J Ophthalmol 2003;87:420–22. https://doi.org/10.1136/bjo.87.4.420
- Vaquero J, Zurita M. Bone marrow stromal cells for spinal cord repair: a challenge for contemporary neurobiology. Histol Histopathol 2009;24:107–16.
- Kim JY, You YS, Kim SH, et al. Epiretinal membrane formation after intravitreal autologous stem cell implantation in a retinitis pigmentosa patient. Retin Cases Brief Rep 2017;11:227–31. https://doi.org/10.1097/ICB.0000000000000327
- Mullen RJ, Buck CR, Smith AM. NeuN, a neuronal specific nuclear protein in vertebrates. Development 1992;116:201–11.
- Lin W, Li M, Li Y, et al. Bone marrow stromal cells promote neurite outgrowth of spinal motor neurons by means of neurotrophic factors in vitro. Neurol Sci 2014;35:449–57. https://doi.org/10.1007/s10072-013-1490-x

Neuromyelitis Optica (NMO, Devic's Disease)

NMO is a demyelinating and degenerative disorder of the central nervous system that affects vision, brain, and spinal cord function. The five-year mortality is approximately 30%. Blindness, respiratory failure, and quadriparesis may result. The majority of cases are caused by autoantibodies to aquaporin 4. There is a subset of aquaporin 4 negative cases associated with antibodies to myelin oligodendrocyte glycoprotein, anti-MOG. NMO may be associated with other autoimmune diseases. Some cases are of unknown etiology.

NMO may be confused with multiple sclerosis (MS) as they may present with similar clinical and radiologic findings; however, it differs from MS in pathogenesis, cerebrospinal fluid findings, disease course, and prognosis.

General Publications

- Iwamoto S, Itokazu T, Sasaki A, Kataoka H, Tanaka S, Hirata T, Miwa K, Suenaga T, Takai Y, Misu T, Fujihara K, Yamashita T. RGMa Signal in Macrophages Induces Neutrophil-Related Astrocytopathy in NMO. Ann Neurol. 2022 Apr;91(4):532–547. https://doi.org/10.1002/ana.26327. Epub 2022 Mar 8. PMID: 35167145.
- Juryńczyk M, Craner M, Palace J. Overlapping CNS inflammatory diseases: differentiating features of NMO and MS. J Neurol Neurosurg Psychiatry. 2015 Jan;86(1):20–5. https://doi.org/10.1136/jnnp-2014-308984. Epub 2014 Sep 23. PMID: 25248365.
- Cho S, Lee H, Jung M, Hong K, Woo SH, Lee YS, Kim BJ, Jeon MY, Seo J, Mun JY. Neuromyelitis optica (NMO)-IgG-driven organelle reorganization in human iPSC-derived astrocytes. FASEB J. 2021 Oct;35(10):e21894. https://doi.org/10.1096/fj.202100637R. PMID: 34460995.
- Zamvil SS, Slavin AJ. Does MOG Ig-positive AQP4-seronegative opticospinal inflammatory disease justify a diagnosis of NMO spectrum disorder? Neurol Neuroimmunol Neuroinflamm. 2015 Jan 22;2(1):e62. https://doi.org/10.1212/NXI.0000000000000062. PMID: 25635259; PMCID: PMC4309526.
- Chen T, Bosco DB, Ying Y, Tian DS, Wu LJ. The Emerging Role of Microglia in Neuromyelitis Optica. Front Immunol. 2021 Feb 19;12:616301. https://doi.org/10.3389/fimmu.2021.616301. PMID: 33679755; PMCID: PMC7933531.
- Wu Y, Zhong L, Geng J. Visual impairment in neuromyelitis optica spectrum disorders (NMOSD). J Chem Neuroanat. 2019 Apr;97:66–70. https://doi.org/10.1016/j.jchemneu.2019.01.012. Epub 2019 Feb 1. PMID: 30716473.
- Nandhagopal R, Al-Asmi A, Gujjar AR. Neuromyelitis optica: an overview. Postgrad Med J. 2010 Mar;86(1013):153–9. https://doi.org/10.1136/pgmj.2009.091389. PMID: 20237009.
- Mader EC Jr, Verdecie O, Losada V, Lovera JF. Autoimmune Myelitis and Myocarditis in a Patient With Anti-Aquaporin-4, Antinuclear, and Antiphospholipid Autoantibodies: The Neuromyelitis Optica-Systemic Lupus Erythematosus (NMO-SLE) Overlap Syndrome. Cureus. 2022 Nov 10;14(11):e31334. https://doi.org/10.7759/cureus.31334. PMID: 36514583; PMCID: PMC9741486.
- Jarius S, Wildemann B, Paul F. Neuromyelitis optica: clinical features, immunopathogenesis and treatment. Clin Exp Immunol. 2014 May;176(2):149–64. https://doi.org/10.1111/cei.12271. PMID: 24666204; PMCID: PMC3992027.
- Drori T, Chapman J. Diagnosis and classification of neuromyelitis optica (Devic's syndrome). Autoimmun Rev. 2014 Apr-May;13(4–5):531–3. https://doi.org/10.1016/j.autrev.2014.01.034. Epub 2014 Jan 11. PMID: 24424197.

Index

J. N. Weiss, *Clinical Trials in Optic Nerve Disease Treatment*,
https://doi.org/10.1007/978-3-031-58815-0

GPSR Compliance

The European Union's (EU) General Product Safety Regulation (GPSR) is a set of rules that requires consumer products to be safe and our obligations to ensure this.

If you have any concerns about our products, you can contact us on ProductSafety@springernature.com

In case Publisher is established outside the EU, the EU authorized representative is:

Springer Nature Customer Service Center GmbH
Europaplatz 3
69115 Heidelberg, Germany

The manufacturer's authorised representative in the EU is Springer Nature Customer Service Centre GmbH, Europaplatz 3, 69115 Heidelberg, Germany. If you have any concerns regarding our products, please contact ProductSafety@springernature.com

Printed and bound by CPI Group (UK) Ltd, Croydon, CR0 4YY
01/10/2026
02225853-0005